Arterial Hypertension

With compliments

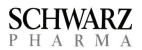

SCHWARZ PHARMA AG · Alfred-Nobel-Straße 10 · 40789 Monheim · Germany

Michael Stimpel

Arterial Hypertension

Foreword by Michael A. Weber

W DE G Walter de Gruyter
Berlin · New York 1996

Michael Stimpel, M. D.
Assistant Professor of Internal Medicine
Medical School, University of Cologne
D-50931 Cologne

Mail address:
Frieding Strasse 13
D-40625 Düsseldorf
Germany

Die Deutsche Bibliothek — Cataloging-in-Publication Data

Stimpel, Michael:
Arterial hypertension / Michael Stimpel. Foreword by Michael
A. Weber. — Berlin ; New York : de Gruyter, 1996
    ISBN 3-11-014176-0

Printed in Germany

Typesetting: Arthur Collignon GmbH, Berlin. — Printing: Gerike GmbH, Berlin. — Binding: Lüderitz & Bauer GmbH, Berlin. — Cover design: Rudolf Hübler, Berlin

Foreword

Hypertension is the most common chronic condition that doctors deal with. Almost one-fifth of the adult population in Europe and the United States has hypertension, and it appears to be even more prevalent in the elderly. Inevitably, the public health and economic implications of this condition have taken it beyond doctors and patients, and have made it a matter of concern for government agencies, organized health plans, insurance companies, and employers.

The management of hypertension is now only rarely the responsibility of specialists and overwhelmingly is undertaken by primary care physicians. But it would be a major error to regard this commitment as a routine matter, for there are many controversies and questions awaiting resolution.

The diagnosis of primary (essential) hypertension is still far from settled. Data from epidemiologic surveys and from the life insurance industry have shown that blood pressure at all levels, ranging from the apparently normal to the obviously elevated, has a clear relationship to the risk of cardiovascular events; in general, the higher the blood pressure, the more likely is a serious clinical result. Committees of experts throughout the world have issued recommendations specifying the levels of blood pressure at which they believe patients make the transition from being "normal" to being "hypertensive". The guidelines in the United States are more aggressive than elsewhere, and physicians tend to start treatment of their patients at lower levels of blood pressure than their colleagues elsewhere. Of course, many factors − including the presence of other risk factors, physical findings, and family history − will influence diagnostic and treatment decisions in individual patients. This new book by Dr. Michael Stimpel provides useful insights and advice on this crucial and still highly debated area of decision making.

It would be foolish of us to be complacent about the management of hypertension in the clinical setting. In the United States, for example, a blood pressure value of 140/90 mmHg has been recommended as the criterion for the diagnosis of hypertension and as the target for antihypertensive therapy. Recent evidence, though, suggests that barely 20% of hypertensive patients in the United States have blood pressures below 140/90 mmHg. Part of the problem is a failure to adequately screen and diagnose hypertension in the community, but by far the greater issue is our failure to adequately treat most hypertensive patients. In many instances patients are taking no treatment whatever, indicating a troublesome inability of physicians to communicate effectively with their patients and explain the need for conscientious long-term therapy. In addition, too many physicians have a casual attitude towards hypertension and are willing to accept mediocre treatment results. There is always a danger that a condition as common as hypertension can be devalued and taken lightly, and it seems that this is occurring, to some extent, on both sides of the Atlantic as well as in most other regions of the world.

This new book has been written by Dr. Stimpel with many of these practical issues in mind. In particular, new knowledge about such basic matters as blood pressure itself is addressed. Most physicians now in practice have been taught that the diastolic blood pressure should be the principal basis for diagnosing hypertension and judging its response to treatment. The systolic blood pressure generally has been seen primarily as a meaningful measurement in the elderly. But growing evidence indicates that the systolic blood pressure – at all ages – appears to be the most accurate predictor of clinical changes and events in the cardiovascular system. Indeed, it is now recognized that the diastolic blood pressure, which is helpful in predicting cardiovascular risks in younger individuals, can be rather difficult to interpret in the middle aged and the elderly.

This book deservedly gives close attention to the technique of ambulatory blood presssure monitoring. This method uses small portable devices that measure blood pressure throughout the full 24 hours of the day, and has allowed us to study patterns of blood pressure in patients or normal volunteers during their routine activities at home and at work. We now know that almost 30% of the patients who appear to have hypertension in the doctor's office or clinic actually have normal blood pressure values when monitored throughout their typical daily activities. This phenomenon of having a blood pressure that is high in the presence of a physician but is normal at other times is sometimes referred to as "office hypertension", "white coat hypertension", or "non-confirmed hypertension". Can we safely assume that these patients are truly normal and do not require treatment? This remains an unresolved question, and for the time being we must recommend that physicians continue to follow these patients even if antihypertensive therapy is not being administered.

A further lesson from ambulatory monitoring is that blood pressure has a distinct pattern throughout the day; it is high during the active morning and afternoon periods, falls during the evening to its lowest values during sleep, and then rises quite sharply to its early morning levels. In some patients the difference between day and night values is blunted, and investigators have claimed that these individuals are at increased risk of cardiovascular changes. Another area of interest is the sharp morning rise in blood pressure, for it is at this time of day that a large number of acute coronary ischemic events and strokes occur. Should we be targeting our antihypertensive therapy to ensure that it is providing maximum efficacy at that apparently critical time of day? Again, we must await carefully performed prospective clinical trials to answer this potentially challenging clinical question.

The growing importance of hypertension in the elderly cannot be overemphasized. Recent clinical trials have provided overwhelming evidence that treatment of the predominantly systolic hypertension in these patients dramatically reduces the incidence of such consequences as strokes and congestive heart failure. When we realize that our populations are aging rapidly, and that hypertension is so prevalent in this group, it comes as no surprise that the demands and opportunities of treating hypertension in older people will become a major part of the practice of most clinicians.

Despite our inevitable focus on blood pressure, hypertension most commonly comprises a syndrome of metabolic and cardiovascular changes. As Dr. Stimpel points out in detail, high blood pressure is commonly associated with such findings as insulin resistance and lipid abnormalities. There is already persuasive evidence that hyperinsulinemia, together with the concomitant alterations in the lipid profile, can directly contribute to the accelerated atherosclerosis that typifies hypertension and almost certainly contributes to disease in the coronaries and other critical arteries. Changes in the structure and function of the left ventricle, early stiffening or loss of compliance of the arterial circulation, and changes in renal function are further intrinsic components of this syndrome. Many of these findings can be demonstrated in the young offspring of hypertensive patients, suggesting that this picture may be part of an inherited process.

Many of us with a special interest in the field of hypertension have been fascinated by recent scientific developments. For the first time we are reading reports of links between clinical hypertension and genetic polymorphisms. Researchers are pointing out, for example, that underlying changes in synthesis of components of the renin-angiotensin system and the sympathetic nervous system can be associated with blood pressure abnormalities and clinical cardiovascular events. Furthermore, the molecular biologists are demonstrating the mechanisms that lead to pathologic changes in the endothelium − with its myriad metabolic and regulatory roles − as well as in the other critical layers of the arterial wall. These breakthroughs surely will govern therapeutic advances in the future.

This comprehensive text by Dr. Stimpel points out, however, that there are many other equally interesting issues for clinicians to ponder. None is more current than the question of treatment outcomes. Traditionally, clinicians have depended almost entirely on short-term outcomes, chiefly the measurements of blood pressure itself. If the blood pressure could be brought down to an acceptable level, if routine clinical tests remained normal, and if patients did not complain of side effects or other symptoms, we were well satisfied. But about 10 or 15 years ago, experts reminded us that the goal of treating hypertension was to protect critical target organs such as the heart and kidneys. They argued that intermediate or surrogate endpoints, for example regression of left ventricular hypertrophy or a reduction in proteinuria and the preservation of renal function, were more important indices of success than simple measures of blood pressure.

Progressively we have come to realize that it is long-term clinical results that must guide us. Which treatments can actually prolong the lives of hypertensive patients? What is the scientifically credible evidence that particular forms of treatment can actually reduce such hard endpoints as strokes and myocardial infarctions? Debate rages over whether the more traditional antihypertensive agents − particularly the diuretics and beta blockers − have the same beneficial effects as the newer drug classes − the angiotensin converting enzyme inhibitors, the calcium channel blockers, and the selective alpha blockers. Although the older agents have been consistently effective in reducing strokes, evidence for meaningful reductions in coronary events have been far less impressive. This is not a minor issue. Coronary outcomes, including acute myocardial infarctions, sudden deaths, the angina syndromes or the need for interventional procedures or surgery, are the most common consequences of hypertension. Will the newer drug classes be more effective in providing protection against coronary disease?

Much research is now being dedicated to even newer drug types. Very recently we have had the benefit of the first of the selective angiotension II receptor antagonists, and we still have much to learn about its hemodynamic and biologic characteristics. Factors involved in regulating the circulation are obvious targets for therapeutic interventions. Drugs that can affect endothelin, nitric oxide, and atrial natriuretic factor — among others — are currently undergoing early development. Despite the abundance of individual antihypertensive agents already available, it is evident that there are still many unmet needs in the treatment of hypertension.

There are several books on hypertension now available, but for the most part they are multi-author volumes composed of collections of chapters each provided by a separate contributor. This provides a certain authority, but only at the sacrifice of continuity. The enormous value of a single author text is that it is complete and, at the same time, avoids redundancy. Most of all, it provides the comprehensive views and experiences of an experienced and thoughtful teacher. Dr. Michael Stimpel is on the faculty of the Department of Internal Medicine at the University of Cologne, and is Head of Cardiovascular Clinical Research at an international pharmaceutical company. This powerful background of teaching and research, coupled with Dr. Stimpel's enviable reputation in publishing scholarly articles in this field, adds much authority to his work. We owe a great deal of gratitude to Dr. Stimpel for making available to us this exceptionally practical, contemporary, and readable treatise on the ever changing subject of hypertension.

New York, March 1996

Michael A. Weber, M. D.
Professor of Medicine
State University Center of New York
Health Science Center, Brooklyn;
Chairman, Department of Medicine
The Brookdale University Hospital
and Medical Center,
Brooklyn, New York

Author's preface

Ever more often, medical textbooks are the product of a group of authors. Due to the rapid pace of scientific and practical advances this trend becomes the only method possible, if a book is aimed at specialists. There are such books available for arterial hypertension which have been written by a more or less large number of competent scientists and clinicians. As an example, the superb, two-volume, and more than 3,000-page textbook "Hypertension: Pathophysiology, Diagnosis and Management", edited by Dr. John Laragh, New York, and Dr. Barry Brenner, Boston, reflects the work of almost 400 authors.

If, however, the textbook is aimed at the non-specialized physician in the clinic or practice, a number of authors may cause difficulties. In such cases the book lacks a uniform diction and the result is frequently such that the individual contributions are too specialized. This bears with it the danger that the reader who is less familiar with the scientific background of the field is left confused.

This book is based on my German-language book "Arterielle Hypertonie – Differentialdiagnose und -therapie", which appeared in 1990. To maintain the claim that the textbook is primarily aimed at the practitioner, I have retained the structure of Fundamentals, Diagnosis and Management, which readers responded to positively. The summary of the most important facts at the end of each chapter makes it possible to obtain a quick overview of the complex material. Furthermore, the text is frequently supplemented with flow charts which should allow for a prudent diagnostic or therapeutic approach in the clinic and practice.

Definite scientific knowledge and generally accepted procedures were dealt with in detail, especially in the diagnostic and management sections of the book. Controversial subjects in arterial hypertension research were only dealt with as an exception. Readers who are interested in such subjects will find a bibliography at the end of each chapter. This bibliography should be viewed more as supplement to the content than as a reference in the normal academic sense. The limited amount of space available required that in many cases older, original publications had to be left out in favor of more current ones. Despite some slight country-specific differences, when the individual guidelines are examined more closely, there is for the most part international uniformity about the diagnostic and management procedures of arterial hypertension. This fact, particularly in view of controversy in the US centering around the JNC V Report published in 1993, was of special importance to me in writing this book.

I would especially like to express my gratitude to Dr. Michael Weber, Chairman of the Brookdale Hospital Medical Center, Brooklyn, New York, and one of the USA's most highly respected experts in the field of hypertension, for the numerous discussions and for his unfailing support in encouraging me in my intention to write an internationally oriented hypertension textbook for the practicing physician. I should also like to thank Ms. Ingrid Ullrich and Dr. Josef Kleine of the Walter de Gruyter publishing house for the close cooperation during the entire process of publishing "Arterial Hypertension".

Cologne, April 1996   Michael Stimpel

Contents

III   Management

I Fundamentals

1 Blood pressure and its regulation

1.1 Anatomy and physiology of the circulatory system

The heart and blood vessels form a self-contained transport system in which the blood serves the body's organs as an agent for provisioning and waste removal, and must, in connection with these needs, be circulated in specific quantities and at an appropriate pressure. The necessary circulatory pressure is generated by the contraction of the left ventricle, and modulated by the reactions of the vascular system. Blood flow during the cardiac atony phase is preserved by the compensatory reaction of large arteries, in particular by the aorta. In this function, the aortic wall, stretched during the systolic phase, contracts again during the diastolic phase, thanks to its elastic qualities, so that the blood can be continually pumped to the periphery along the path of least resistance. The peripheral arterial vascular bed is capable of varying the diameter of the lumen by a contraction or dilatation of the vascular musculature, made possible by a distally increasing responsiveness to neural and humoral impulses. Particularly in the area of the numerous arterioles, changes in vascular (smooth muscle) tone can greatly affect the entire cross-section, and therefore the circulatory resistance, so that the activity of the vascular smooth muscle in these sections is the deciding factor in the compensatory regulation of the visceral capillary blood supply, as well as of the pressure of the dependent blood supply in the entire arterio-vascular system.

In one of its functions, the venous vascular system returns blood to the heart. In another, this portion of the circulatory system serves as the largest reservoir for blood storage. Roughly 65% of the body's total blood volume is located in the venous portion of the circulatory system. While the influence of the venous-vascular tone on total resistance is minimal, its influence on the filling-volume, and, consequently, on stroke volume is nevertheless much higher.

1.2 Blood pressure physiology

Due to the contraction and relaxation of the heart muscle, arterial blood pressure, particularly in the large arteries, is pulsatile in nature. The high point of this fluctuation is dubbed systolic pressure, and the minimum, diastolic pressure. Systolic blood pressure is overwhelmingly determined by means of stroke volume, the myocardial contractility, and myocardial elasticity; while diastolic blood pressure is primarily determined by the peripheral resistance of the smallest arteries and arterioles.

The truly relevant measurement for arterial blood flow is the mean arterial pressure, which is determined by the stroke volume on the one hand and by total peripheral resistance on the other hand. The mean arterial pressure is not identical with the arithmetical mean of the blood pressure amplitude. It can only be precisely determined graphically, by means of planimetry; or electromechanically, through a damping of the pulsatile signal. An approximate value can be obtained by the addition of the value of the diastolic and one third of the pulse pressure value. Although the mean value continuously falls throughout the arterio-vascular system, the difference between pressures measured in the aorta ascendens and in arteries with a rough diameter of 3 mm is only 5 mmHg. Mean arterial pressure first drops significantly in the region of the arterioles as a result of circulatory resistance.

Since the determination of mean arterial pressure – as described – is quite difficult, the measurement of the systolic and diastolic pressures has established itself in practice as an easily accomplished method. When comparing systolic and diastolic pressure measurements in various segments of the arterial vasculature, the varying behavior of the maximum and minimum pressure pulsations must be taken into account in order to avoid misinterpretations. In contrast to the systolic blood pressure – which, proceeding from the aorta, continuously increases and which can be measured, in the femoral arteries, under physiological conditions, at up to 20 mmHg higher than in the aorta ascendens, and in the foot arteries at up to 40 mmHg higher – the diastolic blood pressure continuously falls. The result is an increase in peripheral pulse pressure.

1.3 Factors determining blood pressure regulation: the role of cardiac output and peripheral vascular resistance

The determining factors in arterial blood pressure are cardiac output and total peripheral vascular resistance. It follows that changes in blood pressure can either be affected through a change in cardiac output, through a change in arterial vasotonia, or both. It must be taken into account, on the one hand, that cardiac output is not only an expression of the strength of cardiac contraction and heart rate, but that it is influenced by blood volume as well. It is worth observing, on the other hand, that changes in vascular resistance are not only a reflection of arteriolar vascular tone, but – if only to a minimal degree – of the elasticity of the 'Windkessel' vasculature as well.

A rise in the cardiac output and an increase in peripheral vascular resistance boost blood pressure, whereas a fall in output and dilatation of the arterioles cause a decrease in blood pressure. The increasing loss of aortic elasticity in particular leads to a rise in systolic and a fall in diastolic blood pressure.

1.4 Regulating parameters of blood pressure

The adaptation of blood pressure to needs is achieved through neural, humoral and local factors.

1.4.1 Neuroregulation of blood pressure

Short-term adaptations of blood pressure are predominantly accomplished through neurally transmitted vasomotor changes. The associated, necessary, regulatable parameters are baro- and chemoreceptors, which mediate the autoregulation of the circulation via defined areas (nuclei) located primarily in the medulla oblongata. The objective of these autoregulative processes, which act as a feedback mechanism, is the maintenance of the blood pressure at a specified nominal value; a fall in blood pressure consequently induces blood-pressure-boosting impulses in the vasomotor center – impulses which are directed from there to the periphery and which, by mediation of the adrenergic transmitters norepinephrine and epinephrine, bring about a constriction of the smooth vascular muscle as well as an increase of cardiac contractility and heart rate. A rise in blood pressure, however, impedes central sympathetic activity, so that a preponderance of parasympathetic activity exists, resulting, consequently, in opposite changes to the vascular and cardiac variables.

The transmission of neural impulses through norepinephrine and epinephrine is achieved by the stimulation of organ-specific receptors which are divided into two groups: alpha- and beta-adrenergic receptors. Stimulation of the alpha$_1$-receptors affects a constriction of the vascular smooth musculature; stimulation of the beta-adrenergic receptors (beta$_2$-receptors), a dilatation. The transference of adrenergic impulses to the heart is accomplished primarily through beta$_1$-receptors whose stimulation boosts heart functioning. Neural connections between the vasomotor center and the higher areas of the central nervous system (hypothalamus, limbic system, cortex) shed light on the susceptibility of circulatory regulation to external, emotional stimuli (shock, pain, fear, joy, etc.).

1.4.2 Humoral and local regulation of blood pressure

An increase in intravascular volume and vasoconstriction boost blood pressure, whereas a reduction in intravascular volume and vasodilatation cause a decrease in blood pressure. The modulation of vascular contraction, fluid intake and fluid elimination is accomplished at least in part through endo-, para-, auto-, or intracrine-acting hormones which, as a part of a complex regulatory system, are more or less quickly released or inhibited by changes in volume and/or blood pressure, and so under physiological conditions are capable of maintaining homeostasis. Although a multitude of vasopressor and vasodepressor hormones have been identified (Table 1.1), their physiological role and the intricate details of their interaction are only partially known.

1.4.2.1 Renin-angiotensin system

The systemic renin-angiotensin system (RAS) is central to the regulation of fluid balance and blood pressure. The production, storage and secretion of renin are accomplished in the renal juxtaglomerular cells, which form a functional unit with

Table 1.1: Humoral regulation of blood pressure

Vasopressor hormones	Renin angiotensin aldosterone system
	Arginine vasopressin
	Catecholamines
	Endothelin
Vasodepressor hormones	Natriuretic peptides (ANP, BNP)
	Kinin-kallikrein system
	Medullipine system
	Adrenomedullin
	Nitric oxide (NO)
	Prostaglandins (PGI$_2$, prostacyclin)

the remaining portions of the juxtaglomerular apparatus. Hyponatriemia, hypovo-lemia, hypotension and adrenergic stimuli activate the production and release of renin, which subsequently enzymatically splits the decapeptide angiotensin I from the circulating angiotensinogen. Angiotensin I is not vasoactive, and is only con-verted to the vasoactive angiotensin II (Ang II) by a non-specific converting enzyme and through a further splitting of two C-terminal amino acids. On the one hand, Ang II brings about a constriction of the arteriolar vascular smooth musculature, and on the other, a release of aldosterone from the adrenal cortex with a resultant increase in tubular sodium- and water reabsorption. Consequently, the activation of the RAS, through a direct boosting of peripheral resistance (via Ang II) and through an aldosterone-induced volume expansion, works against a drop in blood pressure.

Since hypervolemia, hypernatriemia, and increases in blood pressure and Ang II-concentrations, under physiological conditions, supplant renin activation in the sense of a negative feedback mechanism, this system can also be understood as a regulatory circuit serving fluid and blood pressure homeostasis (Figure 1.1).

The significance for blood pressure regulation of a tissue-specific, local renin-angiotensin system in the heart, kidney, brain and veins is still unknown. At least for Ang II produced in vascular cells, a separation of para-, auto-, or intracrine activity into regional regulative processes is imaginable.

1.4.2.2 Vasopressin

The peptide hormone vasopressin (arginine-vasopressin; antidiuretic hormone; ADH) is produced in the hypothalamus and stored in the neurohypophysis. Hyper-osmolity and volume decrease are sufficient stimulation for the release of vasopres-sin.

Vasopressin causes a rise in iso-osmotic reabsorption of primary urine in the distal tubule and collecting duct of the kidney. Moreover, isolated vascular preparations could prove vasopressin to have a strong vasoconstrictor effect. Although it is generally accepted that vasopressin is involved in the short-term regulation of blood pressure, the contribution of this peptide hormone to the physiological blood pressure regulation is not yet fully understood.

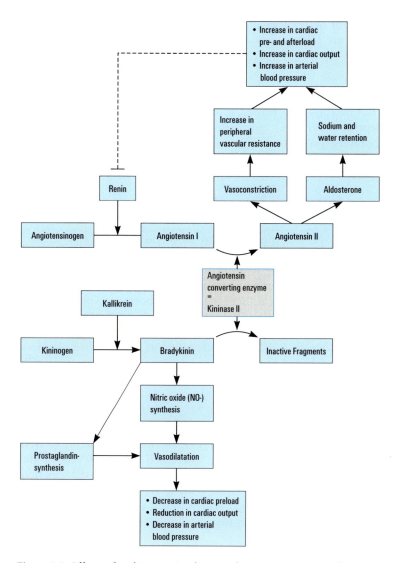

Figure 1.1: Effects of and interaction beween the renin-angiotensin-aldosterone system and the renal kinin system.

|------: Inhibition of renin secretion through negative feedback

1.4.2.3 The kallikrein-kinin-system and prostaglandins

Kinins (bradykinin, kallidin, etc.) serve a vasodilatory, diuretic, and natriuretic function. As so-called tissue hormones, they take effect at the point of synthesis. They are cleaved from the kininogens under the enzymatic effects of kallikrein, and inactivated by the angiotensin-converting-enzyme-identical kininase II (Figure

1.1). Various prostaglandin derivatives (prostacyclin; PGE$_2$), whose synthesis can be stimulated by kinins, are likewise classified as vasoactive, dilatory tissue hormones.

1.4.2.4 Natriuretic peptides

The polypeptides atrial natriuretic peptide (ANP), brain natriuretic peptide (BNP), C-type natriuretic peptide (CNP) and urodilatin form a structurally similar family with natriuretic and diuretic properties. These natriuretic peptides are not identical with the natriuretic hormone (endogenous digitalis-like factor, EDLF) whose existence has for some time been postulated, but which has not yet been isolated (see Chapter 9).

Atrial natriuretic peptide (ANP):

Atrial natriuretic peptide (ANP), formed and stored in the atrium, and released into the plasma through atrial stretching, is a circulatory peptide hormone which may be involved in the regulation of sodium homeostasis and blood pressure. Under physiological conditions, one encounters relatively constant ANP-plasma-levels which, considering the high clearance-rate of this hormone, presuppose a continuous and relatively high production rate. Although an experimental or pathological expansion of extracellular volume prompts an increased production and release of ANP, and although ANP can be classified as a protective hormone against volume overload and blood pressure increase, the significance of its relatively high and largely constant release under physiological conditions is not clear.

Brain natriuretic peptide (BNP):

Brain natriuretic peptide (BNP) was first isolated in porcine brains. In humans, it is found predominantly in the ventricles and atria of the heart. Infusions of BNP − like ANP − induce natriuresis and diuresis. Increased plasma levels of this peptide hormone, along with higher intravascular volume and increased ventricular pressure, have been observed in connection with heart failure, hypertension, and other illnesses. It remains to be clarified whether and to what extent BNP is involved in physiological blood pressure regulation.

C-type natriuretic peptide (CNP):

In contrast to ANP and BNP, whose primary target organ is the kidney, C-type natriuretic peptide (CNP) appears primarily to be a paracrine hormone involved in the regulation of vascular tone. CNP has been detected in various areas of the brain; moreover, it is formed from and secreted by vascular endothelium, among others. A correlation between CNP concentrations circulating in the plasma and blood pressure levels has not been observed.

Urodilatin:

Urodilatin is largely structurally identical with ANP, but nevertheless displays an additional tetrapeptide on the N-terminal end. To date, urodilatin has only been detected in urine.

1.4.2.5 Medullipin system

Medullipin is a substance formed and released in the renal medulla, and converted in the liver to the vasodilatory, blood-pressure-decreasing, circulating hormone medullipin II. Medullipin II lowers intrarenal vascular resistance and increases renal plasma flow, the glomerular filtration rate, diuresis and natriuresis. It is possible that this hormone is a physiological counterpart to Ang II. − Whether or not this hormone system has a physiological significance for the regulation of blood pressure is presently unknown.

1.4.2.6 Endothelial factors

Endothelial cells are involved in the regulation of vascular tone through the secretion of vasoactive substances. Since nitric oxide (NO; identical with "endothelial derived relaxing factor", EDRF) and prostacyclin (PGI_2) bring about a relaxation of vascular smooth musculature, endothelin displays strong vasoconstrictive properties.

Nitric oxide (NO; EDRF):

The formation of NO proceeds from the amino acid L-arginine and is catalyzed by NO-synthase. There is an obvious, basal, continuous release of NO from unstimulated endothelial cells which counteracts vasoconstrictive influences (Ang II, catecholamines) and contributes to vascular dilatation. In the presence of intact endothelium the pharmacological inhibition of NO-synthase induces a constriction of vascular smooth muscle cells. This observation suggests that the endothelial secretion of vasodilatory NO may contribute to the physiological regulation of blood pressure and blood flow.

Endothelin:

The mRNA-encoded precursor of endothelin (ET-1; in all, three additional isoforms of this polypeptide hormone have been isolated) is pre-pro-endothelin, a large molecule, which is converted to "big-endothelin" by proteolytic cleavage. Big-endothelin is converted by a non-specific endothelin-converting enzyme, a neutral metalloendopeptidase (phosphoramidone), to the mature endothelin, the vasoconstrictive properties of which are $10-100$ times stronger than angiotensin II, serotonin, and norepinephrine. Although endothelin is detectable in the blood of the peripheral veins, it may nevertheless be that this peptide hormone functions here as a paracrine-like substance. Although orally administerable, specific endothelin-receptor antagonists are meanwhile available (Chapter 28), it has to date not been established whether and to what degree endothelin is involved, under physiological conditions, in the local and/or systematic regulation of blood pressure. Increased peripheral plasma levels have been observed in humans, up until now, in cases of hemangioendothelioma (Section 14.10), advanced arteriosclerosis, accelerated hypertension, pulmonary hypertension, cardiac ischemia, and toxic shock.

1.4.2.7 Estrogen

A direct vasodilatory effect of estrogen on vascular smooth muscle may be involved in the regulation of blood pressure and blood flow and could at least partially explain the low incidence of hypertension and other cardiovascular illnesses in premenopausal women.

1.4.2.8 Diadenosine phosphates

Vasopressive diadenosin phosphates (diadenosine pentaphosphate and diadenosine hexaphosphate) have been isolated from platelets. They are suspected of potential significance in the local or physiological regulation of blood pressure.

1.5 Blood pressure variability

Arterial blood pressure is not a constant, but a variable parameter which may be influenced by age, time of day, and situational requirements.

1.5.1 Dependency of blood pressure on age

Throughout youth, blood pressure displays a continuous increase. A child's blood pressure can not be assessed by the same standards as an adult's. An age-specific adaptation is called for (Chapter 11).

It is also not clear whether the increase in blood pressure of aging adults in the industrialized western countries is the result of "civilized living" (stress, noise pollution, obesity, alcohol consumption, overuse of salt), or of truly physiological variables. The isolated increase in systolic blood pressure which occurs as age increases is primarily the result of a loss of aortic elasticity.

1.5.2 Diurnal variability of blood pressure

During sleep, a fall in blood pressure is typically observed (Figure 1.2) which is nevertheless not to be interpreted as an intrinsic circadian rhythm, and is therefore observable even in the event of a change in sleeping pattern (change of time zone, shift change etc.). Patients without sleep-related blood pressure drops have been dubbed "non-dippers" to differentiate from the normal "dippers" (Figure 1.2). This differentiation is significant, on the one hand, for prognostic reasons, since "non-dippers" (less than a 10% decrease in blood pressure during sleep) run a greater cardiovascular risk (left ventricular hypertrophy, cerebrovascular damage, first-time cardiovascular event occurrence within 1−5 years). On the other hand, the identification of a "non-dipper" is

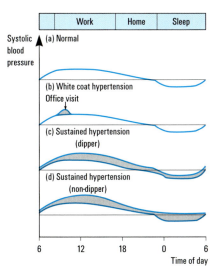

Figure 1.2: Different diurnal blood pressure patterns which may be revealed by ambulatory monitoring in patients with hypertension suspected on the basis of clinic readings. The grey areas show the degree of elevation above normal (adapted from Pickering TG, Ambulatory Monitoring and Blood Pressure Variability, Science Press, London, 1991, p. 9.12).

interesting on (differential-) diagnostic grounds, since a sleep-related decrease in blood pressure is visibly absent in the case of some secondary forms of hypertension — in contrast to primary hypertension. Related publications can be found on renovascular and renoparenchymal hypertension, on primary aldosteronism, on pheochromocytoma, and on Cushing's syndrome. A discontinuance of nocturnal blood pressure decreases has also been observed in patients with cardiac insufficiency, diabetes mellitus with autonomous neuropathy, and malignant primary hypertension; and in a portion of the black (normo- or hypertensive) population of the United States.

1.5.3 Situational fluctuations in blood pressure

A number of daily life influences can cause sometimes considerable fluctuations in blood pressure. Increased physical activity, pain, stress, anxiety and situations of expectancy (first visit to the doctor) lead in this way to blood pressure increases which occasionally match the severity of moderate hypertension (Figure 1.2), but which nevertheless should not be confused with authentic sustained hypertension.

Changes in body position exercise no essential influence on arterial blood pressure. In a healthy patient, one can expect, at the most, a slight increase in diastolic pressure of no more than 5 mmHg when standing.

Summary (Chapter 1)

• Cardiac output, the elasticity of the Windkessel vasculature, and peripheral arterial resistance are the most important determinants in arterial blood pressure.

• An increase in cardiac output and/or of peripheral vascular resistance causes a rise in blood pressure; a decrease in cardiac output and/or of peripheral vascular resistance induces a fall in blood pressure.

• Blood pressure is regulated both neurally and humorally. The objective is the maintenance of a constant, basal blood pressure.

• Short-term blood pressure adjustments are accomplished by way of baro- and chemoreceptors.

• Vasoactive hormones and/or hormone systems are likewise heavily involved in the regulation of blood pressure.

• Blood pressure is not constant, but subject to the various influences of daily life.

Literature (Chapter 1)

Cheung BM, Brown MJ. Plasma brain natriuretic peptide and C-type natriuretic peptide in essential hypertension. J Hypertens 1994; 12: 449−454.

Clozel M, Breu V, Burri K, Cassal JM, Fischli W, Gray GA, Hirth G, Löffler BM, Müller M, Neidhart W, Ramuz H. Pathophysiological role of endothelin revealed by the first orally active endothelin receptor anatgonist. Nature 1993; 365: 759−761.

Inagami T. Atrial natriuretic factor as a volume regulator. J Clin Pharmacol 1994; 34: 424−426.

Level ER. Endothelins. N Engl J Med 1995; 333: 356−363.

London GM, Guerin AP, Pannier B, Marchais SJ, Stimpel M. Influence of sex on arterial hemodynamics and blood pressure. Role of body height. Hypertension 1995; 26: 514−519.

Lowenstein CJ, Dinerman JL, Snyder SH. Nitric oxide: a physiologic messenger. Ann Intern Med 1994; 120: 227−237.

Lüscher TF. The endothelium as a target and mediator of cardiovascular disease. Europ J Clin Invest 1993; 23: 670−685.

MacGregor GA, Markandu ND, Roulston JE, Jones JC. Maintenance of blood pressure by the renin-angiotensin system in normal man. Nature 1981; 291: 329−331.

Margolius HS. Kallikreins and kinins: some unanswered questions about system characteristics and roles in human disease. Hypertension 1995; 26: 230−236.

Michel B, Grima M, Stephan D, Coquard C, Welsch C, Barthelmebs M, Imbs JL. Plasma renin activity and changes in tissue angiotensin converting enzyme. J Hypertens 1994; 12: 577−584.

Mohr E, Richter D. Vasopressin in the regulation of body functions. J Hypertens 1994; 12: 345−348.

Moncada S, Palmer RM, Higgs EA. Nitric oxide: physiology, pathophysiology and pharmacology. Pharmacol Rev 1991; 43: 109−142.

Muirhead EE. Renal vasodepressor mechanisms: the medullipin system. J Hypertens 1993; 11 (suppl. 5): S53−S58.

Nicholls MG, Richards AM, Lewis LK, Yandle TG. Ouabain: a new steroid hormone? Lancet 1995; 346: 1381−1382.

Panfilov VV, Reid JL. Brain and autonomic mechanisms in hypertension. J Hypertension 1994; 12: 337−343.

Ruilope LM, Lahera V, Rodicio JL, Romero JC. Participation of nitric oxide in the regulation of renal function: possible role in the genesis of arterial hypertension. J Hypertens 1994; 12: 625−631.

Schauf CL, Mofett DF, Mofett AB (eds). Human physiology, foundations and frontiers. Times Mirror/Mosby College Publishing 1990.

Schlüter H, Offers E, Brüggemann G, van der Giet M, Tepel M, Nordhoff E, Karas M, Spieker C, Witzel H, Zidek W. Diadenosine phosphates and the physiological control of blood pressure. Nature 1994; 367: 186−188.

Sothern RB, Vesely DL, Kanabrocki EL, Bremner FW, Third JLAC, Boles MA, Nemchausky BM, Olvin JH, Scheving LE. Blood pressure and atrial natriuretic peptides correlate throughout the day. Am Heart J 1995; 129: 907−916.

Swales JD (ed). Textbook of Hypertension. Blackwell Scientific Publishing Oxford 1994. Part 2: Circulation in Hypertension: 60−426.

Volterrani M, Rosano G, Coats A, Beale C, Collins P. Estrogen acutely increases peripheral blood flow in postmenopausal women. Am J Med 1995; 99: 119−122.

Wambach G, Stimpel M, Bönner G. Das atriale natriuretische Peptid und seine Bedeutung für die arterielle Hypertonie. Klin Wochenschr 1989; 67: 1069−1076.

Woolfson RG, Poston L, De Wardener HE. Digoxin-like inhibitors of active sodium transport and blood pressure. Kidney Int 1994; 46: 297−309.

Yanagisawa M. The endothelin system. A new target for therapeutic intervention. Circulation 1994; 89: 1320−1322.

2 Blood pressure measurement

Blood pressure can be measured both directly (invasively) and indirectly (non-invasively).

2.1 Direct (invasive) blood pressure measurement

The direct method of measurement requires the puncturing of a large artery (generally either the radial artery or the femoral artery). With the aid of an electromechanical pressure transformer, pulsations can be directly measured via an intraarterial cannula, so that exceptionally precise values for systolic and diastolic blood pressure can be obtained. To avoid false-positive results, the artery must be punctured and the cannula inserted at least 30 to 60 minutes prior to measurement. All in all, direct blood pressure measurement is coupled with the risks of faulty cannulation (arteriovenous fistula, hematoma, "aneurysm" spurium), of infection, and of arterial embolism; the circumstances under which this reliable measurement method can be applied must, therefore, be precisely defined (e. g. blood pressure monitoring under intensive care conditions).

2.2 Indirect (non-invasive) blood pressure measurement

Indirect methods of measurement have established themselves in practice. The most widely used is the sphygmomanometric determination of arterial blood pressure by the indirect method of Riva-Rocci.

2.2.1 Sphygmomanometric blood pressure measurement

The typical sphygmomanometer is composed of an inflatable cuff, an air pump made of a rubber bulb, and an enclosed mercury- or aneroid-(membrano-)manometer poised on the side. Electronic measuring devices were developed primarily for home blood pressure measurement (Section 2.3.1). To measure, the cuff is applied to the upper arm of the supine, sitting or standing patient and the bladder within the cuff is subsequently pumped up to a pressure roughly 30 mmHg above the patients systolic pressure (disappearance of the radial pulse). The systolic blood pressure can be obtained either palpating or auscultating by means of the attached mercury- or aneoridmanometer.

A variation of the standard mercury sphygmomanometer is the so-called "Hawksley random zero sphygmomanometer" (Hawksley and Sons, Lancing, UK), which finds its greatest application in clinical and epidemiological research, and which prevents the examiner from subjectively influencing test results through the randomized adjustability of the zero point. Comparable tests have nonetheless shown that this device underestimates the true diastolic and systolic blood pressure.

2.2.1.1 Determination of systolic blood pressure by palpation

Systolic blood pressure is established palpatorically when the increasing cuff pressure causes the radial pulse to disappear, or when decreasing cuff pressure allows its reappearance.

2.2.1.2 Auscultatory blood pressure measurement according to the Korotkoff principle

Blood pressure is established by auscultation with the help of a stethoscope whose head is placed over the brachial artery, the position of which is first determined through palpation of the arm in the antecubital space. The auscultatory determination of systolic and diastolic blood pressure values follows the criteria of Korotkoff's sounds phenomenon (Nikolai Korotkoff, Russian surgeon, 1874−1937):

Once the cuff is inflated, the pressure is slowly reduced by the opening of the valve, so that, as the pressure dips below the systolic pressure, the previously compressed brachial artery is once again clear for arterial blood flow. When auscultating, the reintroduction of blood registers as a pulse-synchronous, short, sharp sound. The first occurrence of this sound is labeled phase I of the so-called Korotkoff sounds, and corresponds to the systolic blood pressure.

Through a slow and constant reduction of the cuff pressure, the sound becomes gradually louder. Occasionally, after an initial increase, a temporary decrease in sound intensity can nevertheless be auscultated, which is then followed again by an increase. This potential "auscultatory gap" has practical significance if the cuff, without palpation of the radial pulse, is insufficiently inflated and the renewed increase in noise sound is falsely interpreted as the systolic value.

The distinct rise and fall of the Korotkoff sounds is dubbed "muffling" and corresponds to phase IV. Phase V is characterized by the total disappearance of the Korotkoff sounds and marks the diastolic blood pressure value.

In comparison to direct, intraarterial blood pressure measurement, the indirect method yields systolic values which are slightly too low; and diastolic values which are 5−10 mmHg too high in auscultatory phase IV, and largely identical in phase V. As just mentioned, phase V is used as the auscultatory criterion of diastolic blood pressure. In adolescence, pregnant women, and patients with increased circulatory activity (physical stress, hyperthyroidism), diastolic blood pressure is not equatable with the disappearance (phase V), but with quieting (phase IV) of the Korotkoff sounds. Diastolic blood pressure measured in phase V should nonetheless be noted (Figure 2.1).

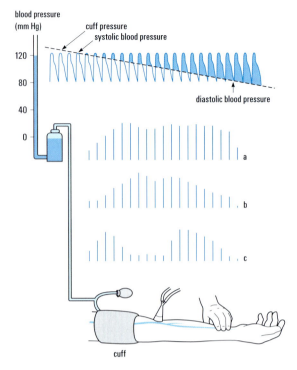

Figure 2.1: Indirect sphygmomanometric measurement of arterial blood pressure using the Riva Rocci method (auscultation according to Korotkoff's method).

After the blood pressure cuff has been inflated, blood flow in the brachial artery is completely cut off. After the cuff pressure has been reduced below the systolic pressure, a short, sharp sound resulting from the inflow can be auscultated following every pulsation (Korotkoff's sound, phase I)(upper portion of Figure 2.1). As cuff pressure is further reduced, the sounds become increasingly louder and then
a) remain at a constant level, or
b) become softer again, or,
c) after an initial increase in volume, decrease temporarily (as so-called "auscultatory gap").

The diastolic blood pressure is arrived at when the sounds become softer (phase IV) and/or disappear entirely (phase V) as the cuff pressure is decreased. Note: the point of auscultation must be level with the heart! (figure adapted from Witzleb E, 1976)

2.2.1.3 Oscillometric method

In this method, blood pressure is determined through measurement of the pulsating pressure fluctuations transmitted from the artery to the cuff. If the cuff pressure exceeds the systolic blood pressure, then only small pressure fluctuations, caused by the beating of the pulse on the constricted artery segment, are registered. At the moment when the cuff pressure falls below the systolic pressure, there is a short systolic opening of the artery and a consecutive increase in oscillation occurs. The oscillations reach their maximum when approaching the mean arterial pressure and subsequently decrease. After a decrease in diastolic pressure and a corresponding uninterrupted opening of the arteries, the pulsations then maintain a constant minimum intensity.

Blood pressure intensity is determined by way of an electronic or mechanical analysis of the registered pulsations. This method allows for the possible determination of mean arterial pressure, thus offering a particular advantage over sphygmomanometric measurement.

2.2.1.4 Doppler-ultrasound method

Systolic blood pressure can be just as well determined in a manner analogous to the Riva-Rocci method by using the Doppler-ultrasound method and a blood pressure cuff placed proximal to the test area (see above). This method is also suited to the measurement of lower blood pressure values, of non-pulsating flow, and of blood pressure in smaller veins. Diastolic pressure values can not be reliably determined using the Ultrasound-Doppler method.

2.2.2 Individual fitting of the blood pressure cuff

The cuff pressure, propagating sphenoidally into the tissue from within the cuff material, must be transmitted to the artery without loss. An individual fitting of the cuff to various extremities is therefore absolutely necessary in order to avoid false measurements. The most widely used cuff size contains an inflatable bladder with a surface measuring 12×24 cm and yields largely reliable blood pressure measurements on upper arms with a circumference of 24 to 32 cm. When applied to larger arm circumferences, this cuff size produces falsely high values; when to smaller, falsely lower. It is therefore indispensable in daily clinical usage to have a variety of cuff sizes available. For upper arms with a circumference of 33 to 41 cm, the inflatable surface should measure 15×30 cm; for larger arms, $18 \times 36-42$ cm. For children, narrower cuffs are available whose width, depending on the individual, should equal two thirds of the length of the upper arm (Table 2.1).

Table 2.1:   Recommendations for the choice of blood pressure cuff size*

	Upper arm diameter	Size of the inflatable rubber portion of the cuff (width × length)
	(cm)	
Small child		5×8
Child (>5 years old)		8×13
Adult	<33	$12 \times 23-24$
	33−41	$15 \times 30-35$
	>41	$18 \times 36-42$

* Modified according to recommendations of the "German Hypertension Society" (1989)

Routine operation may soon be simplified by a new kind of cuff containing three inflatable rubber bags of different sizes, which automatically select the appropriately sized bag in relation to the individual arm circumference (Tricuff, Pressure Group AB, Stockholm, Sweden).

2.2.3 Blood pressure measurement technique

In principal, blood pressure can be measured in a supine, sitting or standing position. The blood pressure cuff should in any case be placed level with the heart in order to prevent hydrostatic effects from influencing the measured values. The sitting position is normally chosen for blood pressure measurement in the examining room or in an ambulance. The patient should be comfortably seated with his/her arm slightly bent and resting on a support. To minimize emotional influences on blood pressure, the measurement is best carried out only after the patient has adapted to the unaccustomed surroundings of the doctor's office. Blood pressure measurements taken "on the run" often lead to high, situationally determined pressure values and are therefore hardly reliable.

Once the patient has assumed the desired position, the uninflated and wrinkle-free cuff is placed approximately in the middle of the exposed upper arm. Shirt and sweater sleeves should not be rolled up, since this could hinder blood flow in the arm and produce false results.

While sensing the radial pulse, the blood pressure cuff is quickly inflated to a pressure roughly 30 mmHg higher than what the pressure should be, at which point the radial pulse disappears. Excessive inflation of the cuff can induce short-term, false-positive increases in systolic pressure, and should therefore be avoided. The cuff pressure is subsequently reduced at a rate of 2−3 mmHg per second.

If the Korotkoff method is followed, the stethoscope should be placed above the pulse point of the brachial artery to enable auscultation. A margin of error no greater than 2 mmHg is critical; (the all-too-common) rounding up or down of results to the nearest multiple of 5 or 10 (e.g. 140/95 mmHg) is too imprecise and therefore not acceptable.

Every first-time blood pressure measurement needs to be carried out on both arms in order to verify or rule out side differences. Ideally, measurement should take place on both arms simultaneously, since serial measurement often yields overestimates of the difference. In the event the pressure on one side exceeds the pressure on the other by more than 20 mmHg when measured serially, a simultaneous measurement should be carried out before recourse to more invasive diagnostic techniques.

It should be noted that in older patients, advanced arteriosclerotic changes of the large arteries may lead to falsely high pressure readings. Blood pressure readings have been taken with the sphygmomanometer which, depending on the degree of the arterial wall rigidity, have exceeded simultaneous, direct, intraarterial readings by as much as 60 mmHg. Such "pseudohypertension" is anticipated where the radial artery remains as palpable as a cord after inflation of the cuff (so-called "Osler's maneuver").

In patients less than 30 years old, coarctation of the aorta (Chapter 16.1) should be excluded by the additional taking of a blood pressure reading on one leg on the occasion of the first test. For this purpose a large upper thigh cuff is necessary. The Korotkoff sounds are then auscultated in the popliteal fossa.

An additional standing blood pressure measurement is required on the occasion of a first visit in order to verify orthostatic reactions. Standing blood pressure measurement is a matter of routine practice with diabetics, elderly patients, and patients receiving vasodilatory treatment.

(For the particulars of blood pressure measurement, see Table 2.2.)

Table 2.2:   Peculiarities of blood pressure measurement

Condition	Peculiarity
Children, adolescents	− Age-related normal ranges, see Figure 11.1 − Cuff size, see Table 2.1 − Diastolic value = phase IV of the Korotkoff sounds
Elderly patients (>65 years)	− Consider "pseudohypertension" − BP measurement in supine and standing position
Pregnancy	− Normal range differs, see Section 15.2 − Diastolic value = phase IV of the Korotkoff sounds
Atrial fibrillation	− Determination of systolic and diastolic BP by calculating the mean of several BP measurements
Shock	− palpatory determination of systolic BP or, if possible, − intraarterial BP measurement
Hyperthyroidism/exercise	− Diastolic value = phase IV of the Korotkoff sounds

2.3 Indirect blood pressure measurement under ambulatory conditions

Although our knowledge of the relationship between blood pressure and the risk of cardiovascular disease is based on studies carried out in private practice or in clinics, this so-called "office blood pressure measurement" is limited in its accuracy. One disadvantage, for example, is the fact that blood pressure values measured in private practice do not necessarily represent those of an individual patient in his usual environment. Blood pressure measurements in patients with or without hypertension tend to be higher when measured by a doctor than when measured by the patient himself, by automatic ambulatory techniques, or by non-medical examiners. This elevation of the blood pressure, most commonly labeled "white coat hypertension," is generally the result of a stressful situation in a medical environment (see Figure 1.2) and can lead — especially in cases of moderate blood pressure elevation — to over-treatment.

As a result, various diagnostic methods have been proposed in recent years which either replace or augment measurements taken in the doctor's office. Increasing consideration is being given to ambulatory blood pressure measurement.

Blood pressure measurement under ambulatory conditions takes two principal forms: self-measurement by the patient in his home environment ("home measurements"), and continuous 24-hour blood pressure monitoring with an automatic measuring device (ABPM).

2.3.1 Ambulatory self-measurement of blood pressure/ home blood pressure measurement

In many instances, ambulatory/home blood pressure measurements obtained by the patient or by a family member enable a more reliable evaluation of average blood pressure than measurements obtained in the doctor's office (Section 2.3). Average daily blood pressure values obtained by home measurement are predominantly lower than those obtained in an office visit, yet hardly distinguishable from values obtained by ABPM (Section 2.3.2).

Home measurement is advisable where a borderline or mild hypertension is suspected, in the presence of mild hypertension with target-organ damage and for therapeutic monitoring in the event of a poor therapeutic response. Moreover, it has been observed that therapeutic compliance improves where the patient is actively involved in treatment through self-measurement.

The blood pressure self-measurement devices available today are predominantly electronic, operating either on the Korotkoff principle, or according to the oscillometric technique. Whereas the cuff of an oscillometric device need not be precisely placed, due to registration of the oscillations over the entire cuff surface, the microphone-bearing cuff of a Korotkoff device must be placed as precisely as possible over the brachial artery. Current microphone quality will nevertheless compensate for small displacements.

On average, oscillometric devices underestimate diastolic (and systolic) blood pressure values. Devices operating on the Korotkoff principle still produce reliable blood pressure measurements. Up to date test results can be found in professional journals and in consumer-oriented publications (e.g. "test", from the Product Testing Foundation [Stiftung Warentest], Berlin, Germany; or "Consumer Reports", in the USA).

With the devices available today, the proper execution of blood pressure measurement should pose no problem. All the same, the fundamentals of measurement ought to be thoroughly explained to the patient. A physician's assistant should provide the patient with a practical introduction and verify his self-reported measurements.

The patient must be further urged to write down self-measured blood pressure test results, and to bring them along when visiting the doctor. A so-called "blood pressure diary," obtainable through many of the national hypertension societies, has been devised for the notation of self-obtained blood pressure measurements.

Devices which measure blood pressure from the finger (e.g. Finger Blood Pressure and Pulse Monitor, Healthteam; VB-211 Finger Blood Pressure Meter, AND Medical Division; Blood Pressure Monitor, Nisseid; HEM-812F, Omron, among others) or from the wrist (Blood Pressure Monitor Watch BP 100, Casio; Blood Pressure Monitor HEM 601, Omron; Blood Pressure Watch, Matsushita, among others) are easy to handle, but underestimate real values. Due to this imprecision, finger measurement devices in particular can not yet be recommended (test, Stiftung Warentest, 2/1994).

2.3.2 Continuous 24-hour ambulatory blood pressure monitoring (ABPM)

Continuous ambulatory recording by means of portable, automatic blood pressure measurement devices ("ambulatory blood pressure monitoring", ABPM) has found increasing application in recent years in private practice, in clinics and in clinical research. The devices currently available work according to the auscultation (Korotkoff) principle with the help of a microphone placed over the brachial artery, according to the oscillometric method, or according to a combination of both methods.

The positioning of a cuff with intermittent compression of the brachial artery can be circumvented by the use of finger measurement devices which also allow for the 24-hour registration of blood pressure values (Finapres; Portapres).

Daytime measurements are normally programmed 15−30 minutes apart, nighttime measurements 30−45 minutes apart. The measurements are stored in a device which the patient carries with him. Upon completion of the tests, the results are analyzed by computer and an average value or percentile determination is made.

To simplify data interpretation, patients should document their activities. Activity level can be alternatively determined by way of an electronic "action graph" attached to the wrist.

ABPM-devices are available today from a number of manufacturers (Table 2.3). Guidelines for the qualitative evaluation of these instruments have been established by the United States Association for the Advancement of Medical Instrumentation (AAMI), and by the British Hypertension Society. Each provides for the incorporation of the latest findings. In Germany, the German Hypertension Society publishes the semiannual "ABPM NEWS LETTER", which addresses fundamental and contemporary issues of blood pressure measurement.

2.3.2.1 Determination of average blood pressure

Average blood pressure is most often calculated either from individual measurements, or from individual average hourly values. To date, the recommendations

Table 2.3:   Devices for ABPM

Device	Mechanism
A & D Engineering Co, Ltd	
TM-2420	
Models 1—5	A
Model 6	A
Model 7	A
TM-2421	O/A
BioAnalogics Systems Inc	
ABP Monitor	A
Biotrac Inc	
Auto-Cuff ABP-1001	O
Circadian Inc	
BP Mate	O
Colin Medical Instruments Corp	
ABPM 630	O
Del Mar Avionics	
Pressurometer IV	A/E (optional)
Disetronic Medical Systems AG	
CH-DRUCK (PressureScan in Germany)	A
Profilomat	A
GH Medical Inc	
ABP 901	O
Healthcare Technology Ltd	
Pulse Time BP-10 monitor/watch	P
BP-50 monitor	P
Hill-Med Corp	
Revelation system	O
IDT France	
Nissei DS-240	A/O/E (optional)
I. E. M. Electromedicina, S. L.	
ACP 2200	O
Adis II	O
I. E. M. GmBH	
Mobil-O-Graph	O
Imex Medical Systems Inc	
ABP 9000	A
Instromedix Inc	
BARO-GRAF 24	A
Kontron Instruments	
AM 5200 Micro Recorder	O/E
AM 5600 Micro Recorder	O
Novacor	
DIASYS 200	A/E (optional)
Oxford Medical, Ltd	
Medilog ABP	A/E
PAR Medizintechnik GmBH	
PAR-PHYSIO-PORT III (TONOPORT II, in Germany)	A/E
PAR-PHYSIO-PORT IIIA (TONOPORT III, in Germany)	O
Pilger Medizin-Elektronik	
Custo Screen	O
Pulse Trend Inc	
Pulse Trend ABP	O

Table 2.3:   (continued)

Device	Mechanism
Save 33 Electronique Medicale	
Mapa 33	O
Schiller AG	
Schiller BR-102	A/O
SpaceLabs Medical Inc	
SL-90202	O
SL-90207	O
First Medic 310	O
Stuart Medical Inc	
SmartLINK ABP 310	A/O/E/R
Suntech Medical Instruments Inc	
Accutracker II	A/E
Accutracker II (version 20−23)	A/E
Accutracker Dx	A/E
Suzuken Co Ltd	
Kenz-BPM AM-200 recorder	O/A
TNO Biomedical Instrumentation	
Portapres Model-2	F/V
Tycos Instruments Inc	
QuietTrak (TENSO24 in Germany)	A/E (optional)
Zewa AG	
Delwa-Star 24	O/A/E (optional)
Zymed Inc	
Multitrak-Plus ABP/ECG	A/E/R

Mechanism codes:

O: oscillometric	P: Pulse wave velocity	F: finger occlusion
A: auscultatory	R: ECG recording	V: vascular unloading
E: ECG gating		

Status 1/1995; from O'Brien E, Atkins N, Staessen J, Hypertension 1995; 26: 835−842

Table 2.4:   Recommendations for normal ranges of blood pressure (BP) as determined by 24-hour ambulatory blood pressure monitoring (ABPM)

Investigator	24-hr. BP	Daytime BP	Nighttime BP
	(mmHg)		
Baumgart et al. (1990)	135/85		
Staessen et al. (1991)	139/87	146/91	127/79
O'Brien et al. (1993)	140/86	148/92	128/77

for blood pressure measurements taken with ABPM devices have been varied but are consistently lower than those accepted for measurements taken sporadically by sphygmomanometer. ($< 140/90$ mmHg) (Table 2.4). The average daily blood pressure norm of $< 135/85$ mmHg proposed at the 1990 International Consensus Conference on Indirect Ambulatory Blood Pressure Monitoring represents a standard value whose validity seems acceptable based on the limited data available to date.

The evaluation of nighttime blood pressure values is more complicated. It has been shown that a minuscule drop (less than 10%) or lack of decrease in nighttime blood pressure correlates with an increased incidence of cardiovascular events within the following 1−5 years, but norms for the measurement of nighttime blood pressure have yet to be defined.

2.3.2.2 Determination of percent increase

Another variant of ABPM evaluation is based on known values established through casual blood pressure measurement. The percent increase over the norm value (> 140/90) is calculated. Percent increase is nevertheless only meaningful for daytime blood pressure values, since normative values for nighttime blood pressure are lacking (see above).

2.3.2.3 Recommended applications of ABPM

Routine, uncritical use of ABPM in the diagnosis and treatment of hypertension is unacceptably costly, whereas its targeted use can actually be economical. ABPM is not only financially practical, but useful as well in detecting "white coat hypertension", and in evaluating a (putatively) therapy-resistant hypertension. In clinical research, and in patients with a poorly controlled hypertension (particularly secondary forms of hypertension), ABPM enables observation − not possible with other methods − of the nighttime and early morning efficacy of antihypertensive agents. The 1993 report of the Joint National Committee on Detection, Evaluation and Treatment of High Blood Pressure (JNC V), moreover, rates episodic hypertension, hypotensive symptoms in association with antihypertensive medication or autonomic dysfunction, carotid sinus syndrome, and pacemaker syndrome as further clinical situations in which the use of ABPM may be helpful.

In spite of the absence of a circadian rhythm to blood pressure under conditions of secondary hypertension (Section 1.5.2), ABPM is not advisable as a routine test to differentiate between primary and secondary hypertension, since an absence of circadian rhythm has been observed in patients with other illnesses (severe heart failure, diabetes mellitus with autonomic neuropathy, malignant hypertension, etc.). Moreover, the lack of a nighttime drop in blood pressure may be attributable to a patient's inability to fall asleep due to contact with the measuring device (Figure 2.2), or to sleep disorders of another kind.

2.3.2.4 Open questions about ABPM

The proof of a reduction in morbidity and mortality due to an antihypertensive therapeutic intervention is based on clinical studies in which the diagnosis of hypertension and the control of therapy were carried out exclusively by use of sporadic blood pressure measurements taken in clinics or private practice. To date

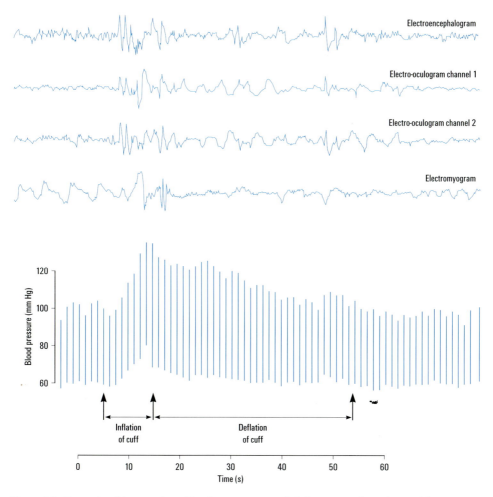

Figure 2.2: Example of beat to beat blood pressure recorded from contralateral arm. Measurement occured during stage 2 sleep. Arousal during cuff inflation is shown in electroencephalogram and electromyogram (From Davies RJO et al., Br Med J 1994; 308: 820).

there are no comparable ABPM-based studies, so that the value of ABPM in the diagnosis and therapy of hypertension can be only indirectly inferred. Future studies will therefore have to clarify whether and to what extent ABPM can produce various diagnostic, therapeutic and/or prognostic findings; and the relationship of ABPM to measurements taken ambulatorily at home and casually in clinics or private practice. It must be determined, in particular, whether ABPM is better suited to the monitoring of therapy and the resulting influences on cardiovascular complications (left ventricular hypertrophy, cardiac events) than casual blood pressure measurements taken in clinics and private practice. It is further unclear which conditions (measurements over a 24-hour period, during the day, during sleep, at home, at work) and which ABPM readings (average or percent increase in blood pressure) provide the best basis for the prognosis of cardiovascular risk.

2.4 Blood pressure: office-visit measurement, ambulatory/home (self) measurement, or ABPM?

In the future, sphygmomanometric blood pressure measurement by the doctor or by medical personnel will remain the method of choice for the routine diagnosis of hypertension and for monitoring the effectiveness of therapy. Ambulatory self-measurement of blood pressure and the associated involvement of the patient in both diagnosis and therapy should be generously prescribed. It is urgently recommended where "white coat hypertension" is suspected, when mild hypertension already exists, or when a recently initiated therapy requires evaluation. Whether or not ABPM offers advantages in these areas is arguable. The question will certainly not be answered before comparative studies (see above) have been concluded. ABPM is presently the only method, however, for measuring nighttime and early morning blood pressure. It can furthermore be helpful in evaluating a questionable resistance to antihypertensive therapy.

2.5 Trough/peak ratio

The ratio of the antihypertensive effect at the end of a dosage interval to the maximum effect (trough/peak ratio) is a parameter which is relatively easy to determine. It has been employed in clinical research to evaluate the safety and 24-hour efficacy of an antihypertensive substance. Proof of at least $50-66\%$ of the maximum antihypertensive effect at the end of a dosage interval is considered to be indicative of a permanent blood pressure reduction without undesired high discrepancy between minimum and maximum effect (example: diastolic blood pressure before intake of the next tablet = -5 mmHg, maximum blood pressure reduction = -9 mmHg; the trough/peak ratio is approximately 0.56). A slight reduction of blood pressure "at trough" with high effect "at peak" results in a quotient < 0.5. A quotient < 0.5 is typical for short-acting substances which only have an antihypertensive effect 24 hours after intake if they were administered in inadequately high dosages.

The determination of the trough/peak ratio as an index for the assessment of substance safety and efficacy is disputed and does contain some methodological weaknesses. In the context of this book however, it is not possible to go into detailed discussion of the subject. For more information other sources are recommended (e.g J Hypertens 1994; 12 (suppl 8): pp 1–119).

2.6 Maintenance of blood pressure measuring equipment

The commonly used blood pressure measurement devices are tested for accuracy and functionality before sale and appropriately stamped with an official seal. Their recalibration must be conducted every two years, and earlier, naturally, in the event of malfunction (e.g. a 3 mmHg deviation of the zero-point on an inflated cuff).

Summary (Chapter 2)

- Routine blood pressure monitoring is normally accomplished through auscultation of the Korotkoff sounds with the help of a mercury sphygmomanometer or oscillometrically.
- Blood pressure must be measured under largely standardized conditions:
  - approximately 5 minutes of rest prior to blood pressure measurement;
  - no clothing between the arm and the blood pressure cuff;
  - a cuff width adjusted to the size of the arm;
  - determination of blood pressure on both arms and on one leg, in both standing and sitting (or supine) positions on the occasion of a first visit;
  - adherence to the chosen body postures (supine or sitting) for repeated measurements;
  - repeated measurement in both standing and sitting (or supine) positions for diabetic patients, elderly patients, and patients undergoing vasodilatory treatment;
  - determination of blood pressure to within a 2 mmHg margin of error.
- Ambulatory self-monitoring of blood pressure ("home measurement") is indicated where "white coat hypertension" is suspected, in cases of mild hypertension, and for the observation of therapeutic progress.
- Automatic, continuous 24-hour blood pressure monitoring (ABPM) is indicated where "white coat hypertension" is suspected, for the evaluation of a questionable resistance to antihypertensive therapy, and in cases of arterial hypertension where the determination of nighttime and early morning blood pressure values is suspected to be of diagnostic and/or therapeutic relevance.
- The true value of ABPM for diagnosis, prognosis and surveillance of therapy in cases of arterial hypertension has yet to be determined.

Literature (Chapter 2)

American College of Physicians. Automated ambulatory blood pressure and self-measured blood pressure monitoring devices: their role in the diagnosis and management of hypertension. Ann Intern Med 1993; 118: 889–892.

Appel LJ, Stason WB. Ambulatory blood pressure monitoring and blood pressure self-measurement in the diagnosis and management of hypertension. Ann Intern Med 1993; 118: 867–882.

Association For The Advancement Of Medical Instrumentation. American national standard for electronic or automated sphygmomanometers. Arlington, Virginia: AAMI; 1987.

Baumgart P, Walger P, Fuchs G, Dorst KG, Vetter H, Rahn KH. Twenty four hour blood pressure is not dependent on endogenous circadian rhythm. J Hypertens 1989; 7: 331–334.

Baumgart P, Schrader J (Hrsg). 24-h-Langzeit-blutdruckmessung. Z Kardiol 1992; 81 (Suppl 2): 1–106.

Davies RJO, Jenkins NE, Stradling JR. Effect of measuring ambulatory blood pressure on sleep and on blood pressure during sleep. Br Med J 1994; 308: 820–823.

Franz IW. ABDM und Ergometrie zur Beurteilung der Hypertonie. Nieren Hochdruckkrkht 1995; 24: 90–92.

Ferrari P, Ostini E, Allemann Y, de Courten M, Weidmann P. Diagnostischer Wert ambulanter Blutdrucktagesprofile: Vergleich mit Messungen durch eine Laborantin. Schweiz med Wschr 1992; 122: 1317–1324.

Davies RJO, Jenkins NE, Stradling JR. Effect of measuring ambulatory blood pressure on sleep and on bood pressure during sleep. Br Med J 1994; 308: 820–823.

De Gaudemaris R, Chau NP, Mallion JM, for the Groupe de la Mesure, French Society of Hypertension. Home blood pressure: variability, comparison with office readings and proposal for reference values. J Hypertens 1994; 12: 831–838.

Fagard R, Staessen J, Thijs L, Amery A. Multiple standardized clinic blood pressures may predict left ventricular mass as well as ambulatory monitoring: a metaanalysis of comparative studies. Am J Hypertens 1995; 8: 533–540.

Gillman MW, Cook NR. Blood pressure measurement in childhood epidemiological studies. Circulation 1995; 92: 1049–1057.

Grin JM, McCabe EJ, White WB. Management of hypertension after ambulatory blood pressure monitoring. Ann Intern Med 1993; 118: 833–837.

Kribben A, Weber F, Anlauf M, Claus M, Hirche H, Simonides R, Philipp T. Elektronische Blutdruck-Selbstmeßgeräte 1990/91. Vergleich von oszillometrischen Geräten mit Korotkow-Geräten. Nieren- und Hochdruckkrkht 1992; 21: 351–357.

Krönig B. ABDM – aktueller Stand der Gerätetechnik. Nieren Hochdruckkrkht 1995; 24: 137–140.

Kugler J, Schmitz N, Seelbach H, Rollnik J, Krüskemper GM. Rise in systolic blood pressure during sphygmomanometer depends on the maximum inflation pressure of the arm cuff. J Hypertens 1994; 12: 825–829.

Mancia G, Di Rienzo M, Parati G. (Clinical Conference) Ambulatory blood pressure monitoring use in hypertension research and clin-

ical practice. Hypertension 1993; 21: 510–524.

Mancia G, Parati G. Commentary on the revised British Hypertension Society protocol for evaluation of blood pressure measuring devices: a critique of aspects related to 24-hour ambulatory blood pressure measurement. J Hypertens 1993; 11: 595–597.

Mancia G, Zanchetti A (eds.). Trough : peak ratio: measurement, limitations and relevance to treatment of hypertension. J Hypertens 1994; 12 (suppl. 8): S1–S118.

Messerli FH, Ventura HO, Amodeo C. Osler's maneuver and pseudohypertension. N Engl J Med 1985; 312: 1548–1551.

Middecke M. Ambulante Blutdruck-Langzeitmessung (ABDM) – Grundlagen und praktische Anwendung. Thieme Verlag, Stuttgart, 1990.

Middeke M, Schrader J. Nocturnal blood pressure in normotensive subjects and those with white coat, primary, and secondary hypertension. Br Med J 1994; 308: 630–632.

O'Brien E, Mee F, Atkins N, O'Malley K. Inaccuracy of the Hawksley random zero sphygmomanometer. Lancet 1990; 336: 1465–1468.

O'Brien, Petrie J, Littler W, De Swiet M, Padfield PL, Altman DG, Bland M, Coats A, Atkins N. The British Hypertension Society pro-tocol for the evaluation of automated and semi-automated blood pressure measuring devices with special reference to ambulatory systems. J Hypertens 1990; 8: 607–619.

O'Brien E, Petrie J, Littler W, De Swiet M, Padfield PL, Altman DG, Bland M, Coats A,Atkins N. Short report: An outline of the revised British Hypertension Society protocol for the evaluation of blood pressure measuring devices. J Hypertens 1993; 11: 677–679.

O'Brien E, Atkins N, Staessen J. State of the market. A review of ambulatory blood pressure monitoring devices. Hypertension 1995; 26: 835–842.

Paky A, Lüscher T, Grimm J, Steiner R, Greminger P, Vetter W. Blutdruckunterschiede an beiden Armen. Ergebnisse serieller und simultaner Blutdruckmessung. Schweiz Rundschau Med (PRAXIS) 1983; 72: 906–913.

Pickering TG. Ambulatory monitoring and blood pressure variability. Science Press, London, 1991.

Pickering TG. How should the diurnal changes of blood pressure be expressed? Am J Hypertens 1995; 8: 681–682.

Staessen JA, Thijs L, Mancia G, Parati G, O'Brien ET. Clinical trials with ambulatory blood pressure measurement: fewer patients needed? Lancet 1994; 344: 1552–1556.

Stolt M, Sjönell G, Aström H, Rössner S, Hansson L. Improved accuracy of indirect blood pressure measurement in patients with obese arms. Am J Hypertens 1993; 6: 66–71.

Wambach G, Jacob R, Treeger A, Stimpel M. Wie zuverlässig ist die oszillometrische Blutdruckmessung mit dem Omron-Gerät? Schweiz Rundschau Med (PRAXIS) 1992; 81: 1258–1261.

White WB, Whelton A, Fox AAL, Stimpel M, Kaihlanen PM. Tricenter assessment of the efficacy of the ACE inhibitor, moexipril, by ambulatory blood pressure monitoring. J Clin Pharmacol 1995; 35: 233–238.

White WB, Berson AS, Robbins C, Jamieson MJ, Prisant LM, Roccella E, Sheps SG. National standard for measurement of resting and ambulatory blood pressures with automated sphygmomanometers. Hypertension 1993; 21: 504–509.

Zweifler AJ, Shahab ST. Pseudohypertension: a new assessment. J Hypertens 1993; 11: 1–6.

3 Determination of the individual blood pressure

The upper norms of arterial blood pressure are arbitrarily set based on the results of epidemiological and interventional studies in which the necessary measurements were carried out almost exclusively on prearranged examination days in clinics or private practices. Future changes in these norms are imaginable, since the increasing integration of continuous 24-hour blood pressure monitoring (ABPM; see Section 2.3.2) in large epidemiological studies may lead to a new understanding of what constitutes "normal" arterial blood pressure.

3.1 Diagnostic value of basal blood pressure and casual blood pressure

As noted in previous chapters, arterial blood pressure presents no constant values, but rather undergoes physiological and situational fluctuations throughout the day and night. The physiological fluctuations possess a characteristic rhythm typified by a nighttime nadir. Situational changes in blood pressure are in contrast determined by the physical, psychic and environmental influences of daily life (see also Section 1.5).

Evaluation of actual, individual blood pressure must therefore be oriented toward blood pressure values repeatedly monitored by a patient in the course of a day. The patient is in danger of blood-pressure-induced target-organ damage, and thereby subject to a diagnosis of chronic hypertension, only after exceeding these norms for a longer period.

ABPM has become a dependable means for determining blood pressure in day-to-day conditions. As a screening procedure for the determination of individual blood pressure, however, this method has proven too expensive. The determination of basal blood pressure, defined as the blood pressure before rising after a night of bedrest under maximum shielding from ambient influences, is also practically impossible at the doctor's office. On the basis of a satisfactory diagnosis with corresponding intraarterial 24-hour blood pressure monitoring, repeated measurement of casual blood pressure under predominantly standardized conditions, has established itself as an easy procedure for determining individual blood pressure. In principle, casual blood pressure can be measured either by medical personnel, or by the patient himself.

3.2 Interpreting blood pressure readings obtained under (ergometric) exercise conditions

Although new studies indicate that the level of increase in blood pressure when under physical stress is an independent variable in the prognosis of cardiovascular mortality, there is to date no uniform international definition of the upper norm of arterial blood pressure under exercise conditions. The values put forth by several authors (Table 3.1) are based on the results of volunteer and patient studies in which the participants' blood pressure was measured while on a treadmill or while riding a bicycle ergometer. No generally binding guidelines yet exist regarding the interpretation of exercise-induced blood pressure increases, since study protocols applied differed significantly in each of the studies mentioned.

Table 3.1:   Upper limits of normal blood pressure during isotonic exercise tests

Criteria	Upper limits
100 W, beginning with 50 W, increasing every minute by 10 W, submaximal exercise intensity (Franz, 1982)	<50 years old: up to 200/100 mmHg >50 years old: up to 215/105 mmHg
All work load levels (Heck et al., 1984)	as above
All work load levels (Jackson et al., 1983; Wilson et al., 1981)	up to 230/110 mmHg
100 W, 6 minutes (Mundal et al., 1994)	up to 200 mgHg systolic

Summary (Chapter 3)

- The upper norms of arterial blood pressure are arbitrary. Their definition is founded on the results of large epidemiological and interventional studies.

- The decisive factor in the development of hypertension-induced end-organ damage is not the level of situational blood pressure increases, but rather the average level of blood pressure over time.

- The measurement of casual blood pressure under largely standardized conditions has in most cases proven itself a satisfactorily reliable indicator of the individual blood pressure.

- There is a positive correlation between exercise-induced blood pressure increases and cardiovascular mortality.

Literature (Chapter 3)

Alam GM, Smirk FH. Casual and basal blood pressure. I. In British and Egyptian men. Br Heart J 1943; 5: 152−155.

Caldwell JR, Schork MA, Aiken RD. Is near basal blood pressure a more accurate predictor of cardiorenal manifestations of hypertension than casual blood pressure? J Chron Dis 1978; 31: 507–512.

Fagard R, Staessen J, Thijs L, Amery A. Prognostic significance of exercise versus resting blood pressure in hypertensive men. Hypertension 1991; 17: 574–578.

Filipovsky J, Ducimetiere P, Safar ME. Prognostic significance of exercise blood pressure and heart rate in middle-aged men. Hypertension 1992; 20: 333–339.

Franz IW. Assessment of blood pressure response during ergometric work in normotensive and hypertensive patients. Acta Med Scand 1982 (suppl 5): 35–47.

Mundal R, Kjeldsen SE, Sandvik L, Erikssen G, Thaulow E, Erikssen J. Exercise blood pressure predicts cardiovascular mortality in middle-aged men. Hypertension 1994; 24: 56–62.

Smirk FH. Observations on the mortality of 270 treated and 199 untreated retinal grade I and II hypertensive patients followed in all instances for 5 years. NZ Med J 1964; 63: 413–443.

4 Definition of arterial hypertension

Blood pressure level alone is an insufficient criterion for evaluating arterial hypertension, since it provides no information concerning recovery, end-organ damage, or the resultant urgency and means of a diagnostic and therapeutic intervention. Arterial hypertension is therefore normally classified depending on:

1. Blood pressure level,
2. course,
3. end-/target-organ damage, and
4. etiology.

4.1 Classification of hypertension according to blood pressure level

Earlier guidelines of the World Health Organization (WHO) defined the upper limits of normal blood pressure as 160 mmHg systolic and 95 mmHg diastolic. In recent years, thanks to the availability of large epidemiological studies, it has been verified that even patients with blood pressure levels below 160/95 mmHg experience higher morbidity and mortality in comparison with the normal, healthy population. It has also been possible to demonstrate that even isolated increases in systolic blood pressure boost the risk of coronary heart disease or cerebrovascular disease. All national and international hypertension associations as well as the WHO have since revised their guidelines to reflect the new information. Although long-term increases in arterial blood pressure to levels of 140 mmHg systolic and/or 90 mmHg diastolic or more are uniformly labeled hypertension, there nevertheless remain differences in the designation of stages as well as in the definition of the normal range (Tables 4.1a and 4.1b).

With an incidence estimated at 20−30% of the population of the western industrialized nations, arterial hypertension is the most common chronic disease. According to the normal ranges defined above, roughly 4/5ths of all hypertensive patients display moderate hypertension or isolated systolic hypertension, while 1/5th displays moderate to severe hypertension.

4.2 Classification of hypertension according to clinical progress

Independently of the blood pressure level, hypertension can also be classified according to its clinical progress.

Table 4.1a: The WHO/ISH* classification of hypertension according to blood pressure level

	SBP** (mmHg)		DBP** (mmHg)
Normotension	<140	and	<90
Mild hypertension	140−180	and/or	90−105
Subgroup: borderline	140−160	and/or	90−95
Moderate and severe hypertension	≥180	and/or	≥105
Isolated systolic hypertension	≥140	and	<90
Subgroup: borderline	140−160	and	<90

    * WHO: World Health Organization
       ISH: International Society of Hypertension
  ** SBP: Systolic Blood Pressure
      DBP: Diastolic Blood Pressure

Table 4.1b: The JNC V classification of hypertension according to blood pressure level (for adults aged 18 years and older)*

Category	Systolic, mmHg	Diastolic, mmHg
Normal**	<130	<85
High normal	130−139	85−89
Hypertension***		
Stage 1 (mild)	140−159	90−99
Stage 2 (moderate)	160−179	100−109
Stage 3 (severe)	180−209	110−119
Stage 4 (very severe)	≥210	≥120

   * Not taking antihypertensive drugs and not acutely ill. When systolic and diastolic pressures fall into different categories, the higher category should be selected to classify the individual's blood pressure status. For instance, 160/92 mmHg should be classified as stage 2, and 180/120 mmHg should be classified as stage 4. Isolated systolic hypertension is defined as a systolic blood pressure of 140 mmHg or more and a diastolic blood pressure of less than 90 mmHg and staged appropriately (eg, 170/85 mmHg is defined as stage 2 isolated systolic hypertension).
     In addition to classifying stages of hypertension on the basis of average blood pressure levels, the clinician should specify presence or absence of target-organ disease and additional risk factors. For example, a patient with diabetes and a blood pressure of 142/94 mmHg, plus left ventricular hypertrophy should be classified as having "stage 1 hypertension with target-organ disease (left ventricular hypertrophy) and with another major risk factor (diabetes)." This specificity is important for risk classification and management.
 ** Optimal blood pressure with respect to cardiovascular risk is less than 120 mmHg systolic and less than 80 mmHg diastolic. However, unusually low readings should be evaluated for clinical significance.
*** Based on the average of two or more readings taken at each of two or more visits after an initial screening.
Adapted from Arch Intern Med 1993; 153: 154−183

4.2.1 Unstable hypertension

The expression "unstable hypertension" is no longer used, since every individual's blood pressure fluctuates (Section 1.5), thus making an exact definition impossible.

Nevertheless, patients whose blood pressure fluctuates repeatedly from normo-tonic to hypertonic should be closely observed in order not to overlook a possible manifestation of stable hypertension.

4.2.2   Stable (manifest) hypertension

4.2.2.1 Borderline hypertension

Hypertension manifests itself in only one third of this group of patients, while in 2/3rds a spontaneous normalization can be observed without the introduction of medication or other antihypertensive therapy. In any case, a diagnosis of borderline hypertension calls for consistent, regular check-ups since the condition could worsen at any time.

4.2.2.2 Benign hypertension

The label "benign" was once used to designate forms of hypertension which ex-hibit no critical exacerbations of blood pressure. From today's standpoint it is no longer useful, since even patients with "benign" hypertension display a marked increase in morbidity and mortality.

4.2.2.3 Malignant hypertension

The expression "malignant hypertension" was coined because this form of hyper-tension so closely resembles the traits of a malignant disease. Without treatment, the constant, massive increases in blood pressure (diastolic mostly > 120 mmHg) lead to death within five years for 95% of those afflicted. Organ damage diagnoses to observe in this phase include arteriolonecrosis of the kidney and a rapidly devel-oping renal insufficiency, progressive insufficiency of the left ventricle, and hyper-tensive encephalopathy. A diagnosis of this form is verified by papillae nodules or by a large exudate in the fundus of the eye (Section 7.3; see also Figure 7.1).

4.3 Classification of hypertension according to the extent of end-/ target-organ damage

The importance of early detection and treatment of arterial hypertension rests in the various types of end-organ damage known to occur over time in the absence of therapy (Chapter 5). The WHO has established a classification of arterial hyper-tension according to the extent of organ damage as a means of morphological evaluation (Table 4.2).

Table 4.2: (WHO-)classification of hypertension according to extent of end organ damage

Stage I:	No demonstrable organ damage to the heart, kidneys and brain; normal eye background
Stage II:	Evidence of at least one of the following signs of organ involvement: − Left ventricular hypertrophy (X-ray, ECG, echocardiography) − Signs of (mild) kidney damage with proteinuria and/or slightly elevated serum creatinine (1.2−2.0 mg/dl) − Generalized and focal narrowing of the retinal arteries − Ultrasonographic or radiological proof of arteriosclerotic plaque (carotid artery, aorta, iliac artery, femoral artery)

Stage III:	Symptoms and clinical signs resulting from end organ damage:
	− Heart
	  − Angina pectoris
	  − Myocardial infarction
	  − Heart failure
	− Brain
	  − Apoplexy
	  − Transient ischemic attack (TIA)
	  − Hypertensive encephalopathy
	− Fundus oculi
	  − Retinal bleeding and exudate, with or without papilledema
	− Kidney
	  − Plasma creatinine concentrations >2.0 mg/dl
	  − Renal failure
	− Vascular system
	  − Dissecting aneurysm
	  − Symptomatic peripheral arterial occlusive disease

WHO = World Health Organization

4.4 Classification of hypertension according to etiology

Arterial hypertension is etiologically classified as

1. primary (essential) hypertension, and

2. secondary hypertension.

The form of hypertension which occurs most frequently and is most often diagnosed is primary hypertension (roughly 95% − including cases of borderline hypertension, 99% − of all cases), whose pathogenesis has yet to be determined. The diagnosis of primary hypertension always requires the exclusion of a clear cause for increases in blood pressure.

Secondary forms of hypertension, at 1−5% (see above), occur much less frequently. Secondary, chronic blood pressure increases are the result of various organ disorders, some of which can be attributed to a causal therapy − hence the need for a differential-diagnostic schema (Table 4.3).

Table 4.3:   Classification of arterial hypertension according to cause

Primary (essential, idiopathic) hypertension

Secondary hypertension
  Renal hypertension
    Renoparenchymal hypertension
    Renovascular hypertension
    Hypertension following kidney transplantation (Post-transplant hypertension)

  Endocrine hypertension
    Pheochromocytoma
    Primary mineralocorticoidism
      − Primary aldosteronism
      − Deoxycorticosterone-producing (DOC-) tumors
      − Adrenogenital syndrome / congenital adrenal hyperplasia
    Glucocorticoidism: Cushing's Syndrome
    Primary hyperreninism
    Acromegaly
    Hyperparathyroidism ·
    Endothelin-producing tumors
    Hypo- and hyperthyroidism

  Pregnancy-specific hypertension
    − Pre-eclampsia/Eclampsia
    − Pre-eclampsia with preexisting chronic hypertension
    − Transient hypertension

  Cardiovascular hypertension
    Coarctation of the aorta
    Systolic cardiovascular hypertension
      − Hyperkinetic heart syndrome
      − Insufficiency of the aortic valve
      − Sclerosis of the aorta ("windkessel" hypertension)
      − Severe bradycardia (i. e. atrioventricular block III°)
      − Arteriovenous fistulae, patent ductus arteriosus

  Hypertension induced by drugs or other substances (drug-induced hypertension)
    − Oral contraceptives ("Pill hypertension")
    − Carbenoxolone and licorice (pseudoaldosteronism)
    − High-dosage glucocorticoid therapy (Pseudo-Cushing's syndrome)
    − Erythropoietin
    − Cyclosporine
    − Alcohol

  Neurogenic hypertension
    Sleep apnea syndrome
    Hypertension caused by neurological disorders

Summary (Chapter 4)

- Arterial hypertension is defined by a sustained increase of diastolic blood pressure above 90 mmHg and/or of systolic blood pressure above 140 mmHg.
- Arterial hypertension is classified by
  - Blood pressure levels (borderline, mild, moderate and severe hypertension; USA: stages 1–4).
  - Clinical progress (borderline, stable [manifest] and malignant hypertension).
  - Extent of end/target-organ damage (Stages I-III of the WHO classification) and
  - Etiology (primary and secondary hypertension).

Literature (Chapter 4)

Burt VL, Whelton P, Roccella EJ, Brown C, Cutler JA, Higgins M, Horan MJ, Labarthe D. Prevalence of hypertension in the US adult population. Results from the Third National Health and Nutrition Examination Survey, 1988–1991. Hypertension 1995; 25: 305–313.

Deutsche Liga zur Bekämpfung des hohen Blutdruckes e.V. Deutsche Hypertonie Gesellschaft. Normwerte des Blutdrucks und Einteilung der arteriellen Hypertonie. Merkblatt, 3. Auflage, Heidelberg 1989.

Guidelines Sub-Committee of the WHO/ISH Mild Hypertension Liaison Committee. 1993 guidelines for the management of mild hypertension: memorandum from a World Health Organization/International Society of Hypertension meeting. J Hypertens 1993; 11: 905–918.

Hypertension Guidelines Committee. Hypertension, diagnosis, treatment and maintenance. Guidelines endorsed by the High Blood Pressure Council of Australia. Royal Australian College of General Practitioner, Adelaide 1991.

Kincaid-Smith P. Malignant hypertension. J Hypertens 1991; 9: 893–899.

Joint Committee on Detection, Evaluation, and Treatment of High Blood Pressure. The fifth report of the Joint Committee on Detection, Evaluation, and Treatment of High Blood Pressure (JNC V). Arch Intern Med 1993; 153: 154–183.

National Advisory Committee on Core Health and Disability Support Services. The management of raised blood pressure in New Zealand. Wellington, New Zealand 1992.

Sever P, Beevers G, Bulpitt C, Lever A, Ramsay L, Reid J, Swales JD. Management guidelines in essential hypertension: report of the second working party of the British Hypertension Society. Br Med J 1993; 306: 983–987.

Swales JD. Editorial Review. Guidelines on guidelines. J Hypertens 1993; 11: 899–903.

Swales JD. Guidelines for treating hypertension. Improved care or retarded progress? Am J Hypertens 1994; 7: 873–876.

WHO Expert Committee. Arterial hypertension. Technical Report Series No. 628. Geneva: World Health Organization, 1978.

5 Clinical significance
of sustained elevated arterial blood pressure

5.1 Hypertension as a cardiovascular risk factor

Diseases of the cardiovascular system are the most common cause of death in the industrialized nations. Beside hypercholesterolemia, nicotine consumption, diabetes mellitus and hyperinsulinemia, arterial hypertension is one of the most important cardiovascular risk factors. On the basis of American life insurance statistics first published in the 1959 "Build and Blood Pressure Study" and later validated by other, larger studies (e.g. the Framingham Studies), it is evident that life expectancy drops as arterial blood pressure increases (Table 5.1). This shortening of life expectancy in the presence of increasing systolic and diastolic blood pressures is apparently the result of an accelerated arterio- and arteriolosclerotic genesis with subsequent organ damage. The appearance of yet other cardiovascular risk factors increases the probability of damage to the cardiovascular system and early death. Nevertheless, the exact atherogenic mechanism of even a single cardiovascular risk-factor-variable has yet to be determined.

5.2 Secondary damage from arterial hypertension

The damages which ensue from an untreated chronically elevated arterial blood pressure make early diagnosis of hypertension a necessity. It manifests itself most

Table 5.1: Life expectancy as a function of blood pressure level for 35-, 45-, and 55-year old men*

Age (years)	Blood pressure (mmHg)	Life expectancy (years)	Life expectancy reduction (years)
35	120/80	41,5	–
	130/90	37,5	4
	140/95	32,5	9
	150/100	25	16,5
45	120/80	32	–
	130/90	29	3
	140/95	26	6
	150/100	20,5	11,5
55	120/80	23,5	–
	130/90	22,5	1
	140/95	19,5	4
	150/100	17,5	6

* Source: Build and Blood Pressure Study (1959)

visibly in the arterial vascular system, particularly that of the kidneys, heart, brain and eyes. Whereas acute end-organ damage is mostly seen in the course of a hypertensive crisis and often takes a very dramatic form (acute decompensation of the left heart, cerebral hemorrhage), the clinical status of chronic, hypertension-induced changes progresses slowly. A single exception to the rule is malignant hypertension, which also leads, in a short span of time and with prior clinical symptoms, to multiple end-organ failure.

5.2.1 Arterio-arteriolosclerosis

Hypertensive patients display arteriosclerotic changes of the small and large arteries earlier and more quickly than the normotensive population. Correspondingly, typical organ manifestations of arterio- and/or arteriolosclerosis are more often, earlier, and more readily detectable in patients with arterial hypertension. The 1975 Framingham Study found hypertensive patients to have a seven-fold greater rate of stroke, a four-fold increase of cardiac failure, a three-fold higher incidence of coronary artery disease, and a doubling of peripheral arterial occlusive disease compared to normotensive patients. Arteriolosclerotic damage of the kidney, which will be addressed separately, is detectable in an autopsy in nearly every patient with a known anamnestic hypertension. Furthermore, arteriosclerosis is found not only in hypertensive individuals, but in normotensive individuals as well − as a normal part, to varying degrees, of their aging process. Although arterial hypertension can not consequently be regarded as the sole causal factor in the development of arteriosclerosis, its role as an accelerating agent is indisputable.

5.2.1.1 Endothelium and the development of arteriosclerosis

The significance of the endothelium in the development of arteriosclerosis has been known since it was observed that its removal advanced the progress of arteriosclerotic changes in hypercholesterol animal experiments. The so-called "response-to-injury" hypothesis, which postulates mechanical, metabolical, toxic or thermal damage to endothelial cells as a primary occurrence in atherogenesis (see below), is derived from these experiments.

The discovery of morphologically intact endothelium in already atherosclerotic vascular layers indicates that dysfunctions of the endothelium can initiate or advance the development of atherosclerosis. These dysfunctions can be summarily described as a loss of the ability to prevent the atherogenic process.

The first indications of an endothelium dysfunction arose from the observation that a dose of the endothelium-dependent vasodilator acetylcholine triggers a dilation in angiographically unremarkable coronary arteries, and, in contrast, a constriction of smooth vascular muscle in stenosized vessels. The endothelial cells apparently lose their ability, under certain conditions, to produce or release the nitric oxide (NO, earlier known as "endothelium-derived relaxing factor," or EDRF), necessary for the vasodilation of the smooth vascular musculature.

The hypothesis that a primary dysfunction of the endothelial cells is the initial occurrence in atherogenesis is therefore especially attractive, since it is capable not only of explaining atherogenesis through pathological damage, but also of conceptually integrating an age-related, physiological dysfunction of the endothelial cells.

5.2.1.2 Hyperlipidemia and arteriosclerosis

It has been known for some time that a close relationship exists between hyperlipidemia and/or disturbed lipoprotein metabolism on the one hand and the development of arteriosclerosis on the other. The exact pathomechanism whereby arteriosclerosis develops, however, has been only partially explained.

It has been possible to demonstrate through animal experiments that endothelial cells exhibit leukocyte-adhesive molecules and chemotactic proteins in the course of a diet-induced hypercholesterolemia. The accumulation of monocytes thus enabled is found primarily in the endothelium of easily-injured vascular areas. The monocytes subsequently permutate in the subendothelial region in order — after transformation into macrophages — to remove superfluous low density lipoprotein (LDL) "packed" cholesterol. The phagocytosis of the LDL-particles and the subsequent mutation of the macrophages into "foam" cells presupposes, however, the prior oxidation of LDL by free oxygen radicals which are excessively produced by endothelial cells as a result of massive cholesterol exposition. Oxidized LDL thereupon stimulates macrophages, endothelial cells, and — in advanced stages — platelets for the purpose of releasing cytokines (chemotactic substances; leukotrienes; platelet derived growth-factor — PDGF; monocyte colony stimulating factor — MCSF), which on the one hand attract further monocytes/macrophages and on the other hand prompt smooth muscle cells to migrate from the media to the intima, and stimulate the production of collagen. The early arteriosclerotic lesions thus arising are described as so-called "fatty streaks."

If the risk factors persist, a retraction of the intravasal, monolayer endothelium results. The partial denudation of the subendothelial tissue leads to an aggregation of thrombocytes with a subsequent release of cytokines (thromboxane; PDGF; serotonin). In connection with similarly accumulating plasma components, these platelets products induce a further proliferation of and collagen production in smooth muscle cells. The microscopic lesions imposing in the first place as fibrous plaques ultimately degenerate into atheroma, which, along with newly formed connective tissue and aggregated platelets, morphologically displays a cell necrosis of all affected cell-types and an accumulation of calcium and lipids (Figure 5.1).

5.2.1.3 Arteriosclerosis: an inflammatory disease?

The endothelial expression of leukocyte adhesion molecules, the release of chemotactic factors and cytokines, as well as the presence of immunocompetent cells in the arterial wall gave rise to the hypothesis that arteriosclerosis is an inflammatory disease. The apparent trigger is hyperlipidemia, which evidently presents an ex-

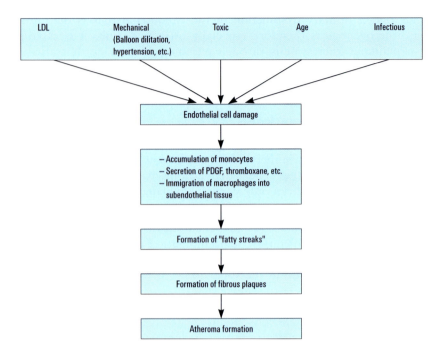

Figure 5.1: Greatly simplified representation of the "response-to-injury" hypothesis on the development of arteriosclerosis (Ross, 1986). LDL = low density lipoproteins; PDGF = platelet derived growth factor.

treme metabolic stimulus for the endothelium and induces excessive production of free oxygen radicals. Free oxygen radicals in turn lead to an release of leukocyte adhesive molecules and a subsequent accumulation of monocyte/macrophage populations. The production of free oxygen radicals may also be responsible for the loss of endothelially-mediated vasodilation, which is typical of arteriosclerotically altered vasculature (see above).

5.2.1.3 Pathogenic role of hypertension in the development of arteriosclerosis

Although according to the "response-to-injury" hypothesis, it is altogether understandable that wall tension increased through a rise in intravasal pressure can, under conditions of arterial hypertension, induce primary damage through an initial endothelial lesion, other factors nevertheless appear necessary in the development of advanced arteriosclerotic vascular changes. It was therefore possible to epidemiologically demonstrate that hypertension alone raises the coronary risk of 40-year-old men only slightly, but when accompanied by hypercholesterolemia, decidedly. The pathogenic point of departure in the development of arteriosclerosis is presently therefore the introduction of a multifactorally determined induction. The role of hypertension, hypercholesterolemia and nicotine consumption is therefore certain, which is to say that their simultaneous appearance multiplies the risk of arteriosclerosis.

New information shows that hypertension also induces the production of free oxygen radicals and therefore exercises a hyperlipidemia-like effect on the arterial wall. The simultaneous appearance of hypertension and hyperlipidemia could therefore lead to an intensified inflammatory reaction of the arterial wall, and provide an explanation for the accelerated development of arteriosclerosis in patients who show both risk factors (Figure 5.2).

Since free oxygen radicals inactivate and/or hinder the release of vasodilating nitric oxide, their pathologically intensified production has also been discussed as a cofactor in the pathogenesis of hypertension.

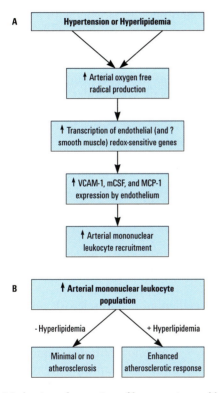

Figure 5.2: Mechanism of synergism of hypertension and hyperlipidemia in the pathogenesis of atherosclerosis. When hypertension accompanies hyperlipidemia, the two act together to trigger a cascade. Increased production of oxygen free radicals leads to increased transcription of redox-sensitive genes, which increases expression of vascular cell adhesion molecule-1 (VCAM-1) by the endothelium, resulting in increased recruitment of monocytes. Both hypertension and hyperlipidemia cause oxidate stress and oxygen free radical production by the arterial wall. By activating redox-sensitive transcriptional control mechanism in the endothelium, a set of genes controlling monocyte recruitment into the arterial wall is activated. Atherosclerosis and foam cell formation occur only in the presence of hyperlipidemia. A synergistic reaction between hypertension and hyperlipidemia, causing or enhancing atherosclerosis, may occur because both states are associated with a common causal mechanism: induction of alterations in vascular redox state. mCSF indicates monocyte colony stimulating factor; MCP-1, monocyte chemotactic protein-1. (Figure and text from Alexander RW, Hypertension 1995; 24: 155−161)

5.3 End-organ damage

5.3.1 Hypertension-related damage to the kidney

Sustained elevated arterial blood pressure leads to either a benign or malignant nephrosclerosis. Despite serious reservations, this morphological distinction is still useful today.

5.3.1.1 "Benign" nephrosclerosis

Pathologists often find changes similar to a benign nephrosclerosis in the course of an autopsy. They are apparently not found only in patients with long-term hypertension, but as well in those with diabetes mellitus or those with general arteriosclerosis but without a known hypertension in their history. In the earliest stages of a "benign" nephrosclerosis, which first strikes a few segments of an interlobular artery and the afferent vessels, accumulations of blood components like C3-complement and IgM are found in the vascular wall. Glomerules, tubules and interstitium are hardly affected at this stage. Through animal experiments it has been possible to demonstrate that these changes manifest themselves in phases in which blood pressure is still normal, so that continuous monitoring is necessary to observe occasional blood pressure extremes. In cases of a longer term hypertension, these initial changes to the vascular wall are followed by an adaptive media hypertrophy, which may be interpreted as a protective reaction of the vessels to elevated intravasal pressure. This wall hyalinosis, which, in contrast to the initial damages, is accompanied by a constriction of the lumen, is reversible after the elevated blood pressure has normalized.

5.3.1.2 Malignant nephrosclerosis

In contrast to benign nephrosclerosis, malignant nephrosclerosis involves an initial stenosis of the arterial wall. Among, and in addition to, other reactive vascular wall processes − such as enlargement of the intima, formation of edema, and accumulation of erythrocyte fragments − a concentric fibrosis, limited at the outset to the interlobular arteries and the afferent vessels, rapidly develops. Soon thereafter glomerules and tubules, initially in places, are damaged. These damages resemble the morphological changes associated with acute kidney failure. Fibrosis of the interstitium as well as atrophy of the glomerules and tubules increase when hypertension is left untreated.

An increase in the number of renin-forming cells of the juxtaglomerular apparatus is often observed, resulting in a renally-determined autonomous hypertension based on increased renin secretion. The degree to which an expansion of the fibrotic remodelling process into the juxtaglomerular apparatus explains the reduction of renin production in patients with so-called "low renin hypertension" is still unknown.

5.3.2 Cardiac damage resulting from hypertension

The cardiac consequences of chronically elevated arterial blood pressure are hypertrophy of the heart, heart dilation, and congestive heart failure. Hypertension is furthermore a substantial cofactor in the development of coronary artery disease.

5.3.2.1 Hypertensive heart disease

Hypertensive heart disease develops in virtually every untreated hypertension patient, and every second patient exhibits manifest cardiac symptoms. The initial phase in the development of hypertensive heart disease is concentric hypertrophy of the heart with thickened myocardial fibers and an increase in interstitial connective tissue. In spite of hypertrophy of both the ventricle wall and -septum with normal or decreased ventricle volume (high mass/volume ratio), this stage − presupposing no disorders of contractility − is in many cases characterized by normal or even increased ventricular function. However, because of the extended oxygen-diffusion path brought on by the hypertrophic myocardium, the oxygen supply to the individual muscle fibers is increasingly poor, so that a discrepancy gradually arises between the amount of oxygen supplied and the amount needed by the hypertrophic cells. Micronecroses, connective tissue replacement ("remodelling"), and further increasing oxygen needs due to decreasing oxygen supply cause a continuous transition to eccentric hypertrophy with increases in the left ventricular radius, the diastolic end-volume, and the systolic wall tension. This dilation coincides with a lower mass/volume ratio, and leads to a reduction in ventricular function. A simultaneously existing, with hypertension, progressive, coronary artery sclerosis accelerates this increasing cardiac failure for all the reasons cited (Figure 5.3).

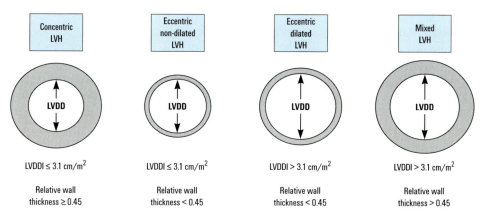

Figure 5.3: Left ventricular architecture characterized by relation of wall thickness to cavity size.

LVDD = left ventricular diastolic cavity dimension in diastole alone and after indexing (LVDDI) for body surface area;
LVH = left ventricular hypertrophy
(From Gottdiener JS et al., JACC 1994; 24: 1492−1498)

Acute danger to the heart due to blood pressure crises results from the abnormal increase of the afterload. This causes a sudden increase of intra- and extracardiac load, because the compensatory capacities of a temporarily dilated heart are fewer than those of an undilated, concentrically hypertrophic heart with a lower basal wall tension and a higher mass/volume ratio (see above).

5.3.3 Hypertensive cerebrovascular disease

On the one hand early arteriosclerotic changes to the basal arteries of the circulus basilii are observable in patients with sustained elevated arterial blood pressure; on the other hand, so is a strong concomitant infestation of the periphery of the arterial system through the cerebral cortex and intracerebrally (putamen of the lenticular nucleus, optical thalamus, gray regions of the cerbellopontine or the cerebellum). Furthermore, there is a demonstrable arteriosclerosis of the intracerebral arterioles in all of these regions. A focal hyalinosis whose spread to the initially unaffected media leads to a constriction of the lumen and thereby to a clear, autoregulatively uncorrectable increase in cerebrovascular resistance, is the primary alteration to the brain arterioles in cases of arterial hypertension.

These changes of the afferent and intracerebral arteries and arterioles also bring about both rheological changes (increased risk of thrombosis) in cerebral circulation and increased rigidity with simultaneous limitation or lack of autoregulation mechanisms of the peripheral arterioles. The consequences are an increased incidence of ischemic and hemorrhagic insults in cases of arterial hypertension. Massive cerebral bleeding, which most often appears in the midst of a hypertensive crisis, is considered the most serious cerebral complication of hypertension.

The concept of hypertensive encephalopathy describes the generalized cerebral consequences of a chronic or acute blood pressure increase. The cause for this symptom is the development of edema and congestion of the brain, mostly at the lower end of an acute blood pressure increase to values exceeding the cerebrovascular, autoregulative compensation mechanisms. Hypertensive encephalopathy is therefore not triggered by infarction or bleeding, and is reversible by means of lowering the blood pressure (Section 32.1).

5.3.4 Peripheral arterial occlusive disease

Peripheral arterial occlusive disease (PAOD) is encountered twice as often in hypertensive patients as in normotensive patients. Although arterial hypertension is therefore considered at least an accelerating atherogenic co-factor in this part of the vascular system, other risk factors seem more significant for the development of PAOD (diabetes mellitus, nicotine consumption).

Summary (Chapter 5)

- The clinical significance of arterial hypertension is derived from the higher morbidity and mortality associated with it.

- The source of this higher morbidity and mortality is arterial hypertension's function as a partial pathogenic factor in the development of arteriosclerosis and of consecutive, prematurely occurring organ damage to the brain, heart, kidneys and peripheral arterial vascular system.

Literature (Chapter 5)

Alexander RW. Hypertension and the pathogenesis of atherosclerosis. Oxidative stress and the mediation of arterial inflammatory response: A new perspective. Hypertension 1995; 25: 155−161.

Brilla CG. Hochdruck und hypertensive Herzkrankheit. Pathophysiologie, Klinik, Diagnostik und Therapie. Walter de Gruyter, Berlin-New York, 1−92, 1994.

Campbell JH, Campbell GR. Cell biology of atherosclerosis. J Hypertens 1994; 12 (suppl 10): S129−S132.

Crawford DW, Blankenhorn DH. Arterial wall oxygenation, oxyradicals, and atherosclerosis. Atherosclerosis 1991; 89: 97−108.

Folkow B. Early structural changes in hypertension: pathophysiology and clinical consequences. J Cardiovasc Pharmacol 1993; 22 (suppl 1): S1−S6.

Franz IW. Hypertonie und Herz. Diagnostische, prognostische und therapeutische Aspekte. Springer-Verlag, Berlin-Heidelberg-New York, 1991.

Frohlich ED, Apstein C, Chobanian AV, Devereux RB, Dustan HB, Dzau V, Fauad-Tarazi F, Horan MJ, Marcus M, Massie B, Pfeffer MA, Re RN, Roccella EJ, Savage D, Shub C. The heart in hypertension. N Engl J Med 1992; 327: 998−1008.

Furchgott RF, Zawadzki JV. The obligatory role of endothelial cells in the relaxation of arterial smooth muscle by acetylcholine. Nature 1980; 288: 373−376.

Gottsdiener JS, Reda DJ, Materson BJ, Massie BM, Notargiacomo A, Hamburger RJ, Williams DW, Henderson WG. Importance of obesity, race and age to the cardiac structural and functional effects of hypertension. J Am Coll Cardiol 1994; 24: 1492−1498.

Helmchen U, Bohle RM. Pathologie der renalen Hochdruckfolgen. In: Ganten D, Ritz E (Hrsg.): Lehrbuch der Hypertonie. Schattauer, Stuttgart-New York 1985.

Klag MJ, Whelton PK, Randall BL, Neaton JD, Brancati FL, Ford CE, Shulman NB, Stamler J. Blood pressure and end-stage renal disease in men. N Engl J Med 1996; 334: 13−18.

Ludmer PL, Selwyn AP, Shook TL, Wayne RR, Mudge GH, Alexander RW, Ganz P. Paradoxical vasoconstriction induced by acetylcholine in atherosclerotic coronary arteries. N Engl J Med 1986; 315: 1046−1051.

Parthasarathy S, Quinn MT, Schwenke DC, Carew TE, Steinberg D. Oxidative modification of beta-very low density lipoprotein: potential role in monocyte recruitment and foam cell formation. Arteriosclerosis 1989; 9: 398−404.

Paulson OB, Strandgaard S. Hypertensive disease and the cerebral circulation. In: Laragh JH, Brenner BM (eds). Hypertension: Pathophysiology, diagnosis and management, 2nd ed. Raven Press New York, 1994.

Reddi AS, Camerini-Davalos RA. Diabetic nephropathy. An update. Arch Intern Med 1990; 150: 31−43.

Quinn MT, Parthasarathy S, Fong LG, Steinberg D. Oxidatively modified low density lipoproteins: a potential role in recruitment and retention of monocyte/macrophages during atherogenesis. Proc Natl Acad Sci USA 1987; 84: 2995−2998.

Ross R, Glomset J, Harker L. Response to injury and atherogenesis. Am J Pathol 1977; 86: 675−684.

Ross R. The pathogenesis of atherosclerosis. N Engl J Med 1986; 314: 488−496.

Safar ME, London GM. The arterial system in human hypertension. In: Swales JD (ed). Textbook of Hypertension. Blackwell Scientific Publishing London 1994, 85−102.

Satriano JA, Shuldiner M, Hora K, Xing Y, Shan Z, Schlondorff D. Oxygen radicals as second messengers for expression of the monocyte chemoattractant protein, JE/MCP-1, and the monocyte colony stimulating factor, CSF-1, in response to tumor necrosis factor-alpha and immunoglobulin G. J Clin Invest 1993; 92: 1564−1571.

Strandgaard S, Paulson OB. Cerebrovascular consequences of hypertension. Lancet 1994; 344: 519−521.

Strauer BE. Das Hochdruckherz. 3. Aufl. Springer, Berlin-Heidelberg-New York 1991.

Sung BH, Lovallo WR, Teague SM, Pincomb GA, Wilson MF. Cardiac adaptation to increased systemic blood pressure in borderline hypertensive men. Am J Cardiol 1993; 72: 407−412.

II Diagnosis

6 The diagnosis of arterial hypertension

The measurement of arterial blood pressure should be a standard component of every physical examination. A single measurement of elevated blood pressure values does not allow, however, for the diagnosis of manifest arterial hypertension, because situation-specific increases in blood pressure can be observed in the physician's practice and especially within the context of the first examination. Every increase in blood pressure should be checked again at the end of the consultation. If elevated blood pressure levels are still found, further monitoring of the blood pressure should be performed at weekly intervals. If the blood pressure does not spontaneously drop to persistent diastolic values under 90 mmHg and/or systolic values under 140 mmHg upon multiple measurement within four weeks (recommendation of the German Hypertension Society: three measurements on at least two different days), then the diagnosis of arterial hypertension is justified.

Patients who give the impression in the physician's practice that they might be subject to a situation-related increase in blood pressure ("white coat hypertension") should be introduced to methods of blood pressure self-measurement ("home measurement") and provided with the necessary equipment. On the basis of self-measured and documented blood pressure values, a more realistic assessment of the actual blood pressure situation will be possible in many cases. If 25% of the self-measured blood pressure values lie over 90 mmHg diastolically and/or over 140 mmHg systolically, a diagnosis of arterial hypertension can also be made according to the definition.

As an alternative to blood pressure self-measurement, one can consider the use of continuous, ambulatory, 24-hour blood pressure measurement (ABPM). An average day-time blood pressure greater than 135/85 mmHg is viewed as hypertensive by most experts (see Section 2.3.2).

The peculiarities of the childhood and pregnancy for the diagnosis of hypertension are dealt with in other sections (Chapters 11 and 15).

Summary (Chapter 6)

- A single measurement of elevated blood pressure values is not enough to justify the diagnosis of chronic arterial hypertension.

- A single measurement of elevated blood pressure values should, however, prompt the implementation of a tight blood pressure monitoring regime.

- If the blood pressure does not spontaneously drop to diastolic values < 90 mmHg and/or systolic values < 140 mmHg upon multiple measurement on several days within a four-week period, arterial hypertension is present.

- If white coat hypertension is suspected, blood pressure self-measurement ("home measurement") or ambulatory blood pressure monitoring (ABPM) should be conducted.

- If more than 25% of the self-measured diastolic and/or systolic blood pressure values lie over 90 mmHg and/or over 140 mmHg, respectively, a diagnosis of arterial hypertension can also be made.

- The blood pressure values gathered through ABPM are considered hypertensive if their day-time average lies over 135/85 mmHg.

Literature (Chapter 6)

Perry HM, Miller JP. Difficulties in diagnosing hypertension: implications and alternatives. J Hypertens 1992; 10: 887−896.

Sinclair AM, Isles CG, Brown I, Cameron H, Murray GD, Robertson JWK. Secondary hypertension in a blood pressure clinic. Arch Intern Med 1987; 147: 1289−1293.

7 Standard diagnostic procedures for confirmed arterial hypertension: contents and significance

The standard diagnostic procedure for confirmed arterial hypertension consists of

- detailed history (family history, patient history, occupational history),
- physical examination,
- laboratory tests and
- additional tests such as ECG, ultrasonography, echocardiography and chest X-ray.

(See the recommendations of the German Hypertension Society, 4th Edition 11/ 1991, Figure 7.3, and the recommendations of the Joint National Committee on Detection, Evaluation, and Treatment of High Blood Pressure, JNC V, 1993).

The goal of the standard diagnostic procedure for confirmed hypertension is to exclude or prove

- the existence of additional cardiovascular risk factors,
- end-organ damage caused by hypertension, and/or
- the underlying existence of a secondary form of hypertension.

7.1 History

7.1.1 The significance of family history for differential diagnosis

Primary hypertension, pheochromocytoma (often in combination with other endocrine organ diseases, e.g., hyperparathyroidism, medullary thyroid carcinoma etc.; see Section 14.1) and polycystic kidney disease are associated with familial clustering. The taking of the family history should therefore be a fundamental component of the standard diagnostic procedure for hypertension, though it is not be overestimated, especially regarding its value as a differential-diagnostic "red flag".

7.1.2 Patient history

The diagnosis of arterial hypertension is often an incidental diagnosis, because in most cases chronic increases in blood pressure do not cause significant complaints and therefore do not lead the patient to the feeling that he is ill.

Headaches and dizziness are more often seen in moderate to severe hypertension. The additional appearance of visual impairments can be a sign of malignant hypertension.

Definite differential diagnostic conclusions on the existence of a secondary form of hypertension are not possible on the basis of information from the patient history. Episodic diaphoresis, tremors, subjective feelings of unrest and headaches reflect the "classic" symptoms of a pheochromocytoma - especially in connection with intermittent blood pressure crises — and therefore also justify a measurement of 24-hour urinary catecholamines as a subsequent investigation. However, it must be remembered that these symptoms are much more likely to be seen or reported in primary hypertension and in hyperthyroidism.

Dysuric complaints are also more often due to a urinary tract infection than to a renoparenchymal disease. A history of repeated infections of the urogenital tract, especially with known previous pyelonephritis, should lead, however, to a careful urinalysis in any case.

Special significance is given to information on the use of medications in the patient history, as various substances can induce hypertension and may thus already represent the initial cause of the increase in blood pressure. In western countries, alcohol consumption and the taking of oral contraceptives may possibly be the most common causes of secondary hypertension (Chapter 17).

The medication history is also of possible diagnostic significance, given that the knowledge on the use of pharmaceutics which deplete potassium (diuretics, laxatives) may offer a further explanation of a hypokalemic hypertension. In conjunction with this, it is important to ask about frequent vomiting or diarrhea.

The connection between alcoholism and hypertension is well known. Asking about the level of alcohol consumption is therefore obligatory as part of the standard diagnostic procedure for hypertension (see above).

In order to evaluate and positively influence additional cardiovascular hazards to the hypertensive patient, the patient should always be asked about possible lipid metabolism disorders, diabetes mellitus and nicotine use.

Progressive decrease in exercise capacity, dyspnea and peripheral edema can, in cases of long-standing hypertension, indicate a decompensating hypertensive heart disease.

The diagnosis of sleep apnea syndrome (Chapter 18) should be considered if patients with hypertension, especially overweight ones, complain of extreme day-time fatigue and morning headaches. The suspicion can be intensified if third parties report that the patient has a history of loud, irregular snoring repeatedly interrupted by pauses to breathe. Because the sleep apnea syndrome is possibly one of the most common causes of secondary hypertension, every hypertensive patient should be asked about sleeping disorders.

7.1.3 Occupational history

It is still not clear to what degree occupational stress is capable of causing and maintaining chronic hypertension. As accelerating factors, however, shift work, continual noise pollution and permanent conflict situations in the work place all seem to have an unfavorable effect on the development of existing hypertension. Heavy physical labor with repeatedly induced blood pressure elevations can lead to a situation of acute cardiac or cerebral danger for patients with a hypertensive blood pressure situation. In the long-term, the already increased risk of hypertensive target-organ damage is undoubtedly further increased by frequent blood pressure elevations.

The goal of an extensive occupational history is to gather information on the work place situation of the hypertensive patient, in order to identify possible influences which may raise blood pressure. Providing practical assistance, however, is not always possible.

7.2 Physical examination

The goal of the physical examination in confirmed hypertension is, on the one hand, the exclusion or verification of the presence of additional organ diseases which may influence the decision on the scope and choice of antihypertensive therapy to be administered. On the other hand, the physical examination may indicate the presence of a secondary form of hypertension. In some cases, the physical inspection can already lead to a tentative diagnosis of Cushing's syndrome (Figures 14.12 a + b, Chapter 14.6) or acromegaly (Figures 14.13 a + b, Chapter 14.8).

A strong pulse in the arm with a weak or missing femoral pulse and the corresponding hypertensive values for the upper and lower blood pressures in the lower extremities are nearly pathognomonic for the presence of a stenosis of the aortic isthmus.

Paraumbilical or abdominal bruits in moderately severe to severe hypertension should lead to consideration of the presence of a renal artery stenosis.

Costovertebral angle tenderness might be indicative of a kidney ailment.

Skin manifestation of liver disease (palmar erythema, spider nevi, lacklipped, etc.) may be signs of alcoholism not admitted to, which is often the cause of (secondary) hypertension.

7.3 Funduscopic examination

Funduscopy should be a standard component of the physical examination of patients with hypertension, as it offers the only possibility to diagnose previously existing vascular damage at low cost and with little effort. This investigation has

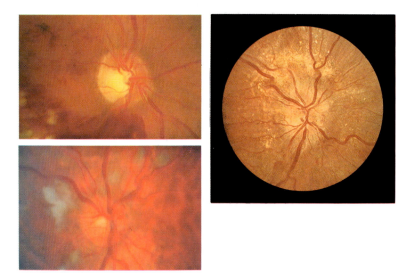

Figure 7.1: Fundus hypertonicus
Left (top):   Late stage with multiple extravasations
Left (bottom):   Late stage with additional complications (Prethrombosis of the central retinal vein, papilledema, cotton-wool spots)
Right: Transition from "red" to "pale" hypertension ("transitional hypertension"); arteries narrowed and progressively stretched ("silver wire arteries"), papilledema (similar to true papilledema due to raised intracranial pressure), degenerative foci, and extravasation (Pschyrembel, Clinical Dictionary, 257th edition, p. 500, 1993).

a decisive significance, especially in the diagnosis of malignant hypertension (Figure 7.1).

Hypertension-induced alterations of the arterial vasculature are most easily diagnosed in the fundus. This procedure also allows for the classification of hypertension according to end-organ damage. The commonly used classification established by Keith, Wagener and Barker allows for a differentiated evaluation of the target-organ damage on the basis of the evaluation of the changes to the fundus (Table 7.1).

Changes in the fundus in stages I and II are not only found in patients who have had hypertension for a longer period of time, but also in normotensive patients with systemic arteriosclerosis. While untreated patients in stages I and II have a 5-year survival rate of more than 80%, the 5-year survival rate for patients in stages III and IV is only 5%. Because of this prognostically clear dividing line between the consequences of hypertension with and without neuroretinal participation, the WHO now differentiates only on the basis of two grades of changes in the fundus:

1. Fundus hypertonicus = grade I and II and

2. fundus hypertonicus malignus = grade III and IV of the previous classification system.

In practice this means that patients with confirmed changes in the fundus of stages III and IV or grade II of the new WHO classification, are in urgent need of

Table 7.1: Classification of hypertensive and arteriosclerotic retinopathy*

| Degree | Hypertension | | | | | Arteriosclerosis | |
| | Arterioles | | Hemor-rhages | Exudates | Papille-dema | Arteriolar light reflex | AV crossing defect**** |
	General narrowing AV ratio**	Focal spasm***					
Normal	3 : 4	1 : 1	0	0	0	Fine yellow line, red blood column	0
Grade I	1 : 2	1 : 1	0	0	0	Broadened yellow line, red blood column	Mild depression of vein
Grade II	1 : 3	2 : 3	0	0	0	Broad yellow line, "copper wire," blood column not visible	Depression or humping of vein
Grade III	1 : 4	1 : 3	+	+	0	Broad white line, "silver wire," blood column not visible	Right-angle deviation, tapering, and disappearance of vein under arteriole
Grade IV	Fine, fibrous cords	Obliteration of distal flow	+	+	+	Fibrous cords, blood column not visible	Distal dilatation of vein Same as grade III

* According to Keith, Wagener and Barker
** This the ratio of arteriolar to venous diameters
*** This is the ratio of diameters of region of spasm to proximal arteriole
**** Arteriolar length and tortuosity increase with severity
(Adapted from Williams GH, Harrison's Principles of Internal Medicine, 1991; 1001–1015)

antihypertensive therapy. In contrast, the significance of changes in the fundus of grades I and II (WHO classification grade I) has not been clearly defined.

7.4 Laboratory tests in standard diagnostic procedure: differential diagnostic screening examination and determination of the overall cardiovascular risk profile

As part of the initial diagnosis of arterial hypertension, the standard diagnostic laboratory tests may provide, on the one hand, indications of the presence of a secondary form of hypertension and, on the other hand, they may uncover previously unknown metabolic disorders as coexisting cardiovascular risk factors. Due to the costs thereby incurred, the scope of the routinely implemented laboratory diagnostic tests should be kept as narrow as possible and made dependent on the specific cases.

Proteinuria and/or microhematuria are often not noticed by the patient. A positive urinalysis requires further diagnostic investigation in order to definitively verify or exclude the existence of renal disease. The same is of course true for evidence of elevated serum creatinine concentrations.

Hypokalemia is often diagnosed in patients with hypertension. Once therapy with diuretics, laxative abuse, diarrhea or vomiting have been definitively excluded, further diagnostic tests are justified, especially with the presence of a moderate, severe or therapy resistant hypertension. The most common secondary form of hypertension associated with hypokalemia is primary aldosteronism. However, it should be remembered that low potassium values in the serum can also be observed in other secondary forms of hypertension, where an increased secretion of aldosterone, in the form of secondary aldosteronism, occurs, due to stimulation of the renin release (renal artery stenoses, pheochromocytoma). The simultaneous appearance of hypertension and hypercalcemia may indicate the presence of a primary hyperparathyroidism. A malignant disorder, however, must definitely be excluded as a cause of the calcium increase.

The measurement of fasting serum glucose, cholesterol (including measurement of HDL and LDL, if possible), triglycerides and uric acid is less important for hypertension diagnosis. However, it is recommended for the evaluation of the total cardiovascular risk and as a basis for making decisions regarding the selection of antihypertensive medications.

7.5 Additional diagnostic examinations for arterial hypertension

The routine performance of an ECG is particularly important upon the initial diagnosis of hypertension, because, to a great degree, the choice of antihypertensive therapy must be guided by the cardiac condition. Electrocardiographic evidence of a cardiac arrhythmia or the suspected presence of a coronary or hypertensive heart disease will, in general, not only lead the attending physician to undertake further diagnostic steps, but also influence his/her choice of anti-hypertensive medication.

Although generally-accepted examination protocols and norms do not currently exist for the bicycle (treadmill) ergometric exercise test for patients with hypertension, an ergometric exercise test is recommended for every patient with borderline-raised, casual blood pressure values. This test enables the attending physician to evaluate, on the one hand, possible cardiac ischemic events and, on the other, the behavior of the blood pressure under exercise-induced stress. We consider the evaluation of the exercising blood pressure particularly appropriate for patients who pursue sports and physical activities. It has been shown that patients with an isolated exercise-induced hypertension demonstrate a significantly increased risk of suffering or dying from a cardiovascular event. The conducting of a bicycle ergometric test at 100 W over six minutes under ambulatory conditions is a reasonable examination for evaluating blood pressure behavior under physical stress. Systolic blood pressure values up to 200 mmHg are considered normotensive under these conditions (see Section 3.2, Table 3.1).

The imperative indication for an ergometric exercise test should generally be considered a matter of course for patients with hypertension who have a reported history of angina pectoris or dyspnea.

If patient history (dyspnea, angina pectoris), clinical (signs of congestion such as auscultatory-detectable wet rhonchi, jugular venous congestion, peripheral edema, etc.) or electrocardiographic signs (dysrhythmias such as arrhythmia absoluta or ventricular ectopy, signs of left ventricular hypertrophy, signs of ischemia, etc.) of cardiac damage are found, an echocardiography is indicated (m-mode, preferably combined with a two-dimensional Doppler investigation). Through a representation in the m-mode in the short parasternal axis or in the parasternal long axis, the scope of left ventricular hypertrophy (LVH) can be best evaluated on the basis of the end-diastolic wall thickness of the intraventricular septum (IVS) and the posterior wall (PW) as well as the left ventricular end-diastolic diameter(LVEDD) (Figure 7.2). A diagnosis of LVH is to be made from these measuring positions when the end-diastolic thickness of the IVS and the PW is > 11 mm (men) or ≥ 11 mm (women). With the help of the parameters ascertained in the m-mode, an LV mass index can also be calculated, in which an LVH is considered present when values lie > 134 g/m^2 in men and > 110 g/m^2 in women (for the calculation of the index see legend to Figure 7.2). Further parameters for the evaluation of cardiac function can be determined through additional Doppler measurements (cardiac output, cardiac index, etc.).

Ultrasonography is one of the routine imaging procedures in medicine. Large adrenal tumors (e.g., pheochromocytoma) and diseases of the kidney (large renal cysts, multiple renal cysts, parenchymal loss, etc.), which may be the cause or consequence of hypertension, can be diagnosed ultrasonographically without any significant inconvenience to the patient.

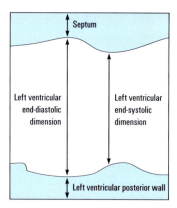

Figure 7.2: Schematic m-mode echocardiogram showing measurements for calculating left ventricular (LV) mass index according to the formula described by Devereux (Am J Cardiol 1986; 57: 450−458):
LV Mass (g) = 0.80 × 1.04 [(VSTd + LVIDd + PWTd)^3 − (LVId)^3] + 0.6 where
VSTd   is ventricular septal thickness at end diastole,
LVIDd   is LV internal dimension at end diastole, and
PWTd   is LV posterior wall thickness at end diastole.
(Figure adapted from Lip GYH et al., Br Med J 1995; 311: 1425−1428).

A radiological representation of the renal arteries, as part of the diagnostic procedures for high blood pressure, is only recommended upon the clinical suspicion of the presence of a renal artery stenosis (paraumbilical bruits in hypertension which is medicinally not well-controlled) and in younger patients (see also Section 13.2.3).

7.6 Additional examinations

If the standard diagnostic procedures (see above) lead to findings which indicate the presence of a secondary form of hypertension, additional testing is called for.

The expense, effort and scope of the investigations must, however, be justifiable from the standpoint of the expected therapeutic consequences. Decisions on additional examinations must thus be made on a case-by-case basis (see also Chapter 8).

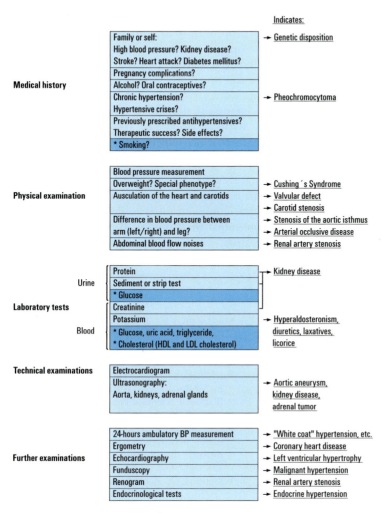

Figure 7.3: Recommendations of the German Hypertension Society (1991) for the diagnosis of hypertension. BP = blood pressure.
* Not necessary in diagnosing hypertension, but useful in establishing the presence of other cardiovascular risk factors.

Summary (Chapter 7)

- Every initial diagnosis of arterial hypertension calls for a supplemental standard diagnostic procedure.

- The standard diagnostic procedure for arterial hypertension consists of the gathering of anamnestic data, physical inspection and examination, laboratory tests, ECG and ultrasonography.

- The goal of the standard diagnostic procedure is to search for
  - coexisting cardiovascular risk factors,
  - target-organ damage caused by hypertension,
  - concomitant disorders/diseases and
  - forms of secondary hypertension.
- Only in exceptional cases does the standard diagnostic procedure provide a definitive diagnosis of secondary hypertension. The standard diagnostic procedure can, however, provide information which acts as a differential diagnostic signpost.

- Additional or more detailed examinations are only indicated if the standard diagnostic procedure leads to the strong suspicion of the presence of hypertension-induced target-organ damages, concomitant disorders/diseases and/or a form of secondary hypertension and if the findings of the investigation are expected to lead to positive therapeutic consequences.

Literature (Chapter 7)

Arnett DK, Rautaharju P, Crow R, Folsom AR, Ekelund LG, Hutchinson R, Tyroler HA, Heiss G. Black-white differences in electrocardiographic left ventricular mass and its association with blood pressure (the ARIC Study). Am J Cardiol 1994; 74: 247−252.

Birkenhäger WH, de Leeuw PW. Determining hypertensive end-organ damage in trials: a review of current methodologies and techniques. J Cardiovasc Pharmacol 1992; 19 (suppl 5): 43−50.

Cooper WD, Glover DR, Hormbrey JM, Kimber GR. Headache and blood pressure: evidence of a close relationship. J Hum Hypertens 1989; 3: 41−44.

Devereux RB, Koren MJ, de Simone G, Roman MJ, Laragh JH. LV mass as a measure of preclinical hypertensive disease. Am J Hypertens 1992; 5: 175S−181S.

McGregor E, Isles CG, Jay JL, Lever AF, Murray GD. Retinal changes in malignant hypertension. Br Med J 1986; 292: 233−234.

Mueller FB, Laragh JH. Clinical evaluation and differential diagnosis of the individual hypertensive patient. Clin Chem 1991; 37: 1868−1879.

Patel V, Kohner EM. The eye in hypertension. In: Swales JD (ed): Textbook of hypertension. Blackwell Scientific Publishing, Oxford 1994, 1015−1025.

Phillips RA. The cardiologist's approach to evaluation and management of the patient with essential hypertension. Am Heart J 1993; 126: 548−666.

Wittenberg C, Zabludowski JR, Rosenfeld JB. Overdiagnosis of hypertension in the elderly. J Hum Hypertens 1992; 6: 349−351.

Zanchetti A, Sleight P, Birkenhäger WH. Evaluation of organ damage in hypertension. J Hypertens 1993; 11: 875−882.

8 Differential-diagnostic aspects of arterial hypertension

The goal of differential diagnostic procedures in confirmed arterial hypertension is to exclude or confirm the existence of secondary hypertension. Because secondary forms of hypertension as a whole make up only a 5% portion of the total hypertensive population (if one includes borderline hypertension, it is probably only 1%), the indication for differential diagnostic clarification must be strictly adhered to due to the time involved and financial costs. In addition, through history, physical examination and inspection, urinalysis, measurement of serum potassium, calcium and creatinine and ultrasonography, it is possible to gain important indicators for the suspected presence of a secondary form of hypertension (Chapter 7). As a rule, the standard diagnostic procedure provides less a definitive proof of a secondary form of hypertension than a more or less high degree of suspicion of one. The intensity and scope of the diagnostic procedures which follow should be oriented on the individual cases and the possible therapeutic consequences. Particularly with younger patients and patients with severe hypertension, given the appropriate indicators, the decision will be made for a complete differential diagnostic clarification, since some secondary forms of hypertension can be cured, thus making a life-long drug therapy unnecessary.

The pathogenesis of primary hypertension is still not known, so that an exact definition of its disease picture has not been possible. This explains why the diagnosis of primary hypertension is only possible through the exclusion of secondary hypertension. The diagnosis of primary hypertension thus represents diagnosis of exclusion.

Summary (Chapter 8)

- The goal of differential diagnostic procedures in confirmed arterial hypertension is to exclude or confirm the existence of a secondary form of hypertension.

- The diagnosis of primary hypertension is only possible through the exclusion of a secondary form of hypertension.

Literature (Chapter 8)

Anderson Jr GH, Blakeman N, Streeten DHP. The effect of age on prevalence of secondary forms of hypertension in 4429 consecutively referred patients. J Hypertens 1994; 12: 609–615.

Sinclair AM, Isles CG, Brown I, Cameron H, Murray GD, Robertson JMK. Secondary hypertension in a blood pressure clinic. Arch Intern Med 1987; 147: 1289–1293.

9 Primary hypertension

9.1 The incidence of primary hypertension

Arterial hypertension was earlier estimated to be present in approximately 10−15% of the adult population of western industrialized countries. However, because this estimate was made on the basis of the earlier definition of hypertension (≥ 160/95 mmHg), a significantly higher incidence of hypertension must be assumed when borderline hypertension (> 140/90 mmHg) is included, as is now commonly done (Table 9.1). Arterial hypertension is the most common diagnosis made for adult patients in general practice.

The most common cause of sustained elevations of blood pressure is primary hypertension. Its portion of the total hypertensive population had previously been estimated to constitute 95%. However, because borderline increases of arterial blood pressure are caused by primary hypertension in nearly all cases, the actual portion constituted by primary hypertension may be nearly 99%.

Table 9.1: Prevalence of hypertension in US adult population

	Percent (SE)	Age-adjusted percent (SE)	Estimated population (SE)*
Overall[+]	24.0 (0.9)	24.2 (0.6)	43186 (2427)
Men[+]	24.7 (1.2)	25.9 (1.0)	21287 (1490)
Women[+]	23.4 (0.9)	22.2 (0.8)	21900 (1238)
Race/ethnicity			
Non-Hispanic black	28.4 (1.4)	32.4 (1.1)	5672 (427)
Men	29.9 (2.0)	34.0 (1.6)	2664 (209)
Women	27.3 (1.5)	31.0 (1.0)	3008 (252)
Non-Hispanic white	24.6 (1.0)	23.3 (0.7)	34697 (2746)
Men	25.6 (1.3)	25.4 (1.2)	17259 (1642)
Women	23.8 (1.1)	21.0 (0.9)	17438 (1334)
Mexican American	14.3 (1.3)	22.6 (0.8)	1143 (124)
Men	14.6 (1.4)	23.2 (1.1)	604 (66)
Women	14.0 (1.3)	21.6 (1.0)	539 (66)

Age-adjusted to the 1990 US civilian, noninstitutionalized population
* In thousands
+ Includes race/ethnic groups not shown separately
SE = standard error
From Burt VL et al., Hypertension 1995; 25: 305−313
Original source: Centers for Disease Control and Prevention, the National Centers for Health Statistics, and the third National Health and Nutrition Examination Survey (NHANES III) conducted during 1988 to 1991

9.2 Hemodynamics in primary hypertension

The initial stage of primary hypertension appears to be characterized hemodynamically by an increased cardiac output. This blood-pressure-increasing mechanism was detected in young patients with hypertension, at least under resting conditions. An additional increase in the peripheral vascular resistance in this disease stage only occurred with dynamic exercise stress.

With increasing age and duration of the hypertension, however, one finds an increase in peripheral vascular resistance independent of exercise stress and a normalization or even lowering of the cardiac output. The development and maintenance of the elevated blood pressure condition in primary hypertension appears therefore to be tied to various pathomechanisms.

9.3 The pathogenesis of primary hypertension

The pathogenesis of primary hypertension has remained unclear. However, there are indications that primary hypertension can not be explained by a single pathomechanism applicable to all affected patients. Rather, it is likely a "multifactorial" disease, set off by various environmental influences in interaction with an as yet undefined genetic predisposition.

A disturbed homeostasis of sodium and sympathetic activity is a component of almost all postulations on the pathogenesis of primary hypertension and even today underlines the significance of these factors in blood pressure regulation.

9.3.1 The significance of psychosocial factors

The high incidence of primary hypertension in industrialized countries indicates possible causal factors, which can be summarized in the term "psycho-social stress". This would include the increasing environmental noise pollution, pressure to succeed, insufficient possibilities for conflict resolution and social isolation caused by urbanization and the simultaneous loss of the extended family. To what degree these external conditions can actually induce primary hypertension can not be definitively answered at the current point in time, because, of course, among other factors, obesity and elevated sodium chloride and alcohol consumption are significantly more common in the industrialized countries.

9.3.2 Heredity

An increased familial frequency of primary hypertension indicates an as yet not more closely definable genetic disposition. This suspicion has been supported by the results of research on twins, which has provided evidence that identical twins develop primary hypertension of a comparable degree of severity, despite different circumstantial and environmental influences.

It is considered confirmed that not a single, but rather about five to eight genes can be responsible for the development of the hypertensive phenotype. Primary hypertension appears therefore to be a poly-genetic disease in which the significance of the genes involved and their potential interaction − to the degree present − have still not been clarified to date.

9.3.3 Sodium chloride

While the presence of arterial hypertension is not observed in some aboriginal peoples (for example, Brazilian Indian tribes) who have a minimal intake of sodium chloride, one finds, particularly in western countries with a high daily intake of sodium chloride, a high positive correlation with the blood pressure level of the population and the frequency of arterial hypertension. This correlation is higher in older people than in younger ones, due to the fact that the kidney function in general and its ability to excrete sodium in particular decreases with increasing age.

Experimental data from rats indicates that the blood pressure raising effect of sodium chloride is not a consequence of increased sodium alone, but rather requires the combination with chloride. As chloride alone, equal molar sodium intake as sodium bicarbonate or sodium ascorbate did not induce hypertension.

An increased intake of sodium does not, however, lead to the development of hypertension in all persons and a normalization of blood pressure levels can not be achieved for all patients with hypertension through the restriction of sodium use. These experiences suggest a "sodium (salt) sensitivity", which is probably hereditary, in a segment of the hypertensive population. Because neither a "marker" (raised ANP-plasma level?) nor a protocol which could be used in routine practice is in existence to identify salt sensitive hypertension, the blood pressure increasing effect of sodium is accounted for "ex iuvantibus". Here a moderate sodium chloride reduction to around 6 g/day (ca. 105 mmol sodium) is recommended for every hypertensive patient as an initial part of the therapeutic non-drug basic measures and − if necessary − as an accompaniment to drug therapy (Section 20.2.2).

9.3.4 Insulin resistance and hyperinsulinemia

Insulin resistance, long recognized in truncal obesity and non-insulin dependent diabetes mellitus, is defined as a (progressive) disorder of insulin-induced glucose uptake, which manifests itself in particular in the skeletal musculature. The hyperinsulinemia found in affected patients is thus to be understood as an attempt by the organism to compensate the declining insulin effect through an increased release of insulin, and thereby maintain the normal glucose tolerance. It should be noted, however, that other insulin effects are not affected by this loss of effectiveness. Otherwise one could not explain the changes observed in hyperinsulinemia, such as an increase in renal sodium retention, the activation of the sympathetic nervous system, the induction of lipid metabolism disorders and accelerated arteriosclerosis. Insulin resistance is occasionally the result of a genetic defect at the (post) receptor level, however, in the majority of all cases it is induced by obesity, lack of physical activity or various medications (beta blockers, thiazide diuretics, steroid hormones, among others). The molecular mechanisms responsible for the induction of insulin resistance have still not been fully explained.

The discovery that insulin resistance is also present in a portion of normal-weight patients with primary hypertension and that this insulin resistance leads to an increased insulin secretion, is relatively recent and has led to speculation about a possible causal relationship between hypertension and hyperinsulinemia. Debate is ongoing, however, about whether the hypertension causes the insulin resistance or whether the development of the hypertension is contingent on the development of insulin resistance with consecutive hyperinsulinemia. Because, on the one hand, good arguments can be found for both hypotheses and, on the other hand, the succession of the actual pathophysiological changes has not yet been explained, the question of which came first, the chicken or the egg, must remain unanswered for now (see also Figure 9.1). However, in no way does a hyperinsulinemia automatically induce hypertension (take, for example, patients with hyperinsulinoma), and not every hypertensive patient develops insulin resistance.

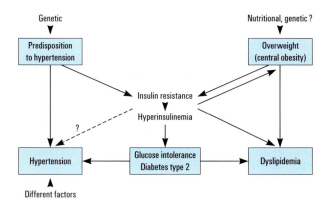

Figure 9.1: Potential causes of insulin resistance and possible effects of insulin resistance and/or hyperinsulinemia on blood-pressure-regulating factors. Acutely, hyperinsulinemia decreases vascular contractility. (From Weidmann P et al., J Hypertens 1995; 13 (suppl 2): S65-S72)

Some authors have coined the terms "metabolic syndrome" or "syndrome X", which try to account for the association observed in many patients between hypertension, hyperinsulinemia and lipid metabolism disorders (reduction of the high-density lipoprotein fraction, HDL, increase in the very-low-density lipoproteins, VLDL). These terms attempt to join this association between various cardiovascular risk factors into one pathogenic entity.

9.3.5 Obesity

As demonstrated by the results of the INTERSALT Study, there exists a positive correlation between body weight and blood pressure. In this study, conducted at a total of 52 centers, this relationship was more significantly pronounced than the relationship between dietary sodium chloride intake and blood pressure level. Approximately 50% of the obese patients exhibited elevated blood pressure, whereas, in contrast, 50% of the patients with primary hypertension were overweight. A loss of weight leads to a drop in blood pressure and therefore constitutes a general therapeutic measure for appropriately disposed patients.

The developing insulin resistance with subsequent hyperinsulinemia is viewed as a significant cause of hypertension in obese patients. Insulin raises the sodium absorption in the distal tubules of the nephron. This leads simultaneously to increased water retention with an increase in the intravascular volume (see above).

In addition, as a result of increased insulin secretion, the sympathetic nervous system is activated. This causes, on the one hand, an increased basal metabolic rate ("dietetic thermogenesis") and on the other, through the increased release of norepinephrine, to an increase in the peripheral vascular resistance with an already increased catecholamine sensitivity of the vessels.

Some investigations were able to show that a decreasing activity of the Na^+/K^+-ATPase may possibly play a role in the development or maintenance of elevated blood pressure values in obesity. A suppression of the Na^+/K^+-ATPase leads to an increase in the free intra-cellularly available calcium (and sodium) and thereby to an increased tone of the vascular smooth musculature with an increase in the peripheral vascular resistance.

In comparison to primary hypertension in persons of normal weight, hypertension in the obese displays some peculiarities. Whereas the peripheral vascular resistance is elevated in hypertensive patients with normal weight and correlates positively to the level of the blood pressure, in obese patients with hypertension there is only a moderate increase in the peripheral vascular resistance. The expansion of the intravascular volume with increased venous return to the heart leads to an increase in the cardiac output. The result is improved organ circulation with reflex (relative) vasodilation, which counteracts the increase in resistance usually associated with primary hypertension. The peripheral vascular resistance in obese patients with hypertension is, however, still significantly higher, compared to normotensive persons.

The heart, which in normal-weight hypertensives has primarily only to compensate the pressure-caused increases in the afterload, is faced with a combined increase in pre- and afterload in obese persons with hypertension. Late consequences are an eccentric/concentric, left-ventricular hypertrophy (Figure 9.2).

9.3.6 Disturbed balance of vasoactive hormones

Attempts to explain primary hypertension as a disturbed homeostasis of the known blood pressure-regulating hormone systems (see also Section 1.4.2) have not delivered satisfactory results.

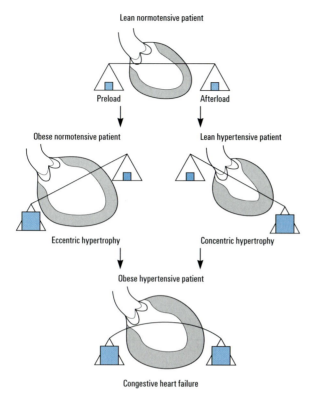

Figure 9.2: Cardiac structural adaptation to obesity (mild wall thickening with chamber dilatation), primary hypertension (wall thickening without chamber dilatation), and combined obesity-hypertension (From Lavie CJ, Ventura HO, Messerli FH, Postgraduate Med 1992; 91: 131−143)

9.3.6.1 Sympathetic nervous system activity

To what degree increased activity of the sympathic nervous system contributes to the development of sustained hypertension can certainly not be definitively judged. While an age-dependent increase in plasma catecholamine levels can be observed in normotensive patients, patients with primary hypertension seem to have plasma catecholamine levels slightly elevated or in the upper normal range for younger patients. It is therefore conceivable that an increased sympathetic tone exists, at least in the development phase of primary hypertension. As was already suggested, the question of whether this constitutes a pathogenic sub-factor, or merely an epiphenomenon, must remain open at this time.

9.3.6.2 The renin-angiotensin system

It has been demonstrated that subpopulations with a differently activated renin-angiotensin system (RAS) can be identified within the total population of primary hypertensives. While an increased plasma renin activity is found on average more frequently among younger patients, the RAS tends on average to be less activated in elderly patients with primary hypertension. The division into "low", "normal" and "high-renin hypertension" has, however, not produced a significant contribution to the pathogenic understanding of primary hypertension or a decisive practical application. Interestingly enough, it was shown that a pharmacological inhibition of the angiotensin-converting enzyme also leads to a decrease in blood pressure, even in cases of "low-renin hypertension". From this, one can conclude that at least additional factors must be participating in the genesis of the increase in blood pressure in primary hypertension.

9.3.6.3 Natriuretic peptides (ANP, BNP)

Elevated plasma levels of ANP (atrial natriuretic peptide) and BNP (brain natriuretic peptide) are only to be expected in hypertensive patients with increased cardiac pre-load (expanded intravascular volume) and/or reduced cardiac function (congestive heart failure, etc.). Normal plasma levels of these natriuretic hormones are found in hypertension without end-organ damage. In contrast to the endogenous digitalis-like factor (see Section 9.3.6.4), an effect on the Na^+/K^+-ATPase could not be demonstrated.

9.3.6.4 Endogenous digitalis-like factor (EDLF)/natriuretic hormone

The increase in intracellular sodium and calcium ions, found in at least a portion of the patients with primary hypertension, has also been repeatedly associated with, among other factors, the existence of a natriuretic hormone. This hormone cross-reacts with digoxin in radioimmunoassay (endogenous digitalis-like factor, EDLF; not identical to the atrial natriuretic peptide) and could be detected in both healthy subjects and patients with hypertension. It is assumed that this hormone, which may be formed in the hypothalamus or in the adrenal glands, is released into the blood stream in higher amounts with increased sodium chloride intake and represents a humoral compensatory mechanism for a genetically-determined disorder of the renal capacity to excrete sodium. Besides an inhibition of the renal sodium transport mechanism with subsequent natriuresis, this hormone is believed to inhibit the membrane-based Na^+/K^+-ATPase of the vascular smooth musculature. The suppression of this transport system causes — according to current speculation — an increase in the intracellular sodium concentration as well as a decrease in the potassium concentration in the resistance vessels. The consequences would be a decrease in the membrane potential with an increase in the influx of free calcium ions through the depolarization (= voltage) operated calcium channels as well as an indirect influencing of the Na^+/Ca^{2+} exchange with consecutive increase in the Ca^{2+} transport in the intracellular space. The resultant increased availability of intracellular free calcium ions would thus explain the elevated arteriolar vascular resistance and resulting increase in blood pressure in primary hypertension (Figure 9.3).

Raised EDLF-plasma levels have been found primarily in hypertensive patients with a suppressed plasma-renin activity and suspected volume expansion. Because hyperinsulinemia is also associated with an increased sodium retention, it

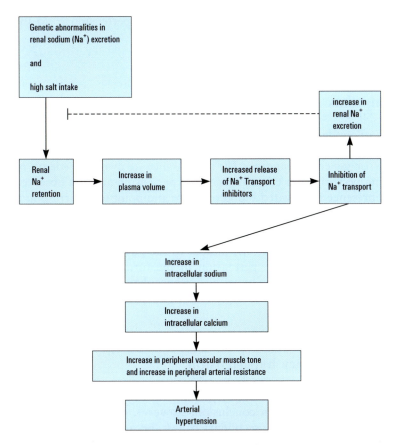

Figure 9.3: Hypothetical pathogenesis of (salt-sensitive) primary hypertension (Blaustein, 1977). |------: Insufficient compensation of renal sodium retention

has been speculated that an increased secretion of EDLF contributes pathogenically to obesity-induced hypertension through consecutive suppression of the Na^+/K^+-ATPase and an increase in the intracellular calcium in the vascular smooth musculature.

9.3.6.5 Endothelin

For patients with primary hypertension, elevated endothelin plasma levels have only been observed with coexisting arteriosclerotic target-organ damage. However, since this strongly vasoconstrictive peptide is primarily a paracrinally or autocrinally acting hormone, the height of peripherally-determined plasma levels may not reflect the local secretion and activity of endothelin. In some animal models of arterial hypertension (e.g., spontaneously hypertensive rats), the administration of endothelin-receptor antagonists caused a decrease in blood pressure. These observations suggest that endothelin contributes — at least under certain conditions and in this animal model of a genetically-determined form of hypertension — to the maintenance of high blood pressure.

9.4 Clinical symptoms

Patients with mild or moderate primary hypertension are frequently completely free of symptoms. Only periodically mentioned are nonspecific symptoms like headache, dizziness or general weakness. The appearance of dyspnea, edema or thoracic pain (angina pectoris) as a consequence of hypertension are first observed after the persistent presence of elevated blood pressure and point to a corresponding damage of the end organs.

In malignant hypertension it is often severe headaches, impaired vision, disturbances of balance or anuria, which lead the patient to the physician.
The acute exacerbation of primary hypertension in the form of a hypertensive crisis is manifested in the picture of the hypertensive encephalopathy and possibly in the symptoms of an acute cardiac decompensation (Chapter 10).

9.5 The diagnosis of primary hypertension

The diagnosis of primary hypertension is only possible through the exclusion of a secondary form of hypertension. This conclusion, however, does not justify an excessive and costly search for possible secondary causes, because on the one hand the probability of a secondary form of hypertension is very slight and, on the other, in many cases, it is only of limited therapeutic relevance. In general, the recommended standard diagnostic program should therefore be strictly followed and only expanded upon thorough supplemental investigations, if the standard diagnostic procedure results in findings, which on the one hand clearly indicate the presence of a secondary form of hypertension and on the other give reason to expect therapeutic consequences (Chapter 7).

Summary (Chapter 9)

- Primary hypertension is the most common chronic disease in industrialized countries.
- The pathogenesis of primary hypertension still remains unclear. However, it is probably a "multifactorial" disease, set off by various environmental influences in interaction with an as yet undetermined genetic predisposition.
- The certain diagnosis of primary hypertension is only possible through the exclusion of a secondary cause.

- The small percentage of secondary forms of hypertension in the total population of patients with hypertension only justifies the targeted search for an organically tangible cause, if a corresponding suspicion has already resulted from the strictly adhered to standard diagnostic procedure, and if therapeutic consequences can be drawn from the expected diagnosis.

- Mild to moderate primary hypertension is usually not accompanied by subjective complaints. Headache, visual disorders and dizziness oftenly first appear in cases of severe or malignant hypertension.

Literature (Chapter 9)

Andronico G, Mule G, Mangano MT, Piazza G, Donatelli M, Cerasola G, Bompiano GD. Insulin resistance and endogenous digoxin-like factor in obese hypertensive patients with glucose intolerance. Acta Diabetol 1992; 28: 203−205.

Blaustein MP. Sodium ions, calcium ions, blood pressure regulation and hypertension: a reassessment and a hypothesis. Am J Physiol 1977; 232: C165-C173.

Burt VL, Whelton P, Roccella EJ, Brown C, Cutler JA, Higgins M, Horan MJ, Labarthe D. Prevalence of hypertension in the US adult population. Results from the third National Health and Nutrition Examination Survey, 1988−1991. Hypertension 1995; 25: 305−313.

Carroll D, Smith GD, Sheffield D, Shipley MJ, Marmot MG. Pressor reactions to psychological stress and prediction of future blood pressure: data from the Whitehall II study. Br Med J 1995; 310: 771−776.

Cutler JA, Kotchen TA, Obarzanek E (eds). The National Heart, Lung, and Blood Institute workshop on salt and blood pressure. Hypertension 1991; 17 (suppl I): I-1-I-221.

Davidson MB. Clinical implications of insulin resistance syndromes. Am J Med 1995; 99: 420−426.

Elliott P. Observational studies of salt and blood pressure. Hypertension 1991; 17 (suppl I): I-3-I-8.

Ferrannini E, Buzzigoli G, Bonadonna R, Giorico MA, Olegini M, Graziadei L, Pedrinellia R, Brandi L, Bevilacqua S. Insulin resistance in essential hypertension. N Engl J Med 1987; 317: 350−356.

Ganten D, Schmidt S, Paul M. Genetics of primary hypertension. J Cardiovasc Pharmacol 1994; 24 (suppl 3): S45-S50.

Goldstein DS. Plasma catecholamines and essential hypertension. An analytical review. Hypertension 1983; 5: 86−99.

Gottsdiener JS, Reda DJ, Materson BJ, Massie BM, Notargiacomo A, Hamburger RJ, Williams DW, Henderson WG. Importance of obesity, race and age to the cardiac structural and functional effects of hypertension. J Am Coll Cardiol 1994; 24: 1492−1498.

Hall JE (ed). The kidney, obesity, and essential hypertension symposium. Jackson, Miss., March 15−16, 1991. Hypertension 1992; 19 (suppl I): I-1-I-135.

Harrap S. Hypertension: genes versus environment. Lancet 1994; 344: 167−171.

Herbold M, Hense HW, Keil U. Effects of road traffic noise on prevalence of hypertension in men: results of the Lübeck blood pressure study. Soz Präventivmed 1989; 34: 19−23.

Hinson JP, Dawnay AB, Raven PW. Why we should give a qualified welcome to ouabain: a whole new family of adrenal steroid hormones. J Endocrinol 1995; 146: 369−372.

Januszewicz A. The natriuretic peptides in hypertension. Curr Opin Cardiol 1995; 10: 495−500.

Kahn CR. Causes of insulin resistance. Nature 1995; 373: 384−385.

Kannel WB, Brand N, Skinner JJ Jr, Dawber TR, Mc Namara PM. Relation of adiposity to blood pressure and development of hypertension: The Framingham Study. Ann Intern Med 1967; 67: 48−59.

Kurtz T. Genetic models of hypertension. Lancet 1994; 344: 167−168.

Landsberg L. Hyperinsulinemia: Possible Role in obesity-induced hypertension. Hypertension 1992; 19 (suppl I): I-61-I-66.

Landsberg L. Diet, obesity and hypertension: An hypothesis involving insulin, the sympathetic nervous system, and adaptative thermogenesis. Q J Med 1986; 236: 1081−1090.

Levine RS, Hennekens CH, Jesse MJ. Blood pressure in prospective population based cohort of newborn and infant twins. Br Med J 1994; 308: 298−302.

Lund-Johansen P. Twenty-year follow-up of hemodynamics in essential hypertension during rest and exercise. Hypertension 1991; 18 (suppl III): III-54-III-61.

Lüscher TF, Seo B, Bühler F. Potential role of endothelin in hy-pertension. Controversy on endothelin in hypertension. Hypertension 1993; 21: 752−757.

Luft FC, Weinberger MH, Grim CE. Sodium sensitivity and resistance in normotensive humans. Am J Med 1982; 72: 726−736.

Morris AD, Petrie JR, Connell JMC. Insulin and hypertension. J Hypertens 1994; 12: 633−642.

Neild GH. Endothelin plasma levels in hypertensive patients with vascular disease. J Hypertens 1994; 12 (suppl 1): S17−S20.

Regecova V, Kellerova E. Effects of urban noise pollution on blood pressure and heart rate in preschool children. J Hypertens 1995; 13: 405−412.

Reisin E. Sodium and obesity in the pathogenesis of hypertension. Am J Hypertension 1990; 3: 164−167.

Reiss U, Stimpel M: Clinical usefulness of atrial peptide measurements. [in German] Schweiz Rundschau Med (PRAXIS) 1993; 82: 755−758.

Ribstein J, du Cailar G, Mimran A. Combined renal effects of overweight and hypertension. Hypertension 1995; 26: 610−615.

Roccini AP. Cardiovascular regulation in obesity-induced hypertension. Hypertension 1992; 19 (suppl I): I-56-I-60.

Schiffrin EL. Endothelin: potential role in hypertension and vascular hypertrophy. Hypertension 1995; 25: 1135−1145.

Sharma AM, Distler A, Luft FC. Strategien zur Erforschung der Genetik des Bluthochdrucks. Dtsch med Wschr 1994; 119: 742−746.

Stamler R, Stamler J, Riedlinger WF, Algera G, Roberts RJ: Weight and blood pressure: Findings in hypertension screening of one million Americans. JAMA 1978; 240: 1607−1610.

Stamler J, Rose G, Elliott P, Marmot M, Kesteloot H, Stamler R. Findings of the international cooperative INTERSALT study. Hypertension 1991; 17 (suppl I): I-9-I-15.

Stamler J. Implications of the INTERSALT study. Hypertension 1991; 17 (suppl I): I-16-I-20.

Stimpel M, Kaufmann W, Wambach G. Atrial natriuretic peptide (ANP) in essential hypertension: humoral marker for salt sensitivity and hypertensive heart disease at a clinically asymptomatic state? [in German] Z Kardiol 1988; 77 (suppl 2): 92−98.

Vanhoutte PM. Is endothelin involved in the pathogenesis of hypertension? Hypertension 1993; 21: 747−751.

Williams B. Insulin resistance: the shape of things to come. Lancet 1994; 344: 521−524.

Williams GH. Essential hypertension as an endocrine disease. Endocrinol Metab Clin N Am 1994; 23: 429−444.

Woolfson RG, Poston L, De Wardener HE. Digoxin-like inhibitors of active sodium transport and blood pressure: the current status. Kidney Int 1994; 46: 297−309.

Zanchetti A. Hyperlipidaemia in the hypertensive patient. Am J Med 1994; 96 (suppl 6A): 3S−8S.

10 Hypertensive crises

Hypertensive crises are characterized by a strong, sudden increase of the systolic and/or diastolic blood pressure with normal or increased initial values. They may be accompanied by symptoms of hypertensive end-organ damage (hypertensive emergency) or without such symptoms (urgency). A hypertensive crisis can not be assessed in the differential diagnostic sense, because it may appear with any form of hypertension. Acute blood pressure exacerbations ("rebound phenomenon") have occasionally been observed following the abrupt discontinuation of some antihypertensive drugs (e.g. clonidine, beta-blockers) (Table 10.1).

Table 10.1: Causes of hypertensive crises

Primary hypertension

Secondary forms of hypertension
   – Renovascular hypertension
   – Renoparenchymal hypertension
   – Pheochromocytoma
   – Primary aldosteronism (rare)
   – Eclampsia

Sudden interruption of antihypertensive drug therapy (esp. with clonidine)
(Dietary) intake of tyramine* during therapy with monoaminooxydase-inhibitors

* Tyramine-containing foods:
  Chocolate, alcoholic beverages, cheese, caviar, chicken liver, yeast extracts

10.1 Complications and symptoms of hypertensive crises

An acute danger for patients results from the possible damage to organs, especially to the brain and heart. When the mean arterial pressure exceeds 150 to 180 mmHg, the autoregulatory compensation mechanisms fail in the region of the cerebral arterial vascular bed. The result is a pressure-related, passive increased blood circulation, which leads to an increased permeability of the vascular basal membrane especially in the cerebral arterioles and capillaries and thus explains the development of cerebral edema and micro-hemorrhages. In later stages, the increasing edema compromises the capillaries, so that the subsequent insufficient cerebral circulation results in the development of local or generalized cerebral ischemia. The acute, hypertension-caused massive hemorrhage is the consequence of a pressure-related rupture of a cerebral vessel and is most often seen with previous severe arteriosclerotic damage.

In the heart, an acute increase in blood pressure causes a spontaneous increase in the afterload with a worsening of the left-ventricular hemodynamics. Especially in the (hypertensive) previously-damaged, dilated heart, the increase in left-ventricular filling pressure, systolic wall tension, myocardial oxygen consumption and the decrease of the coronary flow lead early-on to acute myocardial insufficiency and/or myocardial ischemia. Pulmonary edema and angina pectoris or myocardial infarction are the commonly observed consequences of a hypertensive crisis.

Typical symptoms of hypertensive crises carrying the threat of or with manifest end-organ damage, whose clinical correlate in the form of headache, convulsions, vomiting, nausea, confusion, somnolence, loss of consciousness (hypertensive encephalopathy) and dyspnea and/or angina pectoris symptoms indicate the emergency character, compelling the attending physician to take emergency therapeutic action (hypertensive emergency; Section 32.1.1).

Further possible consequences of an acute blood pressure decompensation are epistaxis, retinal hemorrhage, and the development of a dissecting aortal aneurysma (Table 10.2).

Table 10.2: Complications and symptoms of a hypertensive crisis

Organ damage	Clinical symptoms
Brain	
Hypertensive encephalopathy	− Headaches − Nausea/vomitting − Visual disorders − Convulsions − Transistory neurological incidents − Confusion/sleepness
Heart	
Acute left ventricular insufficiency Pulmonary edema	− Dyspnea
Myocardial ischemia Myocardial infarction	− Stenocardia
Kidneys	
Acute kidney failure	− Oliguria/anuria − Hematuria/proteinuria
Vascular system	
Dissecting aorta Rupture of small arterial vasculature	− Rapid onset of extremely severe thoracic pain

10.2 Differential diagnosis of the hypertensive crisis

The hypertensive crisis must be distinguished from malignant hypertension, in which permanently elevated diastolic blood pressure values of more than

120 mmHg, typical retinal changes (fundus hypertonicus malignus resp. WHO grades III-IV; Figure 7.1) as well as renal damage are present and acute clinical symptoms are usually missing. Still important, but not always easy to make clinically, due to often similar symptoms, is the differentiation between a hypertensive crisis and a reactive blood pressure increase seen in cerebrovascular accident or stroke, as in the latter disease picture, a too rapid or too strong decrease in blood pressure must be prevented. (Section 31.2.1).

Summary (Chapter 10)

- Hypertensive crisis is characterized by an acute increase of the arterial blood pressure with normal or increased initial values; it may or may not be accompanied by threatening or even manifest target-organ damage of the brain, heart, eyes, kidneys and arterial vascular system.

- Hypertensive crisis with clinical symptoms of target-organ damage represents an emergency situation which requires immediate therapeutic intervention with medical supervision under hospitalized conditions.

- If there are no complaints, the blood pressure should be lowered slowly; an emergency hospitalization is generally not necessary ("urgency").

- The hypertensive crisis requires diagnostic differentiation between malignant hypertension and reactive increases in blood pressure (especially in apoplexy).

- The appearance of a hypertensive crisis does not allow, in general, any differential diagnostic conclusions on the etiology of the underlying form of hypertension.

Literature (Chapter 10)

Calhoun DA, Oparil S. Treatment of hypertensive crisis. N Engl J Med 1990; 323: 1177–1183.

Calhoun DA, Oparil S. Hypertensive crisis since FDR – a partial victory. N Engl J Med 1995; 332: 1029–1030.

Gifford RW Jr. Management of hypertensive crisis. JAMA 1991; 266: 829–835.

Kincaid-Smith P. Malignant hypertension. J Hypertens 1991; 9: 893–899.

Kraft K, Kolloch R. Hypertensive Krise und hypertensiver Notfall. Intensiv Notfallbehandlung 1994; 19: 67–72.

Mehta JL, Lopez LM. Rebound hypertension following abrupt cessation of clonidine and metropolol. Treatment with labetalol. Arch Intern Med 1987; 147: 389–390.

Paulson OB, Strandgaard S. Hypertensive disease and the cerebral circulation. In: Laragh JH, Brenner BM (eds). Hypertension: Pathophysiology, diagnosis and management, 2nd ed. Raven Press New York, 1994.

Simon G, Archer SL. Hypertensive urgency due to cholesterol embolization of kidneys. Am J Hypertens 1995; 8: 954–956.

11 Hypertension in children and adolescents

11.1 Definition and classification of hypertension in children and adolescents

The level of the arterial blood pressure during childhood does not allow for strict definitions, as a continual growth-related increase in systolic and diastolic blood pressure takes place. At birth the systolic blood pressure is on average 75 mmHg. In the first weeks of life it rises daily by 1−2 mmHg. A further increase of about 1 mmHg per week is observed until the sixth week of life, thereafter the blood pressure remains constant up to and including the age of four. An extensive diagnostic investigation is recommended for chronic elevations of blood pressure in

− infants (under 1 year) of ≥ 120 mmHg systolic,
− small children (2−5 years) of ≥ 130/80 mmHg,

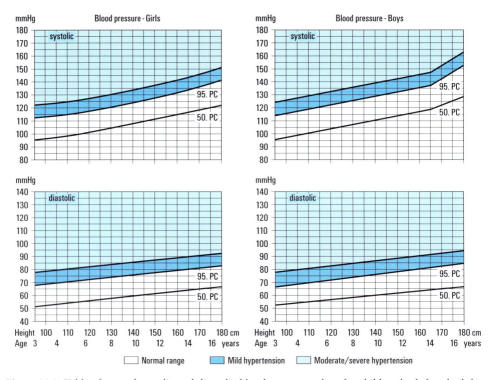

Figure 11.1: Table of normal systolic and diastolic blood pressure values for children both female (left) and male (right). (Source: German Hypertension Society 11/1994)

− primary-school-age children (6−11 years) of ≥ 130/85 mmHg,
− adolescents of ≥ 140/90 mmHg.

Due to the continual increase in blood pressure in children and adolescents, a percentile curve for blood pressure has been established through the evaluation of previously available European studies. Based on this percentile curve, one can make an age-dependent differentiation on the degree of severity of the hypertension (Figure 11.1).

Blood pressure values which lie less than 10 mmHg above the 95th percentile are classified as mild hypertension and those more than 10 mmHg above the 95th percentile are classified as moderate (significant) hypertension. According to this categorization, severe hypertension is present when the blood pressure values are more than 30 mmHg above the 95th percentile.

Normative data on blood pressure from more than 70,000 white, African- and Mexican-American children are provided by the "Report of the Second Task Force on Blood Pressure Control in Children", 1987 (Table 11.1).

Table 11.1: Classification of hypertension in the young by age group*

Age group	High normal (90−94th percentile), mmHg	Significant hypertension (95−99th percentile), mmHg	Severe hypertension (>99th percentile), mmHg
Newborns (SBP)			
7 d	...	96−105	≥106
8−30d	...	104−109	≥110
Infants (≤2 y)			
SBP	104−111	112−117	≥118
DBP	70−73	74−81	≥82
Children			
3−5 y			
SBP	108−115	116−123	≥124
DBP	70−75	76−83	≥84
6−9 y			
SBP	114−121	122−129	≥130
DBP	74−77	78−85	≥86
10−12 y			
SBP	122−125	126−133	≥134
DBP	78−81	82−89	≥90
13−15 y			
SBP	130−135	136−143	≥144
DBP	80−85	86−91	≥92
Adolescents (16−18 y)			
SBP	136−141	142−149	≥150
DBP	84−91	92−97	≥98

* Table adapted from JNC V, Arch Intern Med 1993; 153: 154−183; Original source: Report of the Second Task Force on Blood Pressure Control in Children, 1987

11.2 Techniques for measuring blood pressure in children and adolescents

Even more than is the case with adult patients, before measuring the blood pressure, an effort should be made to allow a child to grow accustomed to the environment of the physician's practice, which is often perceived as being threatening. Nervous excitement and fear of pain lead to "stress-related" increases in blood pressure, which can misrepresent the actual blood pressure condition. Under no circumstances should a routine blood pressure measurement be forced.

The first blood pressure measurement in a child or adolescent has to be performed on both arms, to discover possible hemodynamically relevant vascular malformations. In addition, a measurement of the pressure conditions in the lower extremities is also desirable. The systolic blood pressure is measured via palpation through the inflation of a blood pressure measuring cuff on the lower leg. Thus large differences between the upper and lower extremities can be detected early on. These differences indicate the presence of a stenosis of the aortic isthmus, which appears proportionally more frequently in childhood.

Essentially it does not make a difference whether the blood pressure is measured in a sitting or supine position. However, in order to create comparable conditions, the body position once chosen should be maintained in the subsequent examinations.

The techniques for measuring blood pressure require adjustment to the physical changes in childhood and adolescence. While measuring techniques based on ultrasound-Doppler procedures or on the oscillometric principle are recommended for newborns and infants, the well-known techniques with mercury or membrane manometers according to Riva-Rocci and Korotkoff can be applied with pre-school and primary-school-age children (Chapter 2). In each case, the choice of the cuff width must be suited to the physical size of the child. The American Heart Association recommends a rubber cuff width of at least 2/3rds the length of the individual's upper arm. If one chooses the widest, easily applicable blood pressure cuff for the practice, then, as a rule, three cuff sizes will suffice (5−6 cm, 8−9 cm, and 12−14 cm wide inflatable cuff for infants, children, and adolescents/adults, respectively; Table 2.1).

As in adults, the systolic blood pressure is attributed to phase I of the Korotkoff sounds during auscultation. In the evaluation of the diastolic pressure, the measurements of both phase IV (= beats becoming quieter) and phase V (= disappearance of the sounds) have proven effective, as the Korotkoff sounds often first disappear in children at low pressures or are still auditory after the deflation of the cuff.

11.3 Continuous 24-hour ambulatory blood pressure monitoring (ABPM)

The use of continuous 24-hour ambulant blood pressure monitoring (ABPM) in children is relatively new, so that little data are available. The principal usefulness of this method in a pediatric population and the good reproducibility of the data raised have been verified in a study in which healthy children between the ages of 7 and 14 years of age were each measured twice at 7 month intervals. At the present time, the use of ABPM in children should currently still be restricted to controlled clinical studies, as diagnostic ABPM standards still need to be defined for this population before therapeutic consequences can be recommended based on completed measurements.

11.4 Frequency and causes of hypertension in children and adolescents

Arterial hypertension in children and adolescents is found in approximately 1−3% of all cases. The majority of the patients have a mild form of primary hypertension. Sharp increases in blood pressure indicate, in contrast, the presence of a secondary form of hypertension, whose share of the total patient collective of juvenile hypertensive patients is not likely − according to cautious estimates − to lie higher than in adults (5−10%).

11.5 Standard and differential diagnostic procedures for arterial hypertension in children and adolescents

The scope of the diagnostic measures is based on the blood pressure level. Patient history, clinical examination and the ascertaining of urine status are, however, to be considered part of the standard diagnostic procedures and should be conducted when normal-high and slightly-elevated blood pressure values are encountered. With established hypertension, the standard diagnostic procedure also usual for adults is recommended (see the schema of the German Hypertension Society, Figure 7.3, and the US-JNC V-Report).

As has already been mentioned, sharp increases in the blood pressure in childhood more often indicate the presence of a secondary form of hypertension. The spectrum of possible causes includes all the various disorders which need to be drawn into differential diagnostic consideration as causes in adults. With the exception of the various forms of the adrenogenital syndrome, endocrine forms of hypertension are found even less often in children. 70% of the secondary forms of hypertension are due to renal parenchymal disease, 10% are due to vascular disease and 5−10% are due to a hypertensive disease caused by vascular malformations (Table 11.2). The diagnostic procedure to be followed upon strong suspicion of the presence of a secondary form of hypertension is dealt with in another section (Chapters 7.6 and 13−18).

Table 11.2: Causes and frequency of arterial hypertension in childhood

Clinical picture	Frequency (%)
Primary hypertension	90−95
Secondary hypertension	5−10
Renal hypertension	
− Renal parenchymal hypertension	3−6
− Renovascular hypertension	1
Endocrine hypertension	<1
Cardiovascular hypertension	1−2

Summary (Chapter 11)

- The assessment of the blood pressure level in children and adolescents must be suited to the specific age and growth stage.

- The definition and classification of the degree of severity of arterial hypertension in children and adolescents is made according to a percentile curve.

- The cuff size needs to be adjusted to fit the narrowest arm diameter of the children in order to perform the indirect measurement of the blood pressure.

- The most common cause of arterial hypertension in children and adolescents is (usually mild) primary hypertension.

- The most common cause of secondary hypertension in childhood is renal parenchymal hypertension.

- The (differential) diagnostic procedure for adults with verified hypertension is also applicable to adolescent patients and should be adhered to as restrictively as possible, especially for mild hypertension.

Literature (Chapter 11)

Berenson GS, Cresanta JL, Webber LS. High blood pressure in the young. Ann Rev Med 1984; 35: 535−560.

De Santo NG, Trevisan M, Capasso G, Giordano DR, Latte M, Krogh V. Blood pressure and hypertension in childhood: epidemiology, diagnosis, and treatment. Kidney Int 1988; 34 (suppl 25): S115−S118.

Deutsche Liga zur Bekämpfung des hohen Blutdruckes e.V. Deutsche Hypertonie Gesellschaft. Hypertonie bei Kindern und Jugendlichen, 2. Aufl., 1994.

Hiner LB, Falkner B. Renovascular hypertension in children. Ped Clin N Am 1993; 40: 123−140.

Loggie JMH (ed). Pediatric and adolescent hypertension. Blackwell Scientific Publications, Boston 1992.

Mendoza SA. Hypertension in infants and children. Nephron 1990; 54: 289−295.

Schieken RM. New perspectives in childhood blood pressure. Curr Opin Cardiol 1995; 10: 87−91.

12 Secondary forms of hypertension: classification and incidence

Secondary forms of hypertension are classified into (see also Chapter 4.4):

- Renal hypertension (Chapter 13)
- Endocrine hypertension (Chapter 14)
- Pregnancy-induced hypertension (Chapter 15)
- Cardiovascular hypertension (Chapter 16)
- Hypertension induced by drugs or other substances (Chapter 17)
- Neurogenic hypertension (Chapter 18)

In comparison to primary hypertension, secondary forms of hypertension are uncommon. Their share in the total population of patients with hypertension is about 1−2%. The scope and significance of these in part curable diseases becomes clearer, however, when one notes the actual disease figures. Among an estimated number of approximately 45 million people (Table 9.1) with hypertension in the USA (hypertension is defined as an arterial blood pressure above 140 mmHg systolic or higher than 90 mmHg diastolic) are thus approximately 450,000 to 900,000 patients with a secondary form of hypertension.

Summary (Chapter 12)

1−2% of all patients with hypertension suffer from a secondary form of hypertension. In the United States, therefore, approximately one million patients are thus affected.

13 Renal hypertension

Renal hypertension includes:

- renoparenchymal hypertension,
- renovascular hypertension and
- hypertension following kidney transplant (post-transplant hypertension).

Renal forms of hypertension are by far the most frequent cause (70%) of secondary hypertension.

13.1 Renoparenchymal hypertension

13.1.1 Frequency and causes of renoparenchymal hypertension

Renoparenchymal hypertension is by the far most frequent form of secondary hypertension. In most cases this is the result of bilateral disease of the renal parenchyma, for which it is generally not possible to offer curative therapy. It is generally subject to a more or less progressive course. Primary glomerulonephropathies are more frequently and more readily associated with hypertension than tubulo-interstitial diseases.

Hypertension based on a unilateral renoparenchymal disease is on the other hand to be viewed as potentially curable, because corrective surgery or a nephrectomy of the diseased or altered kidney can remove the responsible pathomechanism. A prerequisite for this is, however, that the mistakenly assumed "healthy" kidney does not exhibit any irreversible, hypertension-related damage, which could contribute to a tertiary maintenance of the hypertension.

13.1.2 Pathogenesis

The progressive loss of functioning nephrons reduces the ability of the diseased kidney to excrete sodium and water. The result is a hypervolemia in the arterial and venous vascular bed with an increase in cardiac output and consequent increase in the arterial blood pressure. In the further course of the disease the hypertension is stabilized by means of an increase in the peripheral arterial resistance. At the same time the cardiac output decreases so that in the stage of "manifest" renoparenchymal hypertension it is a normal or low cardiac output.

The intensifying increase in the peripheral vascular resistance is possibly the result of a disturbed balance between the vasopressive and vasodepressive regulatory mechanisms. The increased formation of the strongly vasoconstrictively acting angiotensin II (Ang II) could offer an important contribution to the shifting of such a balance, because in most patients with renoparenchymal hypertension there is an inadequately stimulated renin-angiotensin-system (RAS), despite hypervolemia and increased whole body sodium. Other changes in vasodepressive factors which are described in parenchymal hypertension and could contribute to the development of elevated arterial resistance are an increased responsiveness of the vascular smooth muscle to Ang II, an increased concentration of free intracellular calcium ions and increased plasma levels of norepinephrine.

Although the hemodynamic and hormonal changes described cause an increased release of atrial natriuretic peptide (ANP; Section 1.4.2.4) as should be expected, this endogenous, vasodepressive compensatory mechanism does not counteract either the hypervolemia and hypernatremia or the vasoconstriction. Renal resistance to ANP apparently sets in as damage to the functional renal tissue increases.

Furthermore, the renal formation and release of vasodilatory hormones appears to decrease. It still needs to be clarified if and to what extent this reduced availability of kinins, prostaglandins (PGE_2 and PGI_2) and endothelial-derived nitric oxide (NO) have an effect on the systemic arterial vascular tone and therefore contribute to the imbalance postulated above. It is possible that these hormones are only involved in the regulation of the intrarenal bloodflow as autocrine or paracrine factors.

Summary (Sections 13.1.1 and 13.1.2)

- Renoparenchymal hypertension is the most frequent form of secondary hypertension.

- Renoparenchymal hypertension is characterized by hypervolemia, hypernatremia, an increase in peripheral arterial vascular resistance and a normal or low cardiac output.

- Hypervolemia and hypernatremia are probably the result of disease-specific, progressive damage to the nephrons with decreasing ability to excrete water and sodium.

- The increasing peripheral vasoconstriction is based at least partially on an inadequately activated renin angiotensin system with increasing formation of angiotensin II.

13.1.3   Causes of renoparenchymal hypertension

13.1.3.1 Bilateral renal diseases

In correlation with the decrease of functioning nephrons almost every bilateral renal parenchymal disease develops into arterial hypertension sooner or later.

Glomerulonephritis:

As mentioned above, hypertension manifests itself earlier and more frequently in primary and secondary glomerular diseases than with tubulo-interstitial nephritides. Of the primary glomerulonephritides, membranoproliferative glomerulonephritis (GN), acute poststreptococcal-GN and rapidly progressive GN are most frequently accompanied by arterial hypertension (Table 13.1).

Table 13.1:   Frequency of hypertension in glomerulonephritis of different causes*

Histological form of glomerulonephritis	Frequency (%)
Membranoproliferative	60
Rapid-progressive	50
Endocapillary of the poststreptococcal type	50
Mesangioproliferative	35
Focal-segmental sclerotic	35
Perimembranous	30
Minimal-proliferating	25

* Modified acc. to Bohle et al. (1976)

Renal diseases which occur as a result of renal involvement in multisystemic diseases (Wegener's granulomatosis, systemic lupus erythematosus) are classified as secondary glomerulonephritides. The frequency of hypertension varies in these diseases between 10 and 50%.

Diabetic nephropathy:

Diabetic nephropathy represents a special form which has a characteristic course in insulin dependent diabetics and leads through an early stage of glomerular hyperfiltration and hypertrophy to a late stage of functional limitation. In the setting of an increased urine albumin excretion with a completely normal glomerular filtration rate (stage III), arterial hypertension develops in almost all patients.

Interstitial nephritis:

Recurrent chronic pyelonephritis leads to damage of the renal parenchyma. Hypertension occurs relatively late in this disease. Analgesic nephropathy is associated with arterial hypertension in 50% of the cases. There is no apparent correlation to the degree of the renal insufficiency.

Polycystic kidney disease:

Polycystic kidney disease appears frequently in a genetic context. The changes develop slowly, so that they frequently only become clinically relevant in middle-age. In advanced stages the destruction of the renal tissue leads to rapid deterioration of the renal function, eventually requiring dialysis treatment. Arterial hypertension develops in 50% of the cases.

13.1.3.2 Unilateral renal diseases

Arterial hypertension which results from a unilateral renoparenchymal disease can be considered to be potentially curable. The most frequent causes of unilateral renal disease accompanied by hypertension are:

- Pyelonephritis,
- solitary renal cysts,
- renal trauma (Page kidney),
- segmental hypoplasia (Ask-Upmark kidney),
- unilateral tuberculous kidney,
- unilateral radiation nephritis and
- renal tumors.

13.1.4   Diagnosis of renoparenchymal hypertension

13.1.4.1 Laboratory diagnostics

Abnormalities in the result of the recommended urinalysis (proteinuria, hematuria, leucocyturia, urinary casts) performed in the routine work-up of arterial hypertension or an increase of the renal retention values in serum lead to the suspicion of a renoparenchymatous genesis of the hypertension. In cases of severe or long-term untreated hypertension, it may be difficult to determine on the basis of this routine test whether the renal damage is the cause or the result of the hypertension.

Indications of the presence of a glomerulonephritis can be derived from the simultaneous proof of microhematuria, red cell casts in the sediment and concomitant proteinuria of more than 2g/day. If the assessment of erythrocyte morphology in cases of isolated hematuria demonstrates more than 10% deformed erythrocytes, a glomerular cause should probably be assumed for the hematuria. It is possible to differentiate between selective and nonselective glomerular proteinuria by cellulose acetate electrophoresis.

The renal clearance rate must be determined in cases of normal renal retention values, so that early functional changes can be detected.

The repeated detection of leucocyturia with concomitant increase in renal retention values in the serum may indicate a chronic pyelonephritis.

13.1.4.2 Imaging procedures

The most important imaging procedure in cases of suspected renoparenchymal disease is ultrasonography. The following diagnostically relevant statements can frequently be made on the basis of ultrasonography:

- Differentiation between uni- and bilateral renal diseases,
- extent of the parenchymal loss

    as well as exclusion or proof of

- hydronephrosis,

- major damage to the calyx system (= indication of a chronic pyelonephritis),

- renal cysts or polycystic kidneys,

- renal tumors,

- encapsulated hematomas.

In some cases (renal tumors, polycystic kidneys, hematomas), a computed tomography (CT) should be included as an additional examination.

13.1.4.3 Renal biopsy

If the laboratory tests indicate the presence of a primary glomerulonephritis as the cause of hypertension, a renal biopsy should be considered. With regard to the indication for renal biopsy it is recommended that nephrology textbooks be consulted.

13.1.4.4 Primary disease

In cases of a multisystem disease with renal involvement, a newly occurring hypertension must be pathogenetically attributed to the primary disease.

Summary (Sections 13.1.3 and 13.1.4)

- Renoparenchymal hypertension can be the result of a unilateral or bilateral kidney disease.

- The most frequent bilateral renal diseases which are accompanied by an arterial hypertension are the glomerulonephrites.

- Hypertension resulting from unilateral disease of the renal parenchyma should be considered as potentially curable.

- A renal genesis of what was originally diagnosed as hypertension is to be assumed if simultaneously a pathological urinalysis and impaired renal function are present.

- Ultrasonography should be considered the most important of the imaging procedures with respect to the screening examination.

13.2 Renovascular hypertension

13.2.1 Cause and incidence

Renovascular hypertension is the most frequent curable form of hypertension. Its portion of the entire hypertensive population is estimated at 0.5%. Approximately

Table 13.2: Causes and frequency of renovascular hypertension

Causative disease	Frequency (%)
Arteriosclerosis	60−70
Fibromuscular dysplasias*	30−40
Infrequent renovascular disorders − Renal arteriovenous fistulas − Aneurysm of the renal arteries − Thrombosis of the renal arteries − Thrombosis of the renal veins	<1
Other lesions or diseases which can cause renovascular hypertension − Coarctation of the aorta − Polyarteritis nodosa − Takayasu's disease − Pheochromocytoma − Growth of metastatic tumors − Neurofibromatosis (Recklinghausen's disease) − Renal cysts − Ergotism	<1

* The various forms of fibromuscular hyperplasia are summarized in Table 13.3

two-thirds of cases are the result of arteriosclerotic changes, one-third result from fibromuscular dysplasia of the renal arteries. Other causes of renovascular hypertension (Table 13.2) are extremely rare (Figure 13.1).

While arteriosclerotic renal arterial stenoses are diagnosed for the most part in elderly male patients, the fibromuscular form is more often found in young, female individuals (Table 13.3).

Fibromuscular dysplasia can be differentiated in a detailed manner using histological criteria (Table 13.3). The most important radiological indication for the presence of a fibromuscular dysplasia is the visualization of "string-of-beads" changes (Figure 13.2), which result from the typical, alternating change between ring-shaped, stenotic and small aneurysmal segments of the diseased vessel and generally allow for easy demarcation of the arteriosclerotically changed renal arteries (Figure 34.1a).

13.2.2 Pathogenesis

Hypertension with renal artery stenosis is the result of reduced renal perfusion with subsequent activation of the renin-angiotensin system (Figure 13.3). The increased formation of Ang II causes an increase in the blood pressure via three mechanisms: 1. direct vasoconstriction with increased peripheral resistance, 2. increased release of aldosterone from the adrenal cortex with consequent sodium retention and increased intravascular volume, and 3. stimulation of the sympathetic nervous system.

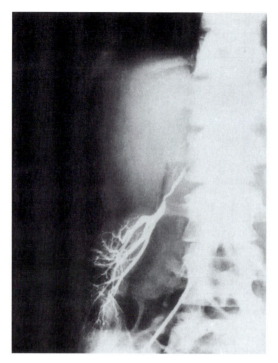

Figure 13.1: An extremely rare cause of renovascular hypertension: A right-sided, hemodynamically effective renal artery stenosis in a patient − aged 50 at the time of diagnosis − with Takayasu's disease. Normalisation of arterial hypertension through high-dosage steroid therapy. (From Stimpel M et al., Cardiology 1985; 72 (Suppl. 1): 1−9)

Table 13.3:   Histological differentiation and frequency of fibromuscular dysplasia

Localization of changes	Histology	Frequency (%)
Intima	Intimal fibrodysplasia	5−10
Media	Medial fibromuscular dysplasia	
	− medial fibroplasia	60−70
	− medial hyperplasia	5−10
	− perimedial fibroplasia	15−25
	− medial dissections	5−10
Adventitia	Periarterial fibroplasia	1

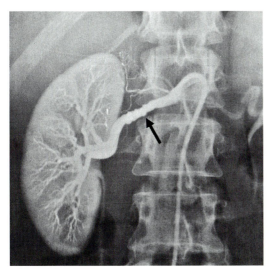

Figure 13.2: Typical 'string of beads' — arteriogram of the right renal artery with stenotic changes of medial fibroplasia (From Stimpel M et al., Cardiology 1985; 72 (Suppl. 1): 1—9)

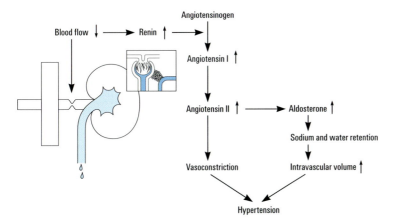

Figure 13.3: Pathogenesis of renovascular hypertension. (From Thomae U, Aktuelles Wissen Hoechst, Reihe Herz-Kreislauf, 1989: Renal failure)

Summary (Sections 13.2.1 and 13.2.2)

- Renovascular hypertension is the most frequent curable form of hypertension.

- It is possible, on the basis of histological (and radiological) criteria, to differentiate between two forms of renovascular hypertension:

- arteriosclerotic changes (about 70%) and
- fibromuscular dysplasia (about 30%)

  of the renal arteries.
- Hypertension caused by renal artery stenoses is the result of a chronically stimulated renin-angiotensin system (RAS). The cause of this RAS stimulation is the stenosis-related hypoperfusion of the kidney(s).

13.2.3   Diagnosis of renovascular hypertension

13.2.3.1 The tentative clinical diagnosis

The tentative clinical diagnosis of renovascular hypertension is performed especially in presence of the following findings: hypertension which is difficult to treat (therapy resistant), sudden deterioration of hypertension which to date had been easily controlled, hypertension and acute renal insufficiency, first diagnosis of hypertension in patients younger than 30 or older than 50 years (30–50 year-olds are, of course, not excluded from suffering from renovascular hypertension) and/ or malignant hypertension.

Abdominal bruits also serve as indications of renovascular hypertension. These are best detected by means of auscultation of the abdomen with the patient supine in a quiet setting. The intensity of arterial bruits may, however, vary, depending on the blood pressure and may decrease when the blood pressure is medicinally controlled or the bloodflow is critically reduced due to increased vascular constriction. Auscultation of the bruit is then no longer possible.

Laboratory findings, which, in conjunction with increased arterial blood pressure values may indicate a renovascular hypertension, are hypokalemia (through stimulation of the renin-angiotensin-aldosterone-system), an inexplicable increase in the renal retention values and proof of a hematuria and/or a proteinuria. It is important to keep in mind that with the differential diagnosis all findings may also be found in patients with primary hypertension. The consequence of this is that the clinical picture and laboratory-chemical investigations may allow for the suspicion of renovascular hypertension, but they do not suffice for a conclusive diagnosis.

Mann and Pickering classified clinical findings according to the probability of the presence of renovascular hypertension into three categories (mild, moderate and severe) (Table 13.4). In accordance with this classification they recommend further diagnostic procedures in patients with arterial hypertension (Figure 13.4).

13.2.3.2 Detailed examinations in suspected cases of renovascular hypertension

The objective of more detailed examinations in cases of clinically based suspected renovascular hypertension is the proof of the corresponding morphological alter-

Table 13.4: Suspected renovascular hypertension (RVH): Categorization of clinical evidence in cases of hypertension as a guideline for further diagnosis*

Degree of suspicion/probability of RVH, in %	Clinical evidence	Further diagnostic procedures
Low/<1%	Mild to moderate hypertension without clinical signs suggestive of RVH	None
Moderate/5−15%	Severe hypertension (diastolic blood pressure >120 mmHg)	Yes, non-invasive
	Hypertension refractory to standard therapy	
	Sudden onset of moderate or severe hypertension in patients <20 or >50 years old	
	Hypertension with a suggestive abdominal bruit	
	Moderate hypertension (diastolic blood pressure >105 mmHg) in smokers, in patients with known occlusive arteriosclerotic vascular diseases (cerebrovascular, coronary, peripheral vascular) or in patients with unexplained, constantly elevated serum creatinine	
	Blood pressure normalization by use of an ACE inhibitor in cases of moderate or severe hypertension (in particular in smokers or patients with newly diagnosed hypertension)	
High/>25%	Severe hypertension with progressive renal insufficiency or refractoriness to aggressive therapy (in particular in smokers or patients with occlusive arterial disease)	Yes, possibly immediately invasive
	Accelerated or malignant hypertension (retinopathy grade III or IV, see figure 7.1)	
	Hypertension with recent serum creatinine elevation, either unexplained or reversibly induced by an ACE inhibitor	
	Moderate or severe hypertension with incidentally discovered asymetry of renal size	

* modified according to Mann SJ and Pickering TG, Ann Intern Med, 1992

ation(s) of the renal artery on the one hand and its hemodynamic relevance for the genesis of the concomitant hypertension on the other hand. The diagnostic procedures for accomplishing this therefore consist of 1. imaging procedures and 2. laboratory-chemical function tests.

Imaging procedures

Ultrasonography:

By means of ultrasonography it is possible to make a reliable assessment of the size of the kidneys and of the parenchyma, so that severe ischemic damages due to stenosed or occluded renal arteries can be readily diagnosed. Ultrasonography therefore represents an easily conducted screening procedure, which − in conjunction with the physical examination and suspicious laboratory-chemical findings (see above) − may serve to solidify the preliminary diagnosis of renovascular hypertension.

Duplex Doppler ultrasonography:

The (color-coded) Doppler ultrasonography makes it possible to non-invasively determine the speed of the bloodflow in the heart and the blood vessels. The continued improvement in the resolution of Doppler ultrasonography in recent years has encouraged the application of this procedure in cases of suspected renovascular hypertension. A criterion for a narrowing in the renal artery was assessed as increased blood flow in comparison to the abdominal aorta. The level of this difference is directly proportional to the extent of the stenosis.

The currently limited importance of duplex ultrasonography for the diagnosis of renal artery stenosis is understandable, if the generally poor visualization of the renal arteries is taken into consideration (40−90% according to data in literature). Especially in cases of obesity, aortic aneurysm or superimposed intestinal gas, it is almost impossible to make a worthwhile assessment. To date, distal segments of renal arteries and side branches can hardly be adjusted ultrasonographically. It is therefore (still) not possible to recommend duplex ultrasonography as a routine diagnostic procedure in cases of suspected renovascular hypertension. This does not, however, hold true for their diagnostic value in the assessment of renal arteries of transplanted kidneys, due to the fact that these are located more superficially (Section 13.3).

Intravenous urography:

The intravenous urogram has increasingly lost importance as a routine examination in cases of suspected renovascular hypertension, in particular because the procedure serves to indicate the disease, but does not prove it. In addition, with the presence of primary hypertension, one must calculate 10−15% false-positive and about 20% false-negative results in the case of renovascular hypertension.

An intravenous urogram is still justified in patients in whom the history or laboratory parameters indicate an additional disease of the parenchyma, the renal pelvis or of the efferent urinary tract. It is however, of essential importance that the diagnostic benefit and the risk of additional damage to the parenchyma from the contrast medium be carefully considered.

Renal scintigraphy:

The advantages of radioisotope examinations consist on the one hand of avoiding intravenous contrast medium injections (which is of particular importance for patients who already have impaired renal function) and the possibility, on the other hand, of obtaining an additional functional parameter on the basis of the bilateral clearance assay. The radionuclides most frequently employed for renal scintigraphy are technetium-99 diethylenetriamine pentaacetic acid (^{99}Tc-DTPA; excretion via glomerular filtration), ^{131}I-hippuran (excretion via tubular secretion and glomerular filtration), and technetium-99-mercaptoacetyltriglycine (MAG$_3$; for the most part via tubular excretion). According to experience, the selection of the radionuclide is not an important factor for the diagnostic certainty of the method.

The essential variables, which can be derived from the time-activity curves, are:

1. The absorption of the radionuclide in the individual kidney in relation to the total renal absorption about one to two minutes after the injection (normal range: 45–55%),

2. the time which is needed to attain the maximum enhancement (peak activity) (normal range 3 to 6 minutes) and

3. the residual activity 20 to 30 minutes after injection in relation to peak activity (the normal value depends on the specific technique and must be individually determined at each examination site).

Findings which indicate the presence of a renal artery stenosis are the decrease in the relative radionuclide absorption, an increased time till the peak activity is reached and an increase in the ratio of residual activity to peak activity.

Scintigraphy combined with ACE inhibition ("ACE-inhibitor renogram"):

The diagnostic value of scintigraphy can be improved considerably by the preapplication of an ACE inhibitor. − In advanced stages of stenosis of a renal artery the perfusion pressure of the blocked kidney decreases continuously. The reactive stimulation of the RAS leads to increased formation of Ang II. By means of an Ang II-mediated constriction of the efferent arterioles, it is temporarily possible to sustain the transcapillary forces necessary for glomerular filtration and the accompanying excretory function of the hypoperfused kidney. An acute ACE inhibition cancels the constriction of the efferent arterioles and thereby causes a reduction in the glomerular filtration in the post-stenotic kidney. This decrease in the renal function can be demonstrated scintigraphically. Qualitative changes following application of the ACE inhibitor, which indicate renovascular hypertension, are a reduced absorption of the isotope in the post-stenotic kidney, a smaller and delayed peak activity and slower wash-out. A normal scintigram following ACE inhibition excludes with a high probability a hemodynamically relevant renal artery stenosis.

An improvement in the contralateral renal function can frequently be observed, because the dramatically increased Ang II in renovascular hypertension systemically decreases following the application of an ACE inhibitor. The scintigraphically detectable differences between normal and stenotic kidneys is therefore more accentuated.

The interpretation of the scintigram can therefore be the result of the comparison between affected and contralateral kidneys following the application of ACE inhibitors or as a comparison of the post-stenotic kidney before and after the ACE inhibitor application.

Captopril, given as a single oral dose of 25 to 50 mg 60 to 90 minutes before the scintigraphic examination, is most widely used. Due to the rapid onset of action the intravenous administration of enalaprilate (the active metabolite of enalapril) is recommended as an alternative.

Previous antihypertensive therapy does not influence the test results and may therefore be continued. Only treatment with ACE inhibitors should be discontinued five days in advance, so as to avoid a false-negative result due to the chronic ACE inhibition. The simultaneous application of furosemide decreases the retention of the radionuclide in the renal pelvis and therefore reduces the probability of a false-negative test result.

The renal scintigraphy in combination with ACE inhibition is the most reliable non-invasive examination for the proof or the exclusion of a hemodynamically relevant renal artery stenosis. In cases of suspected renovascular hypertension (Table 13.4) this examination offers a valuable functional test with high sensitivity and specificity for further diagnosis. The test should not, however, be applied as a universal screening procedure for hypertension.

Intravenous digital subtraction angiography:

Digital subtraction angiography (DSA) did not fulfill the expectations for the diagnosis of renovascular hypertension. The basic disadvantages of this method are the frequently poor visualization of side branches of the renal arteries and the aortic outlet due to the superimposed mesenteric vessels and the relatively high volumes of contrast media needed to improve the quality of the image, in patients who are already suffering from renal insufficiency. Furthermore, a high percentage of images which can not be evaluated have been reported for obese patients or in patients with cardiac dysfunction. In view of the fact that less burdensome and less expensive diagnostic procedures are equal to, or even better than DSA, with regard to diagnostic value, DSA should only be used in cases of suspected renovascular hypertension if a high-degree of arteriosclerotic changes in the femoral arteries and/or the abdominal aorta are present. In such cases, it is necessary to avoid the danger of causing an embolism as a result of arterial injection or an arteriotomy.

Renal arteriography:

While all of the imaging procedures described thus far can be classified as screening methods, the arteriography with a survey aortogram and selective visualization of the renal arteries represents the only certain procedure for detecting a renovascular disease. Beside the differentiation between arteriosclerotic and fibromuscular changes, this method permits a reliable morphological assessment of the peripheral side branches and the aortic outlets (if necessary by means of oblique images). It is, however, not possible to draw conclusions about the hemodynamic relevance of a detected occlusion.

Despite the almost 100% reliability of the diagnosis, the angiographic examination of the renal arteries demands a very strict indication due to the technology involved and the resultant costs and risks (arteriotomy, contrast medium application and complications resulting from the manipulation of the catheter) and the burden on the patient.

Biochemical and pharmacological tests:

Biochemical and pharmacological tests in cases of suspected renovascular hypertension serve to

1. differentiate between primary and renovascular hypertension and

2. detect hemodynamic relevance of an angiographic visualization of renal artery stenosis.

Plasma renin activity (PRA) in peripheral venous blood:

Although, according to the pathogenetic explanation renovascular hypertension is maintained by a chronically stimulated renin-angiotensin system (see above), the determination of the peripheral renin level or the plasma renin activity (PRA) have been shown to be for the most part worthless for differentiation from primary hypertension. Indeed, the PRA is on the one hand normal in 20–50% of the patients with renovascular hypertension and, on the other hand, elevated in about 15% of those with primary hypertension.

Captopril test:

The determination of the PRA in peripheral venous blood before and 60 minutes after oral application of 25 or 50 mg captopril is used to differentiate between renovascular hypertension and hypertension of a different genesis (see Figure 14.7, Section 14.3.4.2). An increase in the PRA of more than 100% of the initial value (or 400% in cases of an initial value of more than 3 ng/ml/hr) indicates a pathologically elevated renin secretion from a chronically stimulated, hyperplastic juxtaglomerular apparatus and therefore makes it possible to reliably diagnose renovascular hypertension in a high percentage of the cases. In patients without concomitant antihypertensive medication and a serum creatinine concentration of less than 1.5 mg/dL, the captopril test has been shown to have a sensitivity of 100% and a specificity of 95%.

Apparently the diagnostic reliability is, however, somewhat poorer in younger patients, in blacks and in patients with renal disorders. The test can also be impaired by previous food intake or medications which have an antihypertensive effect; antihypertensives should therefore be discontinued at least three weeks prior to the test. To avoid a position-related influence of the renin release, the patient should not change his/her body position for 30 to 60 minutes before blood is taken for the determination of the initial PRA value.

Despite this limitation, the captopril test is relatively reliable, inexpensive and can be performed on an out-patient basis. For those reasons it is well-suited as a preliminary test in cases of suspected renovascular hypertension. Section 14.3.4.2 deals with the value of this test for the diagnosis of primary aldosteronism.

Selective, bilateral determination of the PRA in the renal veins (renal vein renin ratio):

The hemodynamic relevance of an angiographically proven renal artery stenosis can be determined by means of a selective, bilateral determination of the PRA in the renal veins. The normal ratio of PRA in the intrarenal vena cava (index for the systemic PRA) is about 1.24 for the two sides. Because renin is released in the kidneys, the PRA in the renal veins is usually higher than in the vena cava.

In patients with renovascular hypertension, the circulating renin stems from the post-stenotic hypoperfused kidney while the renin secretion of the contralateral kidney is suppressed. A quotient of < 1.0 (ratio of PRA in the healthy renal veins to PRA in the vena cava or stenotic renal veins) usually is a sign of suppression of the healthy side.

With a greater than 1.5 times elevated PRA compared to the contralateral side a functional effect of the renal artery stenosis (Table 13.5) and need for interventive therapy can be assumed. Although a positive correlation between the height of the renal venous renin quotients and the degree of stenosis has been described with unilateral disease, it has not been possible to cure the hypertension in every case with elevated quotients by means of correcting the constriction. In contrast, the correction of a renal artery stenosis in patients with a quotient of < 1.5 led to a cure or clear improvement of the hypertension in one third of the cases.

An increase in the diagnostic reliability of this method has been described after the additional renin stimulation by means of salt restriction, hydralazine, nifedipine, captopril or a diuretic. Despite these measures, it is not possible to completely avoid false-positive or false-negative results.

In summary, the selective, bilateral determination of the PRA in the renal veins can be described as a complicated procedure, susceptible to disturbances. If a renal artery stenosis has been angiographically determined, other, less invasive methods with comparable or better sensitivity are preferable for determining the hemodynamic relevance of the constriction.

Table 13.5: Lateralization procedures to determine the functional relevance of renovascular lesions

Calculation from	Ratio
$\dfrac{\text{PRA (stenotic side)}}{\text{PRA (non-stenotic side)}}$	$>1.5^*$
$\dfrac{\text{PRA (non-stenotic side)}}{\text{PRA (Vena cava inferior)}}$	$<1.0^{**}$

*   Ratio suggestive of renovascular hypertension caused by the stenotic side
**   Ratio suggestive of a suppressed renin secretion on the non-stenotic side
PRA = plasma renin activity

13.2.3.3 Diagnosis of bilateral stenoses

Bilateral lesions are present in about 25−30% of the patients with renal artery stenosis. With the aid of renal scintigraphy, combined with acute ACE inhibition, it is possible to identify the functional leading side in most cases. A possible alternative is the more complicated separate, bilateral determination of the PRA in the renal venous blood.

With high-grade, bilateral renal arterial stenoses there is an advanced functional loss of both kidneys with an increase in the serum creatinine. As a result of the increasing sodium retention there is a hypertension which is characterized by an increased intravascular volume, a suppressed separate, bilateral PRA and a poor response to ACE inhibitors. Such patients are clinically ill. The application of ACE inhibitors frequently leads to a further increase in the creatinine and can lead to the suspicion of bilateral renal arterial stenoses. A single functioning kidney should be considered in the differential diagnosis, especially if the ultrasonographic findings display a remarkable difference in the size of the kidneys.

The diagnostic procedure in suspected renovascular hypertension is depicted in Figure 13.4.

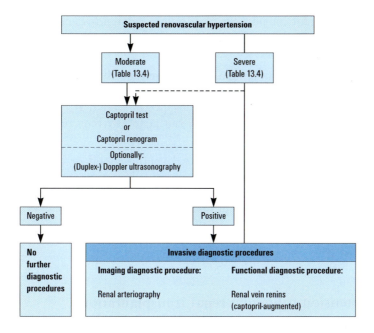

Figure 13.4: Diagnostic procedures in suspected renovascular hypertension.

Summary (Sections 13.2.3.2 and 13.2.3.3)

- Extensive biochemical or imaging diagnostic examinations for the proof or exclusion of renovascular hypertension are only justified with the corresponding clinical suspicion.

- The captopril test is suitable under out-patient conditions as a convenient, easily conducted and relatively inexpensive screening test to differentiate between renovascular hypertension and of hypertension of another genesis.

- An ultrasonographic examination should be conducted as a matter of principle in cases of suspected renovascular hypertension, because it is easy to detect an ischemic related constriction in an under-perfused kidney. Ultrasonography can, however, never serve to confirm the diagnosis, but only to substantiate.

- Duplex Doppler ultrasonography is only indicated in cases of suspected renal artery stenosis of transplanted kidneys.

- Renal scintigraphy in combination with ACE inhibition (ACE inhibitor renogram) is the most reliable non-invasive examination for the proof or exclusion of renovascular hypertension. It is indicated in appropriate cases of clinical suspicion for the purpose of differential diagnosis and in angiography for previously diagnosed stenosis for the assessment of the hemodynamic relevance.

- Arteriography is the only imaging procedure that allows for a definite morphological assessment of the entire arterial vascular supply of the kidneys. An assessment of the hemodynamic relevance of a renal artery stenosis is not possible by means of an angiography, but generally requires that a suitable function test be performed (see above).

- Determination of the PRA in peripheral venous blood or bilaterally in the renal veins, intravenous urogram and digital subtraction angiography (DSA) are examinations for the diagnosis of renovascular hypertension which nowadays are only justified in exceptional cases.

13.3 Hypertension following renal transplantation (post-transplant hypertension)

About half (13−89% in literature) of all kidney transplant patients develop arterial hypertension.

Pathogenetically post-transplant hypertension can be categorized in the following manner:

1. Host/recipient-related pathomechanisms,

2. transplant-related pathomechanisms and

3. immunosuppressive-related pathomechanisms.

It is frequently difficult to etiologically categorize hypertension following renal transplantation, because in most cases it is not possible to precisely differentiate the various causes.

The following constellation of findings does, however, allow for conclusions to be drawn about the genesis and therapeutic consequences of such hypertension:

1. A newly occurring bruit over the transplanted kidney in conjunction with a sudden increase in the blood pressure or an acute deterioration of previously existing hypertension as well as an increase in the creatinine following the application of ACE inhibitors lead to the suspicion of a stenosis of the renal artery of the transplanted kidney. Duplex Doppler ultrasonography is the recommended imaging method for screening, because it is a non-invasive, easily repeatable procedure which does not burden the patient. The high diagnostic value of this method is due to the superficial location of the transplanted kidney. A definitive morphological assessment and localization of the stenosis can only be obtained by means of selective angiography of the arteries of the transplanted kidney.

   Examination methods of the functional relevance of an angiographically detected stenosis by means of the captopril test or renal scintigram are of less importance with post-transplant hypertension. With higher grade stenoses, an angioplastic or surgical revascularization should be performed, if only for reasons of protecting the organs.

2. Elevated plasma concentration of cyclosporine with simultaneous deterioration of the renal function indicate a cyclosporine-induced hypertension (see Section 17.5)

3. The importance of long-term, immunosuppressive therapy with corticosteroids for the genesis of the post-transplant hypertension is somewhat controversial, but should not be ignored.

4. Hypertensive blood pressure values, increasing renal insufficiency, normal or slightly constricted renal artery stenosis and normal cyclosporine concentrations in plasma lead to the suspicion of a transplant rejection. It is the most frequent cause of post-transplant hypertension and is diagnostically determined by means of a renal biopsy.

5. If no changes in the constellation of findings of the transplanted kidney mentioned can be detected, despite the renal biopsy which would serve to explain the development of the hypertension, the native kidney must be assumed to be the pathogenetic cause.

The management of post-transplant hypertension is summarized in Figure 13.5.

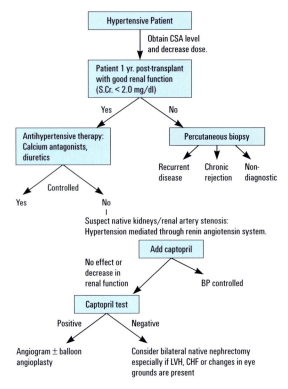

Figure 13.5: Management of post-transplant hypertension.
Abbreviations: CSA = cyclosporine A; S.Cr. = serum creatinine; BP = blood pressure; LVH = left
ventricular hypertrophy; CHF = congestive heart failure
(Adapted from Laskow et Curtis JJ, Am J Hypertens 1990; 3: 721–725).

Summary (Section 13.3)

- Hypertension following kidney transplantation develops in about 50% of patients.

- The pathogenesis of post-transplant hypertension is generally multifactorial.

- As a result of various therapeutic consequences, a distinction should be made
  in the differential diagnosis between

    - renovascular hypertension (stenosis of the transplant artery),

    - cyclosporine-induced hypertension,

    - transplant-related hypertension and

    - hypertension induced by the native kidney.

Literature (Chapter 13)

Renoparenchymal hypertension (Section 13.1)

Beaman M, Adu D. Mesangial IgA nephropathy: an autimmune cause of hypertension? J Hum Hypertens 1988; 2: 139−141.

Brown MA, Whitworth JA. Hypertension in human renal disease. J Hypertens 1992; 10: 701−712.

Grabensee B, Bach D, Heering P, Ivens K. Diagnostik und Verlauf der primären Glomerulonephritiden. Internist 1989; 30: 148−158.

Jacobson SH, Eklöf O, Eriksson CG, Lins LE, Tidgren B, Winberg J. Development of hypertension and uraemia after pyelonephritis in childhood: 27 year follow up. Br Med J 1989; 299: 703−706.

Jacobson HR. Chronic renal failure: pathophysiology. Lancet 1991; 338: 419−423.

Johnston PA, Davison AM. Hypertension in adults with idiopathic glomerulonephritis and normal serum creatinine. A report from the MRC Glomerulonephritis Registry. Nephrol Dial Transplant 1993; 8: 20−24.

Klahr S. Chronic renal failure: management. Lancet 1991; 338: 423−427.

Novick AC, Gephardt G, Guz B, Steinmuller D, Tubbs RR. Long-term follow-up after partial removal of a solitary kidney. N Engl J Med 1991; 325: 1058−1062.

Orofino L, Quereda C, Lamas S, Orte L, Gonzalo A, Mampaso F, Ortuno J. Hypertension in primary chronic glomerulonephritis: analysis of 288 biopsied patients. Nephron 1987; 45: 22−26.

Rambausek M, Rhein C, Waldherr R, Goetz R, Heidland A, Ritz E. Hypertension in chronic idiopathic glomerulonephritis: analysis of 311 biopsied patients. Eur J Clin Invest 1989; 19: 176−180.

Wesson LG. Unilateral renal disease and hypertension. Nephron 1982; 31: 1−7.

Zucchelli P, Zuccala A, Mancini E. Hypertension in primary glomerulonephritis without renal insufficiency. Nephrol Dial Transplant 1989; 4: 605−610.

Renovascular hypertension (Section 13.2)

Davidson R, Wilcox CS. Diagnostic usefulness of renal scanning after angiotensin converting enzyme inhibitors. Hypertension 1991; 18: 299−303.

Davidson RA, Wilcox CS. Newer tests for the diagnosis of renovascular disease. JAMA 1992; 268: 3353−3358.

Degenhardt S, Friedrich H, Wambach G, Fischer JH, Gross-Fengels W, Linden A, Neufang KFR, Hummerich W. Der Stellenwert des Captopriltests in der Hypertoniediagnostik. Klin Wochenschr 1989; 67: 1077−1084.

Mann SJ, Pickering TG. Detection of renovascular hypertension. State of the art: 1992. Ann Intern Med 1992; 117: 845−853.

Müller FB, Sealey JE, Case D'B, Atlas SA, Pickering TG, Pecker MS, Preibisz JJ, Laragh JH. The captopril test for identifying renovascular disease in hypertensive patients. Am· J Med 1986; 80: 633−644.

Rimmer JM, Gennari FJ. Atherosclerotic renovascular disease and progressive renal failure. Ann Intern Med 1993; 118: 712−719.

Semple PF, Dominiczak AF. Detection and treatment of renovascular disease: 40 years on. J Hypertens 1994; 12: 729−734.

Sheps SG, Blaufox MD, Nally JV, Textor SC. Radionuclide scintirenography in the evaluation of patients with hypertension. JACC 1993; 21: 838−839.

Stimpel M, Groth H, Greminger P, Lüscher TF, Vetter H, Vetter W. The spectrum of renovascular hypertension. Cardiology 1985; 72 (suppl.1): 1−9.

Ramsay LE, Waller PC. Blood pressure response to percutaneous transluminal angioplasty for renovascular hypertension: an overview of published series. Br Med J 1990; 300: 569−572.

Hypertension after kidney transplantation/Posttransplant hypertension (Section 13.3)

Laskow DA, Curtis JJ. Post-transplant hypertension. Am J Hypertens 1990; 3: 721−725.

Luke RG. Hypertension in renal transplant recipients. Kidney Int 1987; 31: 1024−1037.

Maia CR, Bittar AE, Goldani JC, Keitel E, Deboni LM, Garcia VD. Doppler ultrasonography for the detection of renal artery stenosis in transplanted kidneys. Hypertension 1992; 19 (suppl II): II-207-II-209.

Olmer M, Noordally R, Berland Y, Casanova P, Coulange C, Rampal M. Hypertension in renal transplantation. Kidney Int 1988; 34 (suppl 25): S-129−S-132.

Raman GV. Post transplant hypertension. J Hum Hypertens 1991; 5: 1−6.

Waltzer WC, Turner S, Frohnert P, Rapaport FT. Etiology and pathogenesis of hypertension following renal transplantation. Nephron 1986; 42: 102−109.

14 Endocrine hypertension

Endocrine hypertension is subdivided into the following forms:

- Pheochromocytoma (Section 14.1),
- Primary mineralocorticoidism (Section 14.2),
    - Primary aldosteronism (Section 14.3),
    - DOC tumors (Section 14.4),
    - Adrenogenital syndromes/congenital adrenal hyperplasia (Section 14.5),
- Glucocorticoidism: Cushing's syndrome (Section 14.6),
- Primary hyperreninism (Section 14.7),
- Acromegaly (Section 14.8),
- Hyperparathyroidism (Section 14.9),
- Endothelin-producing tumors (Section 14.10),
- Hyper- and hypothyroidism (Section 14.11).

The portion of endocrine hypertension in secondary hypertension amounts to about 15%; the frequency of endocrine hypertension in the total population of patients with hypertension is therefore about 0.1−0.2%.

Summary (Chapter 14)

Endocrine hypertension is found in about 0.1−0.2% of all patients with hypertension; this accounts for approximately 15% of the secondary forms of hypertension.

14.1 Pheochromocytoma

14.1.1 Pathogenesis/localization

Pheochromocytomas are catecholamine-producing tumors of the neuroectodermal tissue which are localized in the adrenal medulla in 85% of all cases and in 15% extraadrenally − primarily in the area of the abdominal and thoracic sympathetic trunk. Localizations in the heart, bladder, prostate, pancreas or ovaries are extremely rare. Pheochromocytomas are generally benign tumors, however, 10% do show malignancy. A histological differentiation between benign and malignant pheochromocytomas is not possible with certainty, so the diagnosis of a malignant process requires proof of metastasis or the penetration into blood vessels or neighboring tissue structure. Two-thirds of the tumors secrete epinephrine and norepinephrine, and one-third almost exclusively norepinephrine. An increased secretion of dopamine is observed more commonly in malignant tumors. According to our experience, a relationship between the level of catecholamine secretion and the size of the tumors does not exist.

Pheochromocytomas generally exist alone. Bilateral adrenal or multiple extraadrenal tumors are very seldom seen and when present show an above-average frequency of familial occurrence. The increased occurrence of familial pheochromocytomas with other organ diseases must be included in the diagnostic concept (Table 14.1).

Table 14.1:   Diseases frequently associated with a pheochromocytoma

• Multiple endocrine neoplasia (MEN):	
− MEN type 2A (2):	
Medullary thyroid carcinoma	(>90%)
(Often bilateral) pheochromocytoma	(80−90%)
Hyperplasia of the parathyroids	(ca. 60%)
− MEN type 2B (3):	
Medullary thyroid carcinoma	(>90%)
(Often bilateral) pheochromocytoma	(80−90%)
Hyperplasia of the parathyroids	(rare)
Alimentary tract ganglioneuromatosis	(up to 100%)
Marfanoid habitus	(?)
• Neurofibromatosis (von Recklinghausen's disease)	
• Von Hippel-Lindau's disease (Angiomatosis retinae et cerebri)	
• Tuberous sclerosis	
• Sturge-Weber disease	
• Cholelithiasis	

Summary (Section 14.1.1)

Pheochromocytomas

• are infrequent,
• 85% are located in the adrenal medulla and 15% extraadrenally,
• are usually benign, however, 5−10% are cases of malignant tumors,
• are solitary in more than 90% of all cases,
• show a familial pattern of occurrence, and
• are occasionally associated with other organ diseases.

14.1.2   Diagnosis of a pheochromocytoma

14.1.2.1 Clinical symptoms

The tentative diagnosis of a pheochromocytoma represents a frequent reason for patient transferral to specialized hypertension outpatient clinics. The suspicion of this infrequent disease is founded, in most cases, on the observation of repeatedly occurring hypertensive crises.

The clinical symptoms of this disease — which is often associated with paroxysmal and/or persistent hypertension — are, however, rather non-specific (Table 14.2) and manifest varied levels of intensity. They are therefore often misleading. Sweating, headaches, tachycardia or other ambiguous symptoms can either occur "explosively", may be essentially lacking or may be tolerated by the patient as being not particularly irritating. It thus becomes understandable that pheochromocytomas are frequently overlooked while the patient is alive and not infrequently first diagnosed during the autopsy. In the most optimistic scenario, asymptomatic pheochromocytomas are incidentally discovered during a routine examination or upon the occurrence of tumor-related symptoms of repression (flank pain, upper abdominal pain, feeling of fullness). Where the "classic" symptoms are missing, pheochromocytomas are often mistaken for hormonally inactive tumors ("incidentalomas"). Therefore, for every unclear tumor in the adrenal region or the sympathetic trunk, the necessity arises for a careful endocrinological clarification such as is done in cases of malignant hypertension or hypertension poorly controlled with conventional anti-hypertensives. In addition, hypertensive crises during anesthesia administration, during an operation, as a reaction to a TRH-test (thyrotropin-releasing hormone) or as the result of abrupt physical movement require exclusion or proof of the existence of a pheochromocytoma (Table 14.3). One third of the patients with a pheochromocytoma show catecholamine-related hyperglycemia. In rare cases, the acute decompensation of a catecholamine-induced cardiomyopathy leads to the diagnosis of a pheochromocytoma.

Table 14.2:   Frequency of clinical symptoms and signs in patients with pheochromocytoma

Symptoms	(%)
Hypertension	>90
− sustained	60
− sustained plus paroxysms	50
− intermittent	30 (?)
Headache	80
Orthostatic dysregulation, hypotension	60
Sweating	65
Palpitations, tachycardia	60
Nervousness, anxiety	45
Pallor	45
Tremor	35
Abdominal / flank pain	15
Visual disturbances	15

Table 14.3: Clinical findings requiring additional diagnostic procedures to exclude or confirm the presence of a pheochromocytoma

Clinical finding	Probability to diagnose a pheochromocytoma (%)
New discovered hypertension	<2
Therapy resistant hypertension	<2
Neurofibromatosis Recklinghausen	<5
Repeated hypertensive crises	5–10
Clinical signs and symptoms suggestive of a pheochromocytoma (see Table 14.2)	5–10
Incidentaloma	30
Angiomatosis retinae et cerebri (von Hippel-Lindau)	10–30
Multiple endocrine neoplasia (MEN), type 2A (Sipple's syndrome) and 2B	40–75
Medullary carcinoma of the thyroid	(as with MEN 2A + 2B)

14.1.2.2 Biochemical tests in the diagnosis of pheochromocytoma

Due to this varied manifestation picture, it is understandable that the diagnosis of a pheochromocytoma can never be made solely on the basis of clinical parameters. For every case, the diagnosis requires biochemical proof of a pathologically-increased cathecholamine production. While the physiological catecholamine secretion is under the control of the central nervous system and is stimulated according to the momentary requirements, the synthesis, storage and secretion of the hormones endogenous to the tumor are not subject to a regulated order in the physiological sense. This autonomy causes often strongly fluctuating catecholamine levels in the plasma and must be taken into account in the evaluation of normal or only moderately increased concentrations.

Catecholamines are metabolized partially in the tumor itself or in the liver and excreted through the kidneys in the urine, commonly in the form of vanillylmandelic acid, less-commonly as methylated intermediates (metanephrine) or directly as free catecholamine (Figure 14.1).

Urinary catecholamines:

The measurement of free catecholamines and or the metabolites mentioned above in the 24-hour urine belongs to the standard diagnostic procedure upon the clinical suspicion of a pheochromocytoma. The requirement for an exact measurement is the complete collection of the urine over 24-hours. For ca. 95% of the patients with a pheochromocytoma, the measurement of free catecholamines in the 24-hour urine (preferably by means of high-pressure liquid chromatography (HPLC) followed by chemical electro-detection) allows an exact diagnosis to be made. Moderately increased values (Table 14.4) are, however, generally worthless for differential diagnosis, because they are often also detectable in primary hypertension (Figure 14.2).

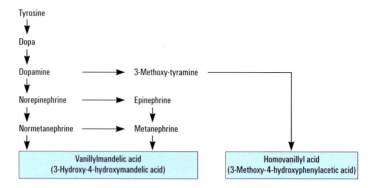

Figure 14.1: Catecholamine metabolism

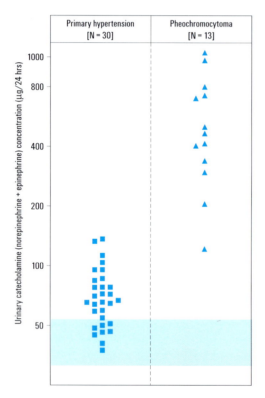

Figure 14.2: Urinary catecholamines (norepinephrine and epinephrine, µg/24 hours) in patients with primary hypertension and pheochromocytoma: It should be noted that among the primary hypertensives with recurring hypertensive crises tested here, more than 60 % display urinary catecholamine concentrations above the normal range (shaded area). (From Stimpel M et al., Dtsch med Wschr 1988; 113: 130−134)

Table 14.4: Normal and abnormal ranges of plasma and urinary catecholamine concentrations

Determination in	Type of catecholamine	Norm	Borderline*	Pheochromocytoma
Plasma	Epinephrine + norepinephrine (ng/l)	<500	500−2000	>2000
Urine	Epinephrine + norepinephrine (µg/24 hr)	<50	51−200	>200
	Vanillylmandelic acid (mg/24 hr)	2−6	7−15	>15
	Total metanephrines (mg/24 hr)	<0.5	0.5−2.5	>2.5

* Borderline catecholamine concentrations necessitate repeated determinations or an expansion of diagnostic procedures (see also Figure 14.6)

Plasma catecholamines:

The measurement of catecholamines in plasma offers an additional possibility for detecting a pathologically increased catecholamines production. However, this examination only makes sense if the blood is extracted via an intravenous cannula which was inserted at least 30 minutes before and if the patient can be placed in a secluded room ca. 30 to 60 minutes before the blood sample is taken. If these − admittedly optimal − conditions can not be met, we recommend that this investigation not be performed, because, on the one hand, false-positive results are common and, on the other hand, as a result, costs are incurred without diagnostic benefit. An "exceptional indication" for blood extraction for the measurement of plasma catecholamines without these preparations being made beforehand is a hypertensive crisis.

14.1.2.3 Suppression tests

If measurements of catecholamines do not lead to conclusive results, a suppression test with clonidine may be recommended. Because the physiological, but not the autonomous catecholamine secretion can be suppressed with clonidine, the comparison of the catecholamine concentrations in the urine or the plasma before and after clonidine administration allows for differential diagnostic conclusions about the underlying disease.

The clonidine-suppression test with the measurement of plasma catecholamines:

The oral clonidine-suppression test with the pre- and post-measurement of the plasma-catecholamines is performed on patients in a supine position. After the administration of 0.15 to 0.3 mg clonidine orally, venous blood is extracted for plasma catecholamine measurements at hourly or half-hourly intervals over a period of three hours.

The diagnostic accuracy of the test is the topic of some discussion. In our own investigations, no increased diagnostic benefit was found in comparison to repeated catecholamine measurement in the urine. While tumors with excessive catecholamine secretion could be clearly identified, this test did not make possible a diagnostic differentiation from primary hypertension in (postoperatively verified) pheochromocytomas with low catecholamine secretion.

We therefore only recommend the clonidine-test with catecholamine measurement in the plasma in patients for whom the reliability of the urine collection is not assured (incontinent patients, children) or not possible (patients with end-stage renal disease). In any event, this function test should only be performed in specialized out-patient clinics or under in-patient conditions, due to the amount of time and financial cost involved.

The clonidine-suppression test with the measurement of catecholamines in the night urine ("overnight" clonidine-suppression test):

An easily performed variation of the suppression test described above is the measurement of the catecholamine concentration in the night urine after the administration of 0.15 to 0.3 mg clonidine (collection period from 9 p.m. to 7 a.m., bed

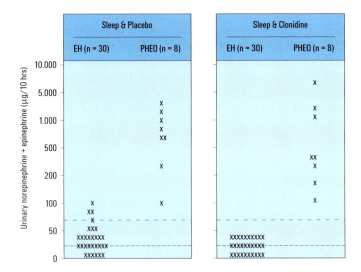

Figure 14.3: Urinary catecholamines after overnight bed rest (9 p.m. to 7 a.m.) in patients with primary hypertension (EH) with recurrent episodes of blood pressure exacerbations ("pseudo-pheochromocytoma") and in patients with (post-operatively) confirmed pheochromocytoma (PHEO).

Left side: Sleep alone does not fully suppress catecholamine secretion in all patients with primary hypertension

Right side: Catecholamines are fully suppressed in primary hypertensives after administration of clonidine prior to bed rest, thus allowing to clearly differentiate primary hypertension from pheochromocytoma with non-suppressible catecholamine secretion.
(From Stimpel M et al., Hypertension 1993; 21: 131)

rest). Due to nightly rest, a significant reduction in catecholamine secretion is expected in normal subjects or patients with primary hypertension. After the evening administration of clonidine, this reduction is accentuated or fully suppressed (Figure 14.3).

If a pheochromocytoma is present, only the physiological, but not tumor-related autonomous catecholamine secretion is suppressed. Thus, despite sleep and clonidine administration, elevated catecholamine concentrations are expected for secreting pheochromocytomas (Figure 14.3). Because this test is simple and can be performed without great cost and effort, it offers an alternative standard diagnostic procedure to the usual catecholamine measurement in the 24-hour urine for hospitalized patients.

Even though no false-negative test results have been published to date, it must be assumed that this function test is also not capable of biochemically differentiating pheochromocytomas with a low level of hormonal activity or hormonally-inactive pheochromocytomas from primary hypertension in a reliable fashion.

14.1.2.4 Stimulation tests

Given the availability of other, diagnostically more accurate methods of detection, provocation tests with histamine or tyramine are today obsolete due to their risk for patients.

In the extremely rare case of a strong suspicion of pheochromocytoma despite normotensive blood pressure values and normal plasma and urine catecholamines, the performance of a glucagon test can be considered, provided intensive medical monitoring is guaranteed.

The (intravenous) administration of glucagon (0.1 to 1.0 mg) leads to an (often massive) increase in blood pressure in patients with pheochromocytoma and to a more than three-fold increase in the release of catecholamines. The previous administration of an alpha-adrenergic receptor blocker or a calcium antagonist should prevent the elevation of the blood pressure without, however, preventing the diagnostically important increase in catecholamines in patients with pheochromocytoma.

14.1.2.5 Non-specific laboratory results with pheochromocytoma

The metabolic and hormonal changes (reduced glucose tolerance, lactate acidosis, secondary aldosteronism), which are often detectable in patients with pheochromocytoma and which should be interpreted as the result of an increased catecholamine release, are only of slight differential diagnostic value.

14.1.2.6 Localization diagnostic procedures

Localization diagnostic procedures in clinically and biochemically proven pheochromocytoma often prove to be equally as difficult as the biochemical proof of a pathognomically increased catecholamine production in clinically asymptomatic pheochromocytoma.

Non-invasive procedures:

While adrenal tumors with a diameter of more than two centimeters can generally be detected without difficulty using ultrasonography, computed tomography (CT; Figure 14.4) or magnetic resonance imaging (MRI), small or extraadrenal tumors escape detection relatively frequently when using these localization procedures.

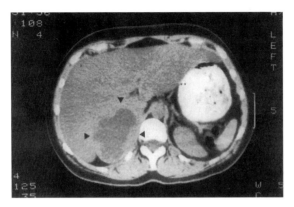

Figure 14.4: Computed tomography of an approximately 6 × 9 cm-large, post-operatively confirmed benign pheochromocytoma of the right adrenal gland in a female patient with sustained hypertension (ca. 180/110 mmHg), aged 39 at the time of diagnosis. Urinary catecholamine (epinephrine + norepinephrine) levels were between 625 and 912 μg/24 hours (normal range: ≤ 55 μg/24 hours).

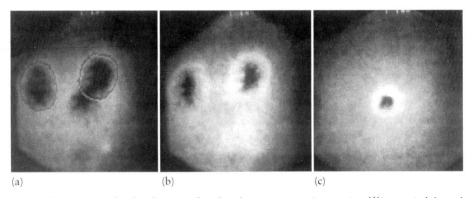

(a)   (b)   (c)

Figure 14.5: Scintigraphic localisation of a pheochromocytoma: Scan, using ^{131}I-meta-iodobenzylguanidine (^{131}I-MIBG), of a 53-year-old male patient with post-operatively confirmed left-sided pheochromocytoma. Over the preceding two years, the patient had experienced recurring headaches, outbreaks of sweat, tachycardia, and chronic arterial hypertension with intermittent hypertensive crises.

(a) Scintigraphic localisation of the pheochromocytoma 72 hours post injection with activity enrichment in projection on the left adrenal gland.
(b) Tagging of the kidneys with [99m]-Tc-DMSA.
(c) Computer-assisted summation of the two static images (a) + (b) with ^{131}I-MIBG and ^{99m}Tc-DMSA in an analogous position of the patient: tagging of the kidneys with the help of an ROI (region of interest). The activity enrichment in (a) projects itself on the left-cranial kidney pole and can be allocated to the adrenal gland.

(Courtesy of Dr. Beate Kozak, Bonn, Germany)

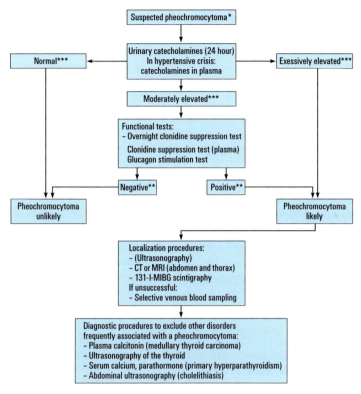

Figure 14.6: Diagnostic procedures in suspected pheochromocytoma

*   See Tables 14.2 and 14.3

**   Clonidine suppression test (urine; "overnight clonidine suppression test"):
   Positive: No or minimal suppression of catecholamines in urine collected from 9 p.m. to 7 a.m.
   Negative: Largely or thoroughly suppressed catecholamines in overnight urine (collected from 9
                      p.m. to 7 a.m.)
   Less recommended:
   Clonidine suppression test (plasma):
   Positive: No significant reduction of plasma norepinephrine and epinephrine
   Negative: Decrease of plasma norephinephrine and epinephrine from (elevated) base-line levels
                      to normal
   Not recommended (for rare exceptions, see text):
   Glucagon stimulation test:
   Positive: 2–3-fold increase of plasma catecholamines from base-line
   Negative: No significant increase of plasma catecholamines

***   See Table 14.4

The performance of scintigraphy with ^{131}I-metaiodobenzylguanidine (after previously conducted "thyroid gland blockage" via sodium perchlorate) is recommended as an additional investigation. Even where pheochromocytomas have already been localized with imaging procedures (CT, MRI), this investigation should be performed additionally to exclude the existence of additional catecholamine - producing tumors (Figure 14.5).

Invasive procedures:

The selective sampling of blood from the vena cava and its side branches for measurements of catecholamines is certainly the most accurate − though invasive − localization procedure. In this procedure the site of the tumor is narrowed in on and localized based on the concentration differences between the junction with the tumor vein and the other extraction sites. Due to the high diagnostic accuracy of the non-invasive imaging techniques now available, selective venous blood sampling to measure catecholamine plasma levels has become outdated; because of it's higher risk for the patient it is only indicated in those extremely rare cases, where non-invasive localization procedures have failed.

14.1.2.7 Obligatory supplemental examinations for proven pheochromocytoma

Pheochromocytomas are sometimes associated with other organ diseases (Table 14.1). Every confirmed diagnosis of a pheochromocytoma therefore requires the exclusion or proof of these diseases. Special consideration should be given to the possibility of a multiple endocrine neoplasia with the frequent combination variation of a medullary thyroid carcinoma and (or) a parathyroid tumor (Table 14.1). Ultrasonography of the thyroid gland and measurement of calcitonin (if necessary, after pentagastrin-stimulation), serum calcium and parathyroid hormone thus represent obligatory supplemental examinations.

The diagnostic procedure in suspected pheochromocytoma is depicted in Figure 14.6.

Summary (Section 14.1.2)

- The clinical symptoms of pheochromocytoma are nonspecific: recurrent hypertensive crises with acute cardiac decompensation have been described, as have fully symptom-free courses.

- The tentative clinical diagnosis of a pheochromocytoma always requires the biochemical proof of a pathologically-increased catecholamine production.

- The measurement of free catecholamines in the urine after a 24-hour collection period is a simple and reliable laboratory test for the biochemical proof of a pheochromocytoma, which can be effectively initiated in out-patient clinics.

- Repeatedly measured, moderately elevated catecholamines represent a very difficult diagnostic 'gray area'. In such cases, a supplemental suppression test with clonidine can be performed.
- Tumors with a diameter of more than two centimeters can frequently be detected with ultrasonography.
- Computed tomography (CT), magnetic resonance imaging (MRI) and ^{131}I-MIBG scintigraphy are the most reliable localization procedures and should be performed whenever biochemical proof or justified suspicion of the presence of a pheochromocytoma exists, in order to exclude the existence of additional tumors.
- The confirmed diagnosis of a pheochromocytoma requires the exclusion or proof of the diseases frequently associated with pheochromocytoma. Because multiple endocrine neoplasias are of particular importance, ultrasonography of the thyroid gland and measurement of calcitonin, serum calcium and parathyroid hormone represent obligatory supplemental examinations.

14.2 Primary mineralocorticoidism

The term "primary mineralocorticoidism" encompasses endocrine disorders associated with arterial hypertension due to an endogenous overproduction of aldosterone or mineralocorticoid-like precursors of the steroid biosynthesis. The following diseases can be included here:

- Primary aldosteronism (Section 14.3),
- DOC-(deoxycorticosterone- and other mineralocorticoid-like precursors of the steroid biosynthesis secreting) tumors (Section 14.4),
- Adrenogenital syndromes/congenital adrenal hyperplasia (Section 14.5).

The common characteristic of mineralocorticoid-related hypertension is the simultaneous appearance of a more or less severe hypokalemia.

14.3 Primary aldosteronism

Primary aldosteronism is characterized by an autonomous overproduction of aldosterone. This should be differentiated from secondary aldosteronism, which is the consequence of an increased, mostly reactive (secondary) renin secretion. Primary reninism as the cause of secondary aldosteronism is a rarity.

The following disorders, which are associated with hypertension and secondary aldosteronism, are discussed in other sections:

- Secondary aldosteronism with primary reninism:
  - Renin-secreting tumors (Section 14.8).
- Secondary aldosteronism with "secondary reninism":
  - primary hypertension treated with diuretics (Section 7.4),
  - oral contraceptive-induced hypertension (Section 16.1),
  - renoparenchymal hypertension (some forms) (Section 13.1),
  - renovascular hypertension (Section 13.2),
  - pheochromocytoma (Section 14.1).

14.3.1 Differentiation of primary aldosteronism

The common characteristic of the etiologically heterogeneous forms of primary aldosteronism is the renin-independent overproduction of the adrenocortical hormone aldosterone, which is formed in the zona glomerulosa, with resultant hypertension, hypokalemia, hyporeninemia and metabolic alkalosis.

While adrenal autonomy of the pathological aldosterone production is considered certain in adrenocortical adenoma (the so-called Conn's syndrome; aldosterone-producing adenoma, APA), adrenocortical carcinoma and primary hyperplasia of the adrenal cortex (primary adrenal hyperplasia, PAH), a primary extraadrenal disorder is strongly suspected in idiopathic bilateral adrenal hyperplasia (idiopathic hyperaldosteronism, IHA) and in dexamethasone-suppressible hyperaldosteronism (DSH). This assumption is based on the detection of a circulating factor in the blood of patients with IHA which is − at least in animal experiments − aldosterone-stimulating as well as on the obvious ACTH-dependency of the aldosterone overproduction in DSH. A further indication of the secondary genesis of this form of aldosterone excess is the experience that the removal of the adrenal gland does not result in normotension. This leads to the conclusion that the previously valid classification of hyperaldosteronism according to pathogenic criteria may possibly require revision. However, because the postulated pathomechanism, which differs from other forms, is still not considered confirmed or fully explained, we currently still favor the previous classification and consider IHA and DSH as variations of primary aldosteronism.

14.3.2 Pathogenesis

The acute hypertensive effect of aldosterone is primarily caused by an initial increase in intravascular volume. The pathogenetic cause is an (aldosterone-related) increased renal reabsorption of sodium, which takes place in the distal tubules in the exchange of hydrogen and potassium. The cause of hypertension in chronic aldosterone overproduction has still not been fully explained, as a persistent increase in extracellular volume is only rarely observed in primary aldosteronism. A direct vasoconstrictive aldosterone effect and an interference of this hormone with a putative hypothalamic cardiovascular regulation center must currently still be viewed as speculative causes of the chronic elevation of blood pressure.

The loss of potassium in primary aldosteronism is slowly progressive. In contrast, the sodium retention is generally of a passing nature, so that a pronounced hypernatremia is rare in patients with primary aldosteronism. Though an elevated plasma level of atrial natriuretic peptide (ANP) is observed in both patients with primary aldosteronism and in drug-induced mineralocorticoidism, the previously known mechanism of action of this hormone, which was first discovered in 1980 and which is secreted by myocardial cells of the atria, can not fully explain the cause of this sodium escape phenomenon.

14.3.3 Clinical symptoms

The clinical symptoms of primary aldosteronism are nonspecific and thus of only very limited value in differential diagnosis. The various symptoms are to be pathologically interpreted as results of the aldosterone overproduction. The relative hyperpolarization of striated (muscle weakness), smooth (constipation) and cardiac musculature (ECG changes: ST-segment depression, T-wave flattening, T and U wave fusion) caused by the progressive loss of potassium as well as hypertension (headaches, visual impairment) may represent the most important causal factors (see also Table 14.5).

Table 14.5:   Clinical signs and symptoms in patients with primary aldosteronism

Symptoms	Frequency (%)
Hypertension	100
Hypokalemia	90
ECG-abnormalities	80
Muscle weakness	80
Polyuria	70
Headache	65
Polydipsia	45
Paresthesia	25
Visual disturbances	20
Tiredness	20
Intermittent paralytic symptoms	20
Intermittent tetany	20
Myalgia	15

Summary (Sections 14.3.1 to 14.3.3)

- The term "primary aldosteronism" can be classified into pathogenetically differing forms:

  - aldosterone-producing adrenocortical adenoma (Conn's syndrome),
  - adrenocortical carcinoma,

- primary hyperplasia of the adrenal cortex (primary adrenal hyperplasia),
- idiopathic bilateral hyperplasia of the adrenal cortex (idiopathic hyperaldosteronism) and
- dexamethasone-suppressible hyperaldosteronism.
- The classic clinical features of primary aldosteronism are hypertension, hypokalemia, hyporeninemia and metabolic alkalosis.
- The loss of potassium in primary aldosteronism is slowly progressive.
- Hypernatremia and increased intravascular volume are infrequent in chronic primary aldosteronism.
- The clinical symptoms of primary aldosteronism are nonspecific and of little use in differential diagnosis.

14.3.4   The diagnosis of primary aldosteronism

14.3.4.1 Tentative and differential diagnosis

The most common cause of hypokalemic hypertension may well be primary hypertension treated with diuretics. However, the joint appearance of hypertension and hypokalemia justifies the tentative diagnosis of a primary aldosteronism, especially when potassium losses via the gastrointestinal tract (diarrhea, laxative abuse, frequent vomiting) or the intake of diuretics can be excluded. The presence of primary aldosteronism should also be considered in patients with hypertension, which is difficult to control with medications or is therapy resistant. Normokalemia does not automatically exclude autonomous aldosterone production: approximately 20% of all patients with primary aldosteronism show potassium concentrations in the plasma that first drop into the hypokalemic category after 3 days of salt loading. Furthermore, an autonomous aldosterone production is to be taken into differential diagnostic consideration in hypertensive patients with incidentally discovered (via ultrasonography, computed tomography or magnetic resonance imaging) unilateral or bilateral adrenal masses (so-called incidentalomas).

14.3.4.2 Laboratory-chemical diagnosis of primary aldosteronism

Testing conditions:

The regulation of the renin-angiotensin-aldosterone system is subject to a number of influencing parameters (Table 14.6), which must be taken into account in the determining the findings. − A prerequisite for the reliable measurement of the required laboratory parameters is optimal testing conditions: withdrawal of any antihypertensive therapy − if possible 14 days before the investigation, balanced diet, available time and space for keeping the patient, monitoring possibility for

Table 14.6: Conditions, drugs and hormones affecting renin secretion

	Renin increased	Renin decreased
Posture:		
• Supine		+
• Standing	+	
Antihypertensive drugs:		
• Diuretics:		
Thiazides	+	
Loop diuretics	+	
Aldosterone antagonists	(+)	
• Sympatholytics:		
Clonidine		+
Moxonidine		+
Guanfacine		+
Alpha-methyldopa		+
Reserpine		(+)
Urapidil		(+)
Alpha-receptor blockers	(+)	(+)
Beta-receptor blockers		+
• Calcium antagonists:		
1,4-dihydropyridines	(+)	
• Inhibitors of the renin angiotensin system:		
ACE inhibitors	+	
AngII receptor antagonists	+	
Renin inhibitors	+	
• Vasodilators:		
(Di-)Hydralazine	+	
Minoxidil	+	
Sodium nitroprusside	+	
Diazoxide	+	
Other medications:		
• Analgesics		+
• Antiphlogistics		+
• Antipyretics		+
• Lithium	+	
* Aminophylline	+	
• Theophylline	+	
Hormones:		
Epinephrine, norepinephrine	+	
Aldosterone		+
ACTH		+
Atrial natriuretic peptide (ANP)		+
Insulin		(+) *
Estrogen	+	
		(+) *

( ): Mild effect
  *: Stimulation of angiotensinogen synthesis leading to increased formation of Ang II; the renin-secretion is only slightly inhibited by negative Ang II-feedback mechanism

several hours as well as quick and proper processing of the samples, especially for the measurement of the hormonal parameters of interest (renin and/or plasma renin activity, aldosterone and/or urine metabolites, possibly cortisol, possibly intermediates of aldosterone biosynthesis). These prerequisites are frequently not to be realized in the out-patient setting, so that hospitalization is less problematic and due to better supervision possibilities, also less hazardous for the patient.

Standard laboratory tests:

The measurement of aldosterone and potassium concentrations in plasma and 24-hour urine are standard laboratory tests in case of suspected primary aldosteronism. The measurement of renin concentrations in the plasma (or plasma-renin activity) can take place before and after the administration of 40 mg furosemide, if necessary.

Salt loading:

In normokalemic patients with a justified suspicion of the presence of primary aldosteronism (see above), Salt (sodium chloride) loading leads to an increased renal sodium/potassium exchange, allowing the unmasking of a latent hypokalemia through this diagnostic maneuver. Close laboratory and ECG monitoring are obligatory due to the resultant forced potassium wastage.

Salt loading also increases the specificity of the plasma aldosterone measurement, because the increased availability of sodium only leads to a suppression of the aldosterone secretion in an intact feedback mechanism of the renin-angiotensin-aldosterone system, not, however, in adrenocortical autonomy.

Captopril test:

Alternatively, the diagnostic value of the basal plasma aldosterone measurement can be improved by previous administration of an ACE inhibitor. After the oral administration of 25 mg of captopril, there is a decreased synthesis of angiotensin II with a resultant drop in arterial blood pressure and plasma aldosterone as well as a reactive increase in renin observed in normal subjects, patients with primary hypertension and patients with renovascular hypertension (Section 13.2.3). Due to its autonomy, no significant change in the production and secretion of aldosterone is expected in primary aldosteronism. A reactive increase in the suppressed renin secretion is thus lacking, so that the ratio of plasma aldosterone concentration to plasma renin activity ("plasma aldosterone/renin ratio") barely changes after captopril administration.

In contrast, in primary hypertension — and even more so in renovascular hypertension — a significant decrease in the ratio (aldosterone decrease, renin increase) is observed.

The specificity of the captopril test can be improved even more if one plots the aldosterone/renin ratio against the level of the plasma aldosterone concentration in a normogram (Figure 14.7).

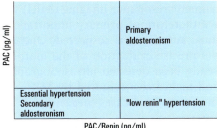

y-axis: PAC (pg/ml)

Primary aldosteronism

Essential hypertension
Secondary aldosteronism

"low renin" hypertension

PAC/Renin (pg/ml)

Figure 14.7: Plasma aldosterone concentrations (PAC) and PAC/renin-quotient, 60 minutes after pharmacologic inhibition of angiotensin-converting enzyme ("captopril test"), in various forms of hypertension. A test sensitivity of appx. 90 % mirrors the "overlapping" casually observed in clinical practice. (From Stimpel M., Dtsch med Wschr 1992; 117: 907–911)

The captropril test shows a high sensitivity and specificity for the presence of primary aldosteronism. The prerequisite for the applicability of this test is, however, that other influences on the renin secretion be avoided, which could falsify the results (see above and also Table 14.6). The captopril test is especially recommended when a sodium chloride loading is too risky or contraindicated (patients with severe hypertension, severe cardiac arrhythmia, congestive heart failure, cardiomegaly).

14.3.4.3 The differential diagnosis of the various forms of primary aldosteronism

Adrenocortical carcinoma, DSH and PAH:

The diagnostic differentiation between the various forms of primary aldosteronism is clinically relevant, because only patients with APA, adrenal carcinoma and PAH profit from an operative removal of the affected adrenal gland(s) (Section 34.5).

Because DSH (diagnosis: suppressibility of aldosterone production with glucocorticoids), PAH (diagnosis: biochemical and functional tests as is done for adenoma) and aldosterone-producing adrenocortical carcinoma (diagnosis: infiltrative growth, metastasis, excessive aldosterone production, rapidly progressing hypokalemia) are very rarely the causes of primary aldosteronism (< 0.1%), further diagnostic efforts will be aimed primarily at the differentiation between the two most common forms of autonomous aldosterone production (APA and IHA).

Differentiating between adenoma and hyperplasia using imaging techniques:

In general, the etiological classification takes place via imaging procedures, where unilateral adrenal gland alterations indicate an adenoma and bilateral alterations of less than 1 cm suggest an idiopathic hyperplasia.

The presence of an adenoma, in particular, can frequently already be classified by differential diagnosis by use of ultrasonography. However, a negative ultrasonographic finding in no way excludes hyperplasia or an adenoma, as APA are relatively small tumors. Approximately 20% measure less than 1 cm.

Computed tomography (CT) and magnetic resonance imaging (MRI) with a significantly higher picture resolution, are therefore of primary importance in the imaging procedures where adrenocortical autonomy is suspected. One of these procedures should be performed for the precise evaluation of the morphology, even in adrenal alteration which has already been detected ultrasonographically. Due, however, to the amount of effort and higher cost required by MRI, we only perform it as a supplemental method in exceptional cases (negative CT finding with biochemically verified primary aldosteronism).

The scintigraphic representation of aldosterone-producing tumors or hyperplasias – either with ^{131}I-19-iodocholesterol or with NP 59 – is a further non-invasive method, whose differential diagnostic power can be increased through the administration of dexamethasone with a resulting ACTH suppression (suppression scintigraphy). In contrast to adenomas, which remain visible, the scintigraphic visualization of idiopathic hyperplasias is increasingly reduced after several days of dexamethasone administration.

The biochemical differentiation between adenoma and idiopathic hyperplasia:

If the imaging procedures do not allow a clear differentiation between APA and IHA due to the anatomical situation or size (< 1 cm) of the adrenal gland changes, an etiological classification must be undertaken based on biochemical parameters.

Findings which indicate rather more the presence of an APA than an IHA, are lower serum potassium concentrations (< 3.0 mmol/L), higher plasma aldosterone and 18-hydroxy-corticosterone concentrations (intermediates in aldosterone biosynthesis, 18-OH-C > 100 ng/dl), a higher 18-OH-C/cortisol ratio after sodium chloride infusion (> 3.0), a higher aldosterone/renin ratio (> 20) after captopril, unchanged high plasma aldosterone concentrations after nightly rest and an aldosterone drop after subsequent, four-hour orthostasis and lack of ability to stimulate renin-secretion with a low-salt diet (see also, Table 14.7). False-positive "outliers" in patients with IHA and false-negative findings in APA, however, have been repeatedly observed.

Due to this overlapping, it is understandable that an absolutely reliable differentiation between adenoma and hyperplasia is not possible on the basis of biochemical parameters.

The greatest differential diagnostic reliability in primary aldosteronism is achieved through selective measurement of aldosterone in the adrenal venous blood on both sides. A unilateral increase in aldosterone indicates the presence of an ipsilateral adenoma, a bilateral increase the presence of an hyperplasia. A simultaneous decrease in the cortisol should always take place before and after ACTH stimulation in order to prevent the incorrect placement of the catheter for blood sampling, on the one hand, and in order to exclude a "secretion depression", on the other. The effort required, the burden on the patient and the risks (damage to the adrenal gland tissue) demand an extremely stringent application of the indication for this invasive investigatory procedure.

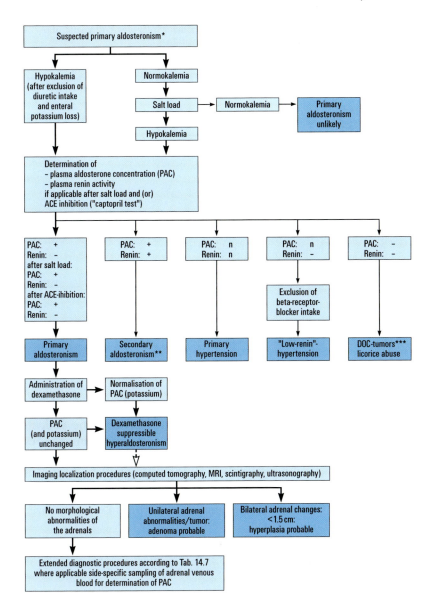

Figure 14.8: Diagnostic procedures in suspected primary aldosteronism
* Suspicion of primary aldosteronism in cases of hypokalemic hypertension, therapy-resistant or difficult-to-treat hypertension and adrenal tumor as incidental findings in a hypertensive patient
** Secondary aldosteronism in cases of renovascular hypertension, primary hypertension treated with diuretics, and pheochromocytoma (optional)
*** DOC tumors = tumors which produce deoxycorticosterone and (or) other mineralocorticoid precursors of the steroid synthesis (localization diagnosis as in primary aldosteronism)
+ = elevated, − = lowered/suppressed, n = normal

(From Stimpel M, Dtsch med Wschr 1992; 117: 907−911)

Table 14.7: Criteria for differentiating between aldosterone-producing adenoma (APA) and idiopathic adrenocortical hyperplasia (idiopathic hyperaldosteronism; IHA)

	APA	IHA
Unilateral adrenal abnormalities	+	−
Bilateral adrenal abnormalities	−	+
Serum potassium <3.0 mmol/l	+	−
PAC elevated	+	−
PAC/renin ratio (after captopril) >20	+	−
Orthostatic reaction		
− PAC-decrease	+	−
− PAC-increase	−	+
S-18-OH-C		
− >100 ng/dl	+	−
− <100 ng/dl	−	+
S-18-OH-C/cortisol (after NaCl-infusion) >3.0	+	−
Sodium chloride infusion	+	−

+ = Diagnosis more probable
− = Diagnosis less probable

PAC: Plasma aldosterone concentration
S-18-OH-C: Serum 18-hydroxy-corticosterone

Despite all efforts, a clear differential diagnostic classification of some patients will not be possible, at least in the short term. In these cases we recommend the initial introduction of drug therapy (Section 34.5), the close observation of the patients over a 6−12 month time period and a subsequent complete diagnostic procedure (Figure 14.8) under hospital conditions, if possible.

The diagnostic procedure upon suspicion of primary aldosteronism is summarized in the flow chart in Figure 14.8.

Summary (Section 14.3.4)

- Hypokalemic hypertension is the classic feature of primary aldosteronism; the most common cause of hypokalemic hypertension is, however, primary hypertension treated with diuretics.

- The diagnosis of primary aldosteronism can be established by increased plasma or urinary aldosterone levels associated with suppressed or lowered plasma renin activity.

- Under out-patient conditions, aldosterone should be measured in the 24-hour urine.

- The basic prerequisite for reliable measurement of renin and aldosterone are constant testing conditions, withdrawal of previous antihypertensive therapy two weeks before and a professional processing of the extracted blood samples.
- The therapeutically relevant differentiation between adenoma and idiopathic hyperplasia of the adrenal cortex organ can be achieved using imaging techniques such as ultrasonography, CT, MRI and/or scintigraphy.
- Unilateral adrenal gland changes larger than 1 cm indicate an adenoma and bilateral changes of less than 1 cm suggest idiopathic hyperplasia.
- The measurement of additional biochemical parameters provides further criteria, which, when taken together with imaging procedures, allow for a reliable differentiation between adenoma and idiopathic hyperplasia in most cases.

14.4 Deoxycorticosterone-producing (DOC) adrenal tumors

14.4.1 Pathogenesis

An extremely rare cause of hypokalemic hypertension is the autonomous production of mineralocorticoid-active precursors of steroid synthesis (usually 11-deoxycorticosterone or 18-hydroxycorticosterone, Figure 14.9, Section 14.5).
In the previously described cases, they were always benign tumors of the adrenal cortex.
Mineralocorticoid-active precursors of the steroid biosynthesis lead – as with aldosterone – to an increased absorption of sodium in the distal tubules of the kidney. A loss of potassium thus takes place in the exchange process. As in the case of primary aldosteronism, one also finds a suppressed renin angiotensin system in the DOC-tumors; however, aldosterone secretion is suppressed (Figure 14.8).

14.4.2 Diagnosis and differential diagnosis

The clinical symptoms are not specific and do not differ from primary aldosteronism.

The diagnosis of autonomous production of mineralocorticoid-active precursors in steroid synthesis results from the typical laboratory constellation of hypokalemia, hypoaldosteronism, suppressed plasma renin activity and the identification of excessive mineralocorticoid production.

"Pseudoaldosteronism" is to be treated separately in the differential diagnosis; it is also characterized by hypokalemic hypertension, hyporeninism and hypoaldosteronism, but is caused by an exogenous intake of glycyrrhetinic acid with the consumption of licorice or through carbenoxolone therapy (Section 17.2).

Localization diagnostics and therapy do not differ from aldosterone-producing adenoma of the adrenal cortex (Sections 14.3.3.2 and 34.5, respectively; see also FIgure 14.8).

Summary (Section 14.4)

- An autonomous production of mineralocorticoid-active precursors in steroid synthesis due to an adrenal cortex adenoma is a possible, but extremely rare cause of a hypokalemic hypertension.

- In chemical analysis, one finds a suppressed plasma renin activity in addition to hypokalemia.

- The most important differential diagnosis is primary aldosteronism (increased aldosterone!) and "pseudoaldosteronism" (decreased aldosterone!).

14.5 Adrenogenital syndromes/congenital adrenal hyperplasia

14.5.1 Pathogenesis

The adrenogenital syndromes (AGS) comprise a group of enzyme defects of steroid synthesis. A number of these inherited disturbances can be accompanied by hypertension since the defect in cortisol synthesis leads to an increased accumulation of mineralocorticoid-active precursors. While the most common form of AGS, 21-hydroxylase deficiency (approximately 95% of all AGS cases), almost always leads to an increased production of testosterone and is not associated with arterial hypertension, 11-hydroxylase deficiency and 17-hydroxylase deficiency lead to an accumulation of mineralocorticoid-active precursors (especially 11-desoxycorticosterone) with a subsequent development of a hypokalemic hypertension (Figure 14.9). As a result of decreased cortisol synthesis, physiological ACTH inhibition no longer occurs, so that an inadequately large amount of ACTH is produced; as a result, this usually leads to an adrenal hyperplasia. The desired cortisol increase is, however, limited by the respective enzyme defect; the result is dependent on the localization of the enzyme defect — an unchecked production of androgens and/or precursors of steroid synthesis.

14.5.2 Diagnosis of AGS

An 11-hydroxylase deficiency leads to an accumulation of 11-deoxycorticosterone and to an increased production of androgens as a result of the decreased pro-

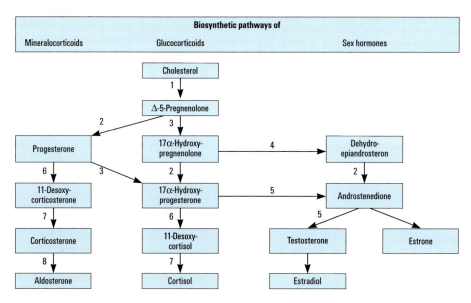

Figure 14.9: Biosynthesis of adrenal steroids
1 = 20,22-desmolase
2 = 5−3ß-hydroxysteroid-dehydrogenase
3 = 17-hydroxylase*
4 = 17,20-desmolase
5 = 17-ketosteroid-oxidoreductase
6 = 21-hydroxylase*
7 = 11ß-hydroxylase*
8 = 18-hydroxylase, 18-dehydrogenase

  * Adrenogenital syndromes/congenital adrenal hyperplasia:
— 21-hydroxylase deficiency syndrome (6):
   most common defect (95 %), no hypertension
— 11-hydroxylase deficiency syndrome (7):
   Increased formation of desoxycorticosterone, hypertension not always present
— 17-hydroxylase deficiency (3):
   Increased formation of mineralocorticoids, hypertension mostly present

duction of aldosterone and cortisol. Male infants often already have macrogenito-somia at birth; girls, common urogenital sinus and hypertrophy of the clitoris. The mineralocorticoid effect of 11-deoxycorticosterone explains the finding of increased retention of sodium, hypokalemic hypertension, the suppression of the renin-angiotensin system and an increased ACTH plasma level.

The consequence of a 17-hydroxylase deficiency is a decreased production of cortisol and sex hormones. The resulting over-production of 11-deoxycorticosterone leads to sodium retention, hypertension, hypokalemia and ACTH over-production. Plasma renin activity is suppressed. Male patients usually have ambiguous genitals or are phenotypically female (male pseudo-hermaphroditism) due to androgen deficiency. Female patients have primary amenorrhea and do not develop secondary sex characteristics.

14.5.3 AGS therapy

Glucocorticoid therapy generally leads to a normalization of blood pressure and to a balancing of electrolyte disturbances.

Normal sexual development can be induced in girls with 17-hydroxylase deficiency through estrogen substitution. The therapy is to be performed for a lifetime in all forms of AGS.

Summary (Section 14.5)

- 11- and 17-hydroxylase deficiency are rare forms of the adrenogenital syndrome (AGS) which is associated with a hypokalemic, hyporeninemic hypertension.

- Hypertension and electrolyte disturbances are a result of the increased production of mineralocorticoid-active precursors of adrenal steroid biosynthesis.

- The administration of glucocorticoids usually leads to a normalization of blood pressure and changes in electrolytes.

14.6 Cushing's syndrome (hypercortisolism)

14.6.1 Pathogenesis

Cushing's syndrome is characterized by an pituitary adrenocorticotrophic hormone (ACTH)-dependent or ACTH-independent hypersecretion of glucocorticoids. The cause in 65–80% of the cases is an increased hypophyseal secretion of ACTH with a secondary hyperplasia of both adrenal glands. In this central type of Cushing's syndrome (so-called "Cushing's disease"), the increased release of ACTH is either caused by a dysfunction of hypothalamic centers with increased production of the corticotropin-releasing hormone (CRH) or by an autonomous anterior pituitary adenoma. In rare cases, the disorder can be associated with an ectopic production of ACTH or CRH. This paraneoplastic ACTH or CRH production is usually associated with a small-cell bronchial carcinoma, but is also observed in other malignant tumors and in neuroendocrine tumors of the carcinoid type.

In ca. 20% of cases, the hypersecretion of glucocorticoids is based on a primary adrenal process. Unilateral findings speak for an adenoma or a carcinoma (Figures 14.10 a + b); changes in both adrenal glands tend to suggest an autonomous micro- or macronodular hyperplasia. – Bilateral adenomas as the cause of hypercortisolism have also been described.

More than 80% of the patients with Cushing's syndrome develop arterial hypertension, the pathogenesis of which is seen as being multifactorial. Possible causes are:

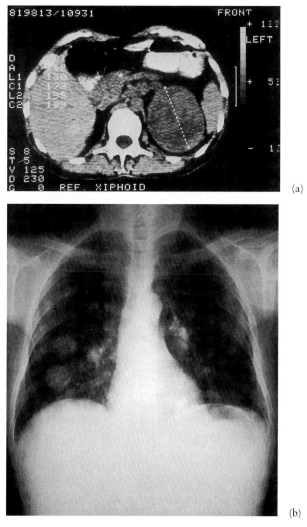

(a)

(b)

Figure 14.10 a and b: CT scan (a) of a malignant, primarily glucocorticoid-producing adrenal carcinoma (confirmed by autopsy) with resulting multiple metastatic dissemination at the time of diagnosis. The a.p. chest X-ray (b) shows numerous pulmonary metastases. 50 year-old patient, moderate hypertension, hypokalemia.

- the mineralocorticoid effect of the high cortisol level with resulting sodium and fluid retention (as well as increased potassium excretion),
- an increased glucocorticoid-induced production of renin substrate with consequent, increased angiotensin II production,
- an increased production and release of mineralocorticoid-active precursors of steroid synthesis (Figure 14.9),
- an increased activity of the sympathetic nervous system,

– an increased response of the vascular musculature to catecholamine and,

– (at least for patients with adrenal Cushing's syndrome) a decreased production of blood pressure-lowering kinins and prostaglandins (PGE_2, PGI_2).

Summary (Section 14.6.1)

- Cushing's syndrome is characterized by a chronic hypersecretion of glucocorticoids.
- The causes of Cushing's syndrome are ACTH dependent or independent:
  – ACTH-dependent (Cushing's disease, ectopic ACTH or CRH syndrome), ca. 80%.
  – ACTH-independent ("Primary hypercortisolism": Adrenal adenoma and carcinoma, micro- and macronodular hyperplasia), ca. 20%.
  – Pseudo-Cushing's syndrome (Major depressive disorders, alcoholism), ca. 1% (Section 14.6.2.2).
  – Arterial hypertension is present in more than 80% of patients with Cushing's syndrome.

14.6.2   Diagnosing Cushing's syndrome

14.6.2.1 Clinical symptoms

The etiological classification of a newly discovered hypertension generally does not present the Cushing's syndrome patients with any differential diagnostic problems since the chronic effect of the glucocorticoid hypersecretion leads to a typical ("cushingoid") distribution of the fat pads. Moon facies, "buffalo hump" and a generally advanced obesity, which is usually distributed over the truncal area, are almost always encountered (Figure 14.11 a + b), though they are often missing in the ectopic form of Cushing's syndrome that is associated with small-cell bronchial carcinoma. Increasing atrophy of the muscles with a subjective feeling of weakness are the result of the catabolic influence of the massively increased glucocorticoid level on the protein metabolism. An extreme decline in performance and fatigue, which in primary adrenal processes and ectopic Cushing's syndrome are worsened by an associated hypokalemia, often characterize the patients' subjective impression. Menstrual disturbances, a loss of libido, an increase in body hair and impotence are further, often existing results of the pathologically increased glucocorticoid production. In the case of advanced hypercortisolism, opportunistic infections can occur as a result of the autoimmune suppression. Disseminated cryptococcosis, aspergillosis, nocardiosis and pneumocystis carinii pneumonia have been reported. An early, high-grade osteoporosis indicates a longer presence of hypercortisolism.

14.6.2.2 Differential diagnosis

The most important clinical differential diagnosis is (diet-induced) obesity, which can also be associated with arterial hypertension (Section 9.3.5) and an increased

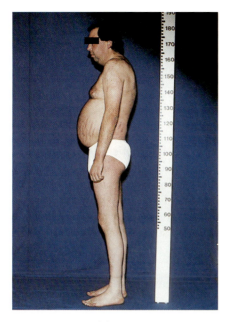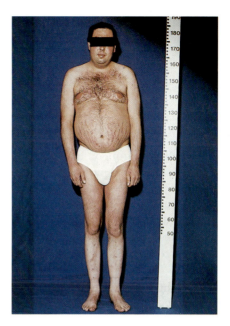

Figure 14.11 a and b: Clinical signs characteristic for Cushing's syndrome (truncal obesity, typical "moon" facies, "buffalo hump" and typical red striae) in a man 36 years of age at the time of diagnosis.

secretion of cortisol and cortiocotropin, and must therefore be excluded by means of additional laboratory diagnostic procedures.

In addition, one must consider a so-called "alcohol-associated pseudo-Cushing's syndrome" in the differential diagnosis that is characterized by heavy alcohol consumption, arterial hypertension, a "cushingoid" appearance and increased plasma and urinary cortisol concentrations which can not be sufficiently suppressed in a single or repeated dexamethasone application ("low-dose dexamethasone suppression test, see Section 14.6.2.3).

An increased secretion of cortisol is also seen in various psychiatric − especially depressive − disorders.

14.6.2.3 Laboratory diagnostics

Proof of hypercortisolism:

Non-specific laboratory parameters:

Hypokalemia, metabolic alkalosis, hyperlipidemia, hyperglycemia (or impaired glucose tolerance) or eosinopenia are non-specific laboratory findings seen, in varying degrees, in many cases of Cushing's syndrome however, in reference to their differential diagnostic value, are of only secondary importance.

Determination of plasma cortisol:

Single cortisol determinations in plasma are not suited as a screening test in suspected Cushing's syndrome, since large variations of cortisol secretions can take place through physiological conditions and pathological glucocorticoid production.

Determination of free cortisol in 24-hour urine:

The determination of free cortisol in 24-hour urine is a generally reliable and unproblematic out-patient test procedure for the overproduction of glucocorticoid. In a patient likely to have Cushing's syndrome, free cortisol should be measured in at least two consecutive 24-hour urine specimens. − Extremely high free cortisol concentrations (and 17-hydroxysteriods and 17-ketosteriods, which can now no longer be recommended on a routine basis) typically suggest a carcinoma of the adrenal cortex.

Overnight 1 mg dexamethasone suppression test (screening test):

A further out-patient screening test for suspected Cushing's syndrome is the determination of the morning plasma cortisol concentration after the intake of 1 mg dexamethasone on the previous evening (between 11 p.m. and midnight). While one would expect a suppression of cortisol release in normal individuals or in patients with obesity, the cortisol secretion in patients with Cushing's syndrome is not influenced by the exogenous glucocorticoid intake. A lack of suppression after a single dose does not, however, justify the diagnosis of Cushing's syndrome, since false positive results are quite often observed (10−20%).

Low-dose dexamethasone suppression test:

The oral administration of 0.5 mg dexamethasone every six hours on two consecutive days (eight doses in total) with a determination of the cortisol concentration in the 24-hour urine before, during and after the test is termed the "low-dose dexamethasone suppression test". Cortisol concentrations of less than 50% of the base line value after and during glucocorticoid intake suggest an ability to suppress the cortisol secretions and speak against the presence of Cushing's syndrome.

Etiological classification of diagnosed hypercortisolism

ACTH determination in plasma:

The evidence of suppressed ACTH plasma levels in proven (i. e., non-suppressible) hypercortisolism allows for the diagnosis of a primary adrenal form of Cushing's syndrome. The differentiation between adenoma, hyperplasia and carcinoma is performed by means of an imaging procedure (ultrasonography, computed tomography, magnetic resonance imaging).

Normal to greatly increased plasma concentrations of ACTH in the case of a lack of cortisol suppression in the low-dose dexamethasone suppression test (see above) are indicative of an ACTH-dependent stimulation of cortisol release. However, a definite differentiation between Cushing's disease (ACTH usually "normal") and an ectopic ACTH or CRH syndrome (ACTH often greatly increased) is not possible.

High-dose dexamethasone suppression test:

In the case of a non-suppressible cortisol and ACTH release without an imaging localization of the disease process, the "high-dose" dexamethasone suppression test can supply further information for the etiological classification of the Cushing's syndrome. The pathophysiological basis for this test is, in contrast to an ectopic ACTH-producing tumor, a principally retained possibility to influence the hypophyseal ACTH release in Cushing's disease with high dose of dexamethasone.

Thus 2 mg dexamethasone are administered orally in six-hour intervals (8 mg daily) on two consecutive days. A reduction of cortisol excretion in the urine suggests the presence of Cushing's disease (hypothalamic-pituitary related hypercortisolism); the lack of suppression on the other hand suggests the presence of an ectopic (or adrenal) form of Cushing's syndrome.

Despite a generally good differential diagnostic reliability of this function test (introduced in 1960), both false negatives (lack of suppression of cortisol secretion in approximately 10−20% of patients with Cushing's disease) as well as false positives (suppression in ectopic ACTH-syndrome) have been reported.

Corticotropin-releasing hormone (CRH) stimulation test:

A differentiation between central and ectopic Cushing's syndrome is also possible with the determination of the ACTH and cortisol plasma concentrations after an intravenous injection of 100 µg CRH (corticotropin releasing hormone). While a marked increase of the recorded parameter is observed in Cushing's disease, ACTH and cortisol secretion are not influenced by the CRH application for ectopic ACTH-producing tumors.

The CRH stimulation test as well as the "high-dose" dexamethasone suppression test should be used for applicable differential diagnostic problems, since concurring results in both functional tests increase diagnostic reliability.

CRH test and catheterization of the inferior petrosal sinuses:

The most reliable method for the etiological clarification of Cushing's syndrome is the simultaneous, bilateral catheterization of the inferior petrosal sinuses for the determination of the ACTH plasma concentration after CRH stimulation. The ACTH plasma concentration in a peripheral vein serves as a reference. When the ACTH concentration in the petrosal sinus is at least three times more than in the peripheral vein, a pituitary origin of the hormone is indicated. A ratio of >1.4 between the two sinuses is considered a suitable criterion to lateralize an adenoma within the pituitary gland. However, this interpretation was only postoperatively supported in 71 of 105 examined patients.

The bilateral catheterization of the inferior petrosal sinuses demands that the examining physician have a high level of technical expertise, and it should only take place in centers that have corresponding experience in diagnosing and localizing Cushing's syndrome.

Summary (Sections 14.6.2.1−14.6.2.3)

- A visual diagnosis is possible in most patients with Cushing's syndrome due to the typical ("cushingoid") habitus.

- However, the lack of truncal obesity, "moon facies", "buffalo hump" and other characteristic clinical features never exclude Cushing's syndrome.

- The diagnosis of Cushing's syndrome is ensured by proof of a non-suppressible cortisol hypersecretion.

- Primary adrenal causes of a non-suppressible hypercortisolism are proven by a suppressed ACTH plasma level and are localized with the use of CT or MRI.

- A suppressibility of cortisol through a high-dosage application of dexamethasone (high-dose dexamethasone test) and/or a stimulation of ACTH and cortisol through CRH (CRH stimulation test) suggests a pituitary, ACTH dependent Cushing's syndrome (Cushing's disease).

- In the case of ectopic ACTH or CRH-producing tumors and in the case of primary adrenal causes of Cushing's syndrome, the secretion of ACTH and cortisol is not influenced by the application of dexamethasone or CRH.

- The most reliable, though invasive, procedure for the etiological determination of Cushing's syndrome is the bilateral measurement of ACTH in the inferior petrosal sinuses after a preceding CRH stimulation. A pituitary process is present when the ACTH concentration is at least three times greater than in a peripheral vein.

14.6.2.4 Localization procedures

Primary adrenal Cushing's syndrome:

Evidence of cortisol-producing adrenal tumors is usually determined using CT or MRI (see above). − One can scintigraphically represent cortisol-producing adenomas of the adrenal gland after the application of ^{131}I-cholesterol. A negative scintigraphic result in the case of a biochemically and computed tomographically proven adrenal Cushing's syndrome suggests the presence of an adrenal gland carcinoma.

Pituitary ACTH-dependent Cushing's syndrome (Cushing's disease):

A microadenoma of the anterior pituitary lobe with an average diameter of 5 mm is in most cases a morphological correlate to Cushing's disease. A pre-operative, pictorial representation of these tumors is most successful using high resolution MRI, though it is often not at all possible. A number of research groups additionally suggest the attempt at a functional localization of the adenoma within the pituitary gland in every case. − The necessary bilateral simultaneous catheterization of both inferior petrosal sinuses was already described in Section 14.6.2.3.

Ectopic Cushing's syndrome:

A paraneoplastic ACTH or CRH secretion was observed in small-cell bronchial carcinomas, carcinoid tumors and in rare cases in malignant tumors of other organs (see above).

In cases in which a localization of the tumor is not possible using chest X-ray and/ or CT or MRI examination of the thorax and abdomen, the site of paraneoplastic ACTH or CRH production can be more closely determined and represented using a targeted angiographic or CT examination with step-by-step, selective venous blood sampling. The search can be very frustrating, especially in the case of slow-growing carcinoid tumors, since these tumors are often very small despite their high endocrine activity. − The role of somatostatin receptor scintigraphy in the localization of occult ectopic ACTH-secreting or CRH-secreting tumors has not yet definitely been determined.
(For diagnostic procedures see also flow chart Figure 14.12)

Summary (Section 14.6.2.4)

- A primary adrenal Cushing's syndrome is best represented using CT or MRI.

- The localization of a pituitary ACTH-dependent Cushing's syndrome (Cushing's disease) results using a combination of imaging (MRI) and functional (simultaneous, bilateral ACTH determination in the petrosal sinuses after a CRH application) examination procedures.

- After an unsuccessful routine radiological search for an ectopic ACTH-producing tumor, one can attempt to narrow the localization using a selective, step-by-step venous blood sampling to determine ACTH levels and then identify the site with a targeted angiographic or MRI examination.

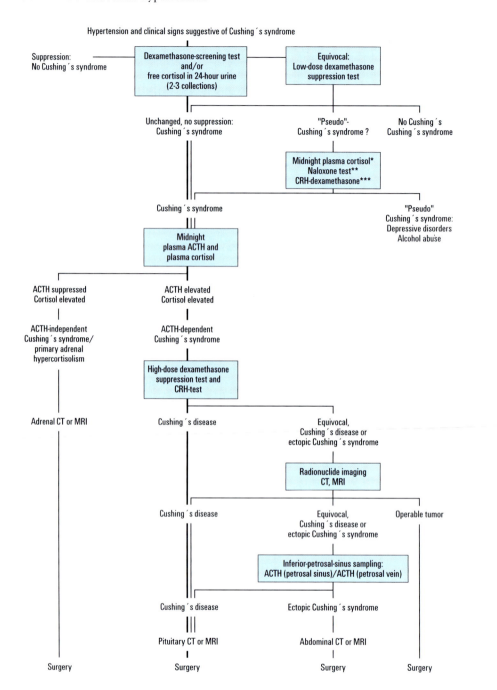

14.7 Primary hyperreninism

The autonomous production and secretion of renin with resultant secondary aldosteronism is an extremely rare cause of arterial hypertension. Less than 50 cases have been described to date in the literature world-wide. Most of these cases consisted of intrarenally located tumors displaying various histological characters, such as juxtaglomerular cell tumors, hemangiopericytomas, hamartomas, Wilms' tumors or renal cell carcinomas. An ectopic renin production was observed in carcinomas of the liver, the pancreas, the ovaries, the bronchial system and other organs.

Because at least the intrarenal renin-producing tumors are overwhelmingly benign, hypertension can generally be cured by the removal of the tumor. The possibility of autonomous renin secretion should be considered in cases of secondary aldosteronism with hypokalemic hypertension where a pathophysiological explanation of the increased renin secretion (therapy with diuretics, stenoses of the renal artery, pheochromocytoma, renal cysts, etc.), is lacking.

Summary (Section 14.7)

- The extremely rare possibility of autonomous renin production should be considered in differential diagnosis when both secondary aldosteronism and hypokalemic hypertension are present and after stenosis of the renal artery, pheochromocytoma and therapy with diuretics have been excluded.

14.8 Acromegaly

14.8.1 Pathogenesis

The overproduction of growth hormone (GH) before epiphyseal closure leads to gigantism, after the end of the growth period it leads to acromegaly. An adenoma of the pituitary gland is the cause of the autonomous overproduction of GH in almost all cases. Arterial hypertension is observed in patients with acromegaly more frequently than it is in the general population. This hypertension can be at

Figure 14.12: Diagnostic procedures and management of patients with clinical signs suggestive of Cushing's syndrome.
  * Midnight plasma cortisol is usually low in pseudo-Cushing's syndrome (in contrast to Cushing's syndrome)
 ** Naloxone stimulates the release of CRH more in pseudo-Cushing's syndrome than in Cushing's disease
*** Sequential administration of dexamethasone and CRH and determination of plasma cortisol:
    Pseudo-Cushing's syndrome: Plasma cortisol low after both dexamethasone and CRH
    Cushing's syndrome: Plasma cortisol not as low after dexamethasone and increased after CRH
(Adapted and modified from Orth DN, N Eng J Med 1995; 332: 791—803)

least partially explained by the sodium-retentive effect of the highly increased GH and the consecutively increased intravascular volume. The left ventricular hypertrophy associated with acromegaly is partially a result of the hormone influence and not exclusively a result of the hypertension.

14.8.2 Diagnosis

The clinical features of established acromegaly are highly suggestive of the definite diagnosis: roughness of the facial features (prognathism, prominence of the supraorbital eminence, enlarged nose), often massive enlargement of the hands and feet as well as a general bone enlargement are all typical changes associated with this endocrine disorder (Figure 14.13 a + b). In less pronounced cases, a comparison with relatives or older photographs of the patient may be diagnostically helpful. To confirm the diagnosis, the proof of raised plasma levels of insulin-like growth factor I (IGF-I) and GH are required. Characteristically, they are not suppressible through an oral dosage of 100 g glucose (GH suppression test).

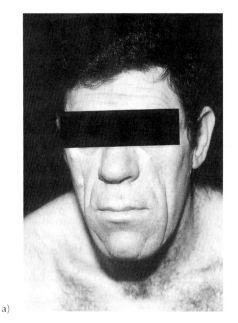
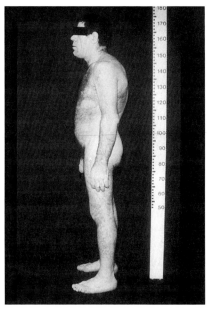

a)   b)

Figure 14.13 a and b: Characteristic features in an acromegalic patient with a postoperatively confirmed GH-producing pituitary adenoma. Note the increased size of the nose, the jaw and the nasolabial skin fold (a) as well as the enlarged feet (so-called "Yeti-like" feet) and hands (b).

14.8.3 Antihypertensive therapy in acromegalics

The drug therapy of acromegaly-associated hypertension does not show any peculiarities, so that the general guidelines for antihypertensive treatment (Chapters

19–30) can be referred to. A successful treatment of the underlying disease by radiation or transsphenoidal operation of the hypophyseal tumor leads to a normalization or decrease in the elevated blood pressure, at least in part of the patient population. Whether the medicinal lowering of GH secretion by the somatostatin analogue octreotide can normalize blood pressure over the long term is not known.

> **Summary (Section 14.8)**
>
> - Arterial hypertension with acromegaly is common and possibly the result of an GH-related sodium retention.
> - The general recommendations for the treatment of hypertension apply to the drug therapy of acromegaly-related hypertension.

14.9 Primary hyperparathyroidism

The diagnosis of arterial hypertension and the simultaneous proof of hypercalcemia should lead to the consideration of a possible underlying primary hyperparathyroidism (HPT), as this disease is approximately ten times more common among hypertensive patients than among the average population. Conversely, arterial hypertension is present in 10–70% of patients with primary HPT.

Increased plasma concentrations of parathyroid with hormone (PTH) concomitant hypercalcemia indicate HPT. HPT-related arterial hypertension is likely not caused by a uniform pathomechanism. On the one hand, the development of hypertension after a long-term history of the disease can be easily explained as a consequence of increasing renal dysfunction. On the other hand, the normalization of blood pressure after the surgical correction of the HPT in patients with healthy kidneys gives rise to the conjecture that a causal relationship may exist between hypertension and pathologically increased parathyroid hormone secretion in these cases. It is possible that the hypertension of a part of the patient population with HPT may be explained by the existence of a hypertension-inducing factor (parathyroid hypertensive factor, PHF), which is also produced by the parathyroid gland. PHF has been detected in spontaneously hypertensive rats and recently also in the plasma of a few hypertensive patients with HPT. The proof of an endocrine-related genesis of hypertension with HPT is, however, still lacking. Because primary HPT occasionally arises within the context of a multiple endocrine neoplasia, one must consider the possible concomitant existence of a pheochromocytoma in hypertensive patients with HPT (MEN 2A, see also Section 14.1). The most important consideration in the differential diagnosis of "hypercalcemic hypertension" is the coincidental association of primary hypertension with a malignant disease. Antihypertensive therapy with HPT does not follow any specific guidelines.

Summary (Section 14.9)

• Primary hyperparathyroidism (HPT) is accompanied by arterial hypertension with above-average frequency. This hypertension is presumably not to be explained by a uniform pathogenic mechanism.

• Hypercalcemic hypertension leads to the suspicion of HPT. The coincidental association of two different diseases (e.g., primary hypertension and malignant disease) should, however, be considered in differential diagnosis.

• The laboratory-chemical diagnosis of primary hyperparathyroidism is achieved by the proof of normal or raised plasma levels of parathyroid hormone with hypercalcemia and hypophosphatemia.

14.10 Endothelin-secreting tumors

Endothelin I (ET-1) is a polypeptide with strong vasoconstrictive properties that is formed and released by the endothelial cells and which was only recently discovered and isolated (Yanagisawa, 1988). The physiological significance of this hormone, which may only be autocrinally effective, is currently still unknown. An endothelin-dependent hypertension was suspected in two patients with malignant, endothelin-secreting hemangioendothelioma. The plasma endothelin concentrations and arterial blood pressure normalized after surgical removal of the tumor.

14.11   Hypo- and hyperthyroidism

14.11.1 Hypothyroidism

Patients with hypothyroidism often develop an increase in diastolic blood pressure that is reversible in some of the patients after sufficient thyroid hormone substitution. This primary increase in the diastolic blood pressure is the consequence of a reactive activation of the sympathetic nervous system with consequent increase in the peripheral vascular resistance. This is obviously a compensation mechanism, which seeks to maintain the required tissue perfusion despite a metabolism-related decrease of the heart rate and cardiac output.

14.11.2 Hyperthyroidism

Increased blood pressure with hyperthyroidism is the consequence of an increased cardiac output. It is characterized by an isolated systolic hypertension with normal or lower diastolic blood pressure values. An increase in the diastolic blood pressure in endocrinologically confirmed hyperthyroidism indicates the simultaneous existence of primary hypertension. Because the mean arterial pressure is normal in hyperthyroidism, hyperthyroid hypertension does not actually represent a form of hypertension which requires therapy. The significance of hypertension with hyperthyroidism in the context of the differential diagnosis of arterial hypertension comes from its similarity with the clinical symptoms of hyperkinetic heart syndrome, Windkessel hypertension of older hypertensive patients and pheocromocytoma (the latter, however, is generally associated with an additional increase in the diastolic blood pressure). Where an antihypertensive therapy has been considered, beta-adrenergic receptor blockers led to a normalization of the heart rate and the increased systolic blood pressure.

Summary (Section 14.11)

- Hypertension with hypothyroidism is primarily associated with increased diastolic blood pressure values. The initial cause is a reactive increase in the peripheral vascular resistance.

- Increased systolic and often decreased diastolic blood pressure values are frequently present in hyperthyroidism. Because the mean arterial pressure is not elevated, antihypertensive therapy is normally not required.

- Increased diastolic blood pressure values in hyperthyroidism point to another cause of the hypertension.

Literature (Chapter 14)

Pheochromocytoma (Section 14.1)

Bravo EL, Tarazi RC, Gifford RW, Stewart BH. Circulating and urinary catecholamines in pheochromocytoma. N Engl J Med 1979; 301: 682−686.

Bravo EL, Tarazi RC, Fouad FM, Vidt DG, Gifford RW Jr. Clonidine-suppression test: a useful aid in the diagnosis of pheochromocytoma. N Engl J Med 1981; 305: 623−626.

Gagel RF. Multiple endocrine neoplasia. In: Wilson JD, Foster DW (eds). Williams Textbook of Endocrinology, 8th ed. WB Saunders, Philadelphia, 1992: 1537−1553.

Gifford RW, Manger WM, Bravo EL. Pheochromocytoma. Endocrinol Metab Clin N Am 1994; 23: 387−404.

Grossman E, Goldstein DS, Hoffman A, Keiser HR. Glucagon and clonidine testing in the diagnosis of pheochromocytoma. Hypertension 1991; 17: 733−741.

Hamada M, Shigematsu Y, Mukai M, Kazatani Y, Kokubu T, Hiwada K. Blood pressure response to the valsalva maneuver in pheochromocytoma and pseudopheochromocytoma. Hypertension 1995; 25: 266−271.

Krane NK. Clinically unsuspected pheochromocytomas. Experience at Henry Ford Hospital and a review of the literature. Arch Intern Med 1986; 146: 54−57.

Manelli M. Diagnostic problems in pheochromocytoma. J Endocrinol Invest 1989; 12: 739−757.

Manger WM, Gifford RW. Phaeochromocytoma: a clinical overview. In: Swales JD (ed), Textbook of Hypertension, Blackwell Scientific Publications London 1994: 941−958.

Neumann HPH, Berger DP, Sigmund G, Blum U, Schmidt D, Parmer RJ, Volk B, Kirste G. Pheochromocytomas, multiple endocrine neoplasia type 2, and von Hippel-Lindau disease. N Engl J Med 1993; 329: 1531−1538.

Schürmeyer TH, Engeroff B, von zur Mühlen A, Dralle H. Symptomatik und endokrinologische Befunde bei katecholamin-sezernierenden Tumoren. Ergebnisse bei 106 konsekutiven Patienten. Dtsch Med Wschr 1994; 119: 1721–1727.

Scully RE, Mark EJ, McNeely BU. Weekly Clinicopathological Exercises. Case 6–1986. N Engl J Med 1986; 314: 431–439.

Shapiro B, Copp JE, Sisson JC, Eyre PL, Wallis J, Beierwaltes WH. 131-Iodine metaiodoben-zylguanidine for the locating of suspected pheochromocytoma. Experiences in 400 cases. J Nucl Med 1985; 26: 576–85.

Stimpel M, Wambach G. Diagnostik des Phäoch-romozytoms. Dtsch Med Wschr 1987; 112: 1422–1425.

Stimpel M, Schürmeyer TH, Ivens K, Wambach G, Volkmann HP, von zur Mühlen A. Diagnos-tic value of the clonidine suppression test in suspected phaechromocytoma. [in German] Dtsch med Wschr 1988; 113: 130–134.

Stimpel M, Reiss U, Volkmann HP, Wambach G. The overnight clonidine suppression test (OCST) in the diagnosis of pheochromocy-toma. Hypertension 1993; 21: 131.

Vincent D, Pradalier A. Pheochromocytoma-like catecholamine levels induced by clonidine ces-sation. Europ J Med 1993; 2: 313.

Primary mineralocorticoidism
(Sections 14.2–14.5)

Biglieri EG. Spectrum of mineralocorticoid hy-pertension. Hypertension 1991; 17: 251–261.

Biglieri EG, Schambelan M. The significance of elevated levels of plasma 18-hydroxy-cortico-sterone in patients with primary aldosteron-ism. J Clin Endocrinol Metab 1979; 49: 87–91.

Bravo EL, Tarazi RC, Dustan HP, Fouad FM, Textor SC, Gifford RW, Vidt DG. The chang-ing clinical spectrum of primary aldosteron-ism. Am J Med 1983; 74: 641–651.

Dluhy RG, Lifton RP. Glucocorticoid-remediable aldosteronism. Endocrinol Metab Clin N Am 1994; 23: 285–297.

Fallo F, Sonino N, Boscaro M, Armanini D, Mantero F, Dörr HG, Knorr D, Kuhnle U. Dexamethasone-suppressible hyperaldosteron-ism: Pathophysiology, clinical aspects, and new insights into the pathogenesis. Klin Wochenschr 1987; 65: 437–444.

Gross MD, Shapiro B. Scintigraphic studies in adrenal hypertension. Semin Nucl Med 1989; 19: 122–143.

Irony I, Biglieri EG, Perloff D, Rubinoff H. Pathophysiology of deoxycorticosterone-secre-ting adrenal tumors. J Clin Endocrinol Metab 1987; 65: 836–840.

Kater CE, Biglieri EG. Disorders of steroid 17-alpha-hydroxylase deficiency. Endocrinol Metab Clin N Am 1994; 23: 341–357.

Melby JC. Primary aldosteronism. Kidney Int 1984; 26: 769–778.

Melby JC. Clinical review 1: endocrine hyperten-sion. J Clin Endocrin Metab 1989; 69: 697–704.

Stimpel M. Diagnosis of primary aldosteronism. [in German] Dtsch med Wschr 1992; 117: 907–911.

Stimpel M, Grimm U, Degenhardt S, Krone W, Wambach G. Captopril-test in the diagnosis of primary aldosteronism. [in German]. Nieren Hochdruckrkht 1992; 21: 582–584.

Wambach G, Homburg H. Der primäre Hyperal-dosteronismus: Differenzierung zwischen Conn-Syndrom und idiopathischem Hyperal-dosteronismus. Akt Endokr Stoffw 1989; 10: 170–180.

Weinberger MH, Fineberg NS. The diagnosis of primary aldosteronism and separation of two major subtypes. Arch Intern Med 1993; 153: 2125–2129.

White PC, New MI, Dupont B. Congenital adre-nal hyperplasia (First of two parts). N Engl J Med 1987; 316: 1519–1524.

White PC, New MI, Dupont B. Congenital adre-nal hyperplasia (Second of two parts). N Engl J Med 1987; 316: 1580–1586.

Cushing's syndrome (Section 14.6)

Danese RD, Aron DC. Cushing's syndrome and hypertension. Endocrinol Metabol Clin N Am 1994; 23: 299–324.

Gold PW, Loriaux DL, Roy A, Kling MA, Cala-brese JR, Kellner CH, Nieman LK, Post RM, Pickar D, Galluci W, Avgerinos P, Paul S, Old-field EH, Cutler GB, Chrousos GP. Responses to corticotropin-releasing hormone in the hyp-ercortisolism of depression and Cushing's dis-ease. Pathophysiologic and diagnostic implica-tions. N Engl J Med 1986; 314: 1329–1335.

Hermus ARMM, Pieters GFFM, Pesman GJ, Smals AGH, Benraad TJ, Klop-penborg PWC. The corticotropin-releasing-hormone test ver-sus the high-dose dexamethasone test in the differential diagnosis of Cushing's syndrome. Lancet 1986; 2: 540–544.

Kaye TB, Crapo L. The Cushing syndrome: an update on diagnostic tests. Ann Intern Med 1990; 112: 434–444.

Leinung MC, Young WF, Whitaker MD, Schei-thauer BW, Trastek VF, Kvols LK. Diagnosis of corticotropin-producing bronchial carcinoid tumors causing Cushing's syndrome. Mayo Clin Proc 1990; 65: 1314−1321.

Liebl R. Störfaktoren beim Dexamethason-Hemmtest. Klin Wochenschr 1986; 64: 535−539.

Müller J. Sinnvolle und sinnlose Steroidbestimmungen: Zweckmässige Labordiagnostik der Nebennieren-Funktion. Schweiz med Wschr 1991; 121: 482−487.

Nieman LK, Chrousos GP, Oldfield EH, Avgerinos PC, Cutler GB Jr, Loriaux DL. The ovine corticotropin-releasing hormone stimulation test and the dexamethasone test in the differential diagnosis of Cushing's syndrome. Ann Intern Med 1986; 105: 862−867.

Oldfield EH, Doppman JL, Nieman LK, Chrousos GP, Miller DL, Katz DA, Cutler GB, Loriaux DL. Petrosal sinus sampling with and without corticotropin-releasing hormone for the differential diagnosis of Cushing's syndrome. N Engl J Med 1991; 325: 897−905

Orth DN, Kovacs WJ, DeBold CR. The adrenal cortex. In: Wilson JD, Foster DW (eds). William's Textbook of Endocrinology, 8th ed. WB Saunders, Philadelphia, 1992: 489−619.

Orth DN. Cushing's syndrome. N Engl J Med 1995; 332: 791−803.

Saruta T, Suzuki H, Handa M, Igarashi Y, Kondo K, Senba S. Multiple factors contribute to the pathogenesis of hypertension in Cushing's syndrome. J Clin Endocrin Metab 1986; 62: 275−279.

Primary hyperreninism (Section 14.7)

Corvol P, Pinet F, Galen FX, Plouin PF, Chatellier G, Pagny JY, Bruneval P, Camilleri JP, Menard J. Primary reninism. In: Laragh JH, Brenner BM (eds): Hypertension. Pathophysiology, diagnosis, and management, 2nd ed. Raven Press, New York 1994.

Baruch D, Corvol P, Alhenc-Gelas F, Dufloux MA, Guyenne TT, Gaux JC et al. Diagnosis and treatment of renin-secreting tumors. Hypertension 1984; 6: 760−766.

Kreutz R, Zhou H, Pfeifer U, Gasc JM, Ganten D, Kessler FJ. Primary reninism, a rare cause of secondary arterial hypertension [in German]. Dtsch med Wschr 1993; 118: 1110−1114.

Acromegaly (Section 14.8)

Deray G, Rieu M, Devynck MA, Pernollet MG, Chanson P, Luton JP, Meyer P. Evidence of an endogenous digitalis-like factor in the plasma of patients with acromegaly. N Engl J Med 1987; 316: 575−580.

Melmed S. Acromegaly. N Engl J Med 1990; 322: 966−977.

Primary hyperparathyroidism (Section 14.9)

Diamond TW, Botha JR, Wing J, Meyers AM, Kalk WJ. Parathyroid hypertension. A reversible disorder. Arch Intern Med 1986; 146: 1709−1712.

Lewanczuk RZ, Pang PK. Expression of parathyroid factor in hypertensive primary hyperparathyroid patients. Blood Pressure 1993; 2: 22−27.

Endothelin-producing tumors (Section 14.10)

Yokokawa K, Tahara H, Kohno M, Murakawa K, Yasunari K, Nakagawa K, Hamada T, Otani S, Yanagisawa M, Takeda T. Hypertension associated with endothelin-secreting malignant hemangioendothelioma. Ann Intern Med 1991; 114: 213−215.

Hypo- and Hyperthyroidism (Section 14.11)

Saito I, Ito K, Saruto T. Hypothyroidism as a cause of hypertension. Hypertension 1983; 5: 112−115.

Saito I, Saruto T. Hypertension in thyroid disorders. Endocrinol Metab Clin N Am 1994; 23: 379−386.

Streeten DH, Anderson GH, Howland T, Chang R, Smulyan H. effects of thyroid function on blood pressure. Recognition of hypothyroid hypertension. Hypertension 1988; 11: 78−83.

15 Hypertension during pregnancy

Arterial hypertension during pregnancy is found in 15−20% of all nulliparous women. Roughly 1/3rd of those affected have already registered a chronic blood pressure increase before pregnancy with a primary (primary hypertension) or secondary (renovascular or renoparenchymal hypertension, endocrine hypertension, etc.) genesis. This hypertension, which is not specific to pregnancy, must be differentiated from blood pressure increases which first appear after the 20th week of pregnancy and which are triggered by pregnancy-related changes. Although the pathogenesis of pregnancy-specific hypertension has still not been fully explained, due to its demonstrable hemodynamic and hormonal changes, it can be clearly differentiated from other forms of hypertension and − through delivery − is causally treated. By definition, pregnancy-specific increases in blood pressure are thus secondary forms of hypertension.

15.1 Prognostic significance of hypertension during pregnancy

The dangers to a mother from arterial hypertension are for the most part no different from the potential cardiovascular risks which arise from chronically elevated blood pressure outside of pregnancy. Furthermore, in cases of preeclampsia, there is always a danger of eclampsia, which can be defined as hypertensive encephalopathy, accompanied by seizures and which can lead to cerebral edema and cerebral hemorrhage with lethal consequences.

The growth of a fetus can be hindered by arterial hypertension, especially when accompanied by renal insufficiency or an underlying preeclampsia. The consequence is increased perinatal morbidity and mortality.

15.2 Definition and classification

Hypertension during pregnancy is defined as chronically increased blood pressure values of 135/85 mmHg (2nd trimester) or 140/90 mmHg (3rd trimester) or more, or an increase in the systolic blood pressure of 30 mmHg and/or an increase in the diastolic blood pressure of 15 mmHg or more. − With reference to the "Working Group Report on High Blood Pressure in Pregnancy (8/1990, published by the U.S. Department of Health and Human Services), sustained blood pressure increases, which appear during pregnancy, can be classified as follows:

- Pregnancy-specific hypertension:
  - preeclampsia/eclampsia,
  - preeclampsia with pre-existing chronic hypertension (superimposed pre-eclampsia),
  - transient hypertension.
- Non pregnancy-specific hypertension:
  - chronic primary or secondary hypertension.

15.3 Pregnancy-specific hypertension

15.3.1 Preeclampsia/eclampsia

The pregnancy-specific constellation of hypertension, proteinuria and/or edema after the 20th week of pregnancy is referred to as preeclampsia. It is diagnosed by fulfilling one or more of the following criteria:

1. Increase in the systolic blood pressure of 30 mmHg or more
   and/or
2. increase in the diastolic blood pressure of 15 mmHg or more.

The average blood pressure values before the 20th week of pregnancy are used as a reference parameter. If no initial values are available, then blood pressure values $\geq 140/90$ mmHg after the 20th week of pregnancy fulfill the blood pressure-related criteria for a preeclampsia. Proteinuria is present when the protein secretion in the 24-hour urine is 0.3 g or higher. – Edema can be detected during physical inspection. Fluid retention, however, can also occur without the development of edema.

Although preeclampsia always represents a possible risk for mother and child, the following findings are to be interpreted as particularly unfavorable signs:

- Systolic blood pressure above 160 mmHg and/or diastolic blood pressure above 110 mmHg,
- proteinuria of 2.0 g/24 hours or more,
- new increase in the serum creatinine (> 1.2 mg/dl),
- decrease in platelets to less than 100.000 µl and/or evidence of a microangiopathic hemolytic anemia (with increase in the LDH) (the concurrence of hemolysis, elevated liver enzymes and low platelet count has been termed HELLP syndrome),
- increase in hepatic enzymes,
- headache or other neurological irregularities (visual impairment, etc.),
- epigastric pain,
- pulmonary edema,
- pronounced retardation of fetal growth (ultrasonography),
- pathological results from cardiotocography.

If seizures occur in a patient diagnosed with preeclampsia, this is referred to as eclampsia.

15.3.2 Preeclampsia with pre-existing chronic hypertension

The diagnosis of preeclampsia in patients with pre-existing chronic hypertension is based on evidence of an increase in blood pressure (more than 30 mmHg systolic and/or 15 mmHg) in association with proteinuria or generalized edema. The prognosis for mother and child is significantly worse than it is upon the isolated appearance of arterial hypertension or preeclampsia.

15.3.3 Transient (transitory) hypertension

Pathological blood pressure increases which occur in the last trimester up to a maximum of 24 hours post delivery at the latest are termed transient hypertension, as long as no other signs of preeclampsia are present and no hypertension existed prior to pregnancy. In most cases, the blood pressure normalizes again by the 10th day post partum. The probability of developing arterial hypertension later in life is significantly increased in patients with transient high blood pressure.

15.3.4 Pathogenesis of pregnancy-specific hypertension

The course of a normal pregnancy is characterized by a primary vasodilatation of unclear genesis (increase in vasodilative prostaglandins like prostacyclin, PGI_2? arteriovenous fistulas of the placenta?). This leads to a reduction above all in the diastolic blood pressure of about $5-10$ mmHg, to stimulation of the renin angiotensin aldosterone system (RAAS) and to hypervolemia. The increase in plasma volume is accompanied by a relatively slight increase in the erythrocyte count which is apparently an important prerequisite for the normal development of the fetus. In contrast to this, one finds a reduced intravascular volume, vasoconstriction with a resulting increased peripheral vascular resistance and paradoxically little stimulated RAAS (preeclampsia, but not with transitory or pre-existing hypertension) in patients with pregnancy-specific hypertension.

The rationale for the currently most accepted hypothesis on the development of preeclampsia is the assumption of a hypoperfusion of the placenta, for which there is likely a genetic predisposition with an autosomal-recessive hereditary pattern. The reduced placental perfusion may possibly lead to the release of circulating factors (anaphylaxins type C3a, C5a? lipid peroxides? "mitogens"? "cytotoxic substances"?) from trophoblasts. These may have direct vasoconstrictive effects, increase peripheral vascular resistance and thus cause an increase in blood pressure and also induce endothelial lesions. The damage to the endothelial cells leads to a decrease in vasodilatory-acting prostacyclins, an increased release of endothelin and of fribronectin. Fibronectin promotes the aggregation of thrombocytes, which in turn also secrete vasoactive substances like thromboxane and serotonin. Intravascular coagulation, fibrin deposit, generalized vasospasm and endothelial cell damage — so runs the conjecture — might also explain the multi-organ damage observed in severe preeclampsia. Hypertension with preeclampsia is thus only to be viewed as an accompanying symptom of a systemic disease.

15.4 Non pregnancy-specific hypertension

15.4.1 Chronic hypertension

Chronic hypertension during pregnancy is defined as consistently elevated blood pressure values of more than 140/90 mmHg, which were already known before the pregnancy, which are diagnosed during but also before the 20th week of pregnancy or which persist after the 42nd day post partum. Primary or secondary hypertension (renal, endocrine) may be the cause. In general, only the simultaneous finding of renal insufficiency (serum creatinine > 2 mg/dl) with the therefore increased risk of developing preeclampsia (superimposed preeclampsia) have an influence on the prognosis for mother and child.

15.5 Diagnosis and differential diagnosis

The diagnosis of hypertension during pregnancy is performed by comparison with the blood pressure values measured before or at the beginning of the pregnancy, taking into account the pregnancy-specific definitions of hypertension (see above). In contrast to the otherwise common measurement of the diastolic values by the disappearance of the Korotkoff sounds (phase V, see Section 2.2.1.2), the significant quieting of the sounds (phase IV) is taken as the auscultatory criterion for the diastolic blood pressure during pregnancy. In addition, a change in the diurnal rhythm of the blood pressure is typical for late pregnancy, so that measuring blood pressure only in the morning is insufficient. Measuring in the evening is thus recommended, even for routine monitoring. For patients with known, previous renal or hypertensive diseases, multiple measurements at various times of day should be performed alongside particularly close blood pressure monitoring. The prescription of a blood pressure measuring device for patient self-measurement may be advisable, though it should be noted that electronic measuring devices are not suited for this task.

An increase in blood pressure found first in the 20th week of pregnancy is a differential diagnostic indication of pregnancy-specific hypertension. The symptom triad — hypertension, proteinuria and edema — is characteristically observed in primary gestosis and is referred to as preeclampsia. However, proteinuria, in particular, is often initially absent, generally first occur in the third trimester and then normalizing with the blood pressure again around 1 to 2 weeks post-partum and which are subsumed under the term "transient or transitory pregnancy-specific hypertension"

It is not uncommon for the first blood pressure measurements and urine tests a patient ever receives are those performed during pregnancy. For this reason, a clear differentiation between pregnancy-specific and pre-existing renal or hypertensive disease is often not possible on the basis of patient history and laboratory diagnostic tests.

The performance of costly differential diagnostic examinations during the pregnancy is very difficult and is only therapeutically relevant in exceptional cases. Most authors thus recommend that a differentiated diagnostic work-up for hypertension be performed first a few months post-partum.

One should not pass up the opportunity, however, of supplementing routinely performed ultrasonographic monitoring with a careful sonographic inspection of the mother's renal and suprarenal region. During pregnancy as well, the ultrasonographic demonstration of an adrenal tumor, in particular, demands the definitive exclusion or inclusion of a pheochromocytoma, as the appropriate therapeutic measures must be initiated (see Section 14.1).

Summary (Chapter 15)

- Hypertension during pregnancy is present when the following are measured:
  - persistently increased systolic blood pressure values of 135 mmHg (2nd trimester) or 140 mmHg (3rd trimester) or more,
  - persistently increased diastolic blood pressure values of 85 mmHg (2nd trimester) or 90 mmHg (3rd trimester) or more,
  - an increase in the blood pressure during pregnancy of 30 mmHg systolic or more and/or 15 mmHg diastolic or more.
- Hypertension during pregnancy is either
  - due to a pregnancy-specific cause (preeclampsia/eclampsia, preeclampsia with pre-existing hypertension, transitory/transient hypertension) or
  - is based on a pre-existing, non pregnancy-specific cause (primary hypertension, renal or endocrine hypertension, etc.).
- The diagnosis of preeclampsia is probable, when hypertension develops after the 20th week of pregnancy and is accompanied by proteinuria and edema.
- The most dangerous complication of preeclampsia is eclampsia, which is to be viewed as a hypertensive encephalopathy, the course of which is frequently lethal.
- Preeclampsia is characterized by increased peripheral vascular resistance, a paradoxically lowered activity of the RAAS, hemoconcentration and an activation of the intravascular coagulation system. Hypertension is only a concomitant symptom to this presumably autosomally recessive inherited, systemic disease.
- Transient hypertension is not accompanied by proteinuria and edema formation.

All pregnancy-specific increases in blood pressure are reversible and the therapy of choice is delivery. Preeclampsia/eclampsia, superimposed preeclampsia and transient hypertension are thus to be categorized as secondary forms of hypertension.

Literature (Chapter 15)

August P, Mueller FB, Sealey JE, Edersheim TG. Role of renin-angiotensin system in blood pressure regulation in pregnancy. Lancet 1995; 345: 896–897.

Cunningham FG, Lindheimer MD. Hypertension in pregnancy. N Engl J Med 1992; 326: 927–932.

Deutsche Liga zur Bekämpfung des hohen Blutdruckes e.V. Hochdruck in der Schwangerschaft, 2. Aufl. Heidelberg 1991.

Friedberg V. Pathophysiologie des Schwangerschaftshochdrucks. Gynäkologe 1992; 25: 370–385.

Ginsburg J, Duncan S. Direct and indirect blood pressure measurement in pregnancy. J Obstet Gynaecol Br Commonw 1969; 76: 705–710.

Girndt J. Ursachen der Hypertonie in der Schwangerschaft. Nieren Hochdruckkrkh 1993; 22: 602–604.

Lyall F, Greer IA. Pre-eclampsia: a multifaceted vascular disorder of pregnancy. J Hypertens 1994; 12: 1339–1345.

Kaplan NM. Hypertension induced by pregnancy, oral contraceptives, and postmenopausal replacement therapy. Cardiol Clin 1988; 6: 475–482.

National High Blood Pressure Education Program (NHBPEP). Working group report on high blood pressure in pregnancy. US Department of Health and Human Services, National Institutes of Health, National Heart, Lung, and Blood Institute. NIH Publication No. 90–3029, 1990.

Roberts JM, Redman CWG. Pre-eclampsia: more than pregnancy-induced hypertension. Lancet 1993; 341: 1447–1454.

Robillard PY, Hulsey TC, Perianin J, Janky E, Miri EH, Papiernik E. Association of pregnancy-induced hypertension with duration of sexual cohabitation before conception. Lancet 1994; 344: 973–975.

WHO Study Group. The hypertensive disorders of pregnancy. WHO Tech Rep Ser 1987; 758: 1–114.

16 Cardiovascular hypertension

All chronic increases in blood pressure, which have a primary cardiac and/or a primary aortic cause, are considered cardiovascular forms of hypertension. Differentiation can be made between diseases associated with a combined systolic/diastolic hypertension (coarctation of the aorta) and those associated with an isolated increase in systolic blood pressure (Table 16.1).

Table 16.1: Classification of cardiovascular hypertension

Primary cardiac causes (hypertension following increased cardiac output):

 – Hyperkinetic circulation
 – Aortic valvular insufficiency
 – Atrioventricular block III°

Primary aortic causes:

 – Sclerosis of the aorta ("windkessel hypertension")
 – Congenital stenoses of the aorta (coarctation of the aorta)
  – Stenosis of the aortic isthmus/arch
  – Atypical localizations of aortic coarctation

16.1 Coarctation of the aorta

Congenital constrictions of the aorta are referred to as coarctation of the aorta. In 98% of all cases they affect the isthmus section of the aorta (stenosis of the aortic isthmus). Other, atypical localizations are the aortic arch, the throracic aorta and the abdominal aorta (see below). In all forms of coarctatio aortae, one finds a more-or-less strongly pronounced arterial hypertension in the prestenotic sections. The intrarenal constriction of the abdominal aorta is generally accompanied by normotone blood pressure values and thus represents an exception.

16.1.1 Pathogenesis of hypertension

The prestenotic increase in the arterial blood pressure is, above all, to be interpreted pathogenetically as a reactive adaptation to the increase in vascular resistance.

It is possible, however, that reduced renal perfusion leads to an activation of the renin angiotensin aldosterone system (RAAS). Thus this humoral mechanism may also contribute to the maintenance of hypertension at least in the forms of coarctation of the aorta located proximal to the suprarenal arteries.

The existence and extent of the hypertension are determined by the degree of aortic coarctation.

16.1.2 Stenosis of the aortic isthmus: pathological-anatomical differentiation

The constriction of the aorta in the isthmus region is by far the most common localization of a congenital aortic coarctation. A pathological-anatomical differentiation is made between two principally different forms of stenosis of the aortic isthmus: the preductal (previously referred to as "infantile type") form with stenosis of the aorta and the postductal (previously referred to as "adult") form with constriction of the aortic vessel distal to the junction with the ductus arteriosus (ligamentum arteriosum) (Figure 16.1). Additional malformations are frequently present in both forms: in the preductal form, these are generally ventricular septal defects, severe changes in the aortic valve and a persistent ductus arteriosus. As a compensatory short circuit, the latter leads to a mixed cyanosis of the lower half of the body. The resulting complaints are the symptoms of a severe heart failure, already found in newborns and infants, which, if untreated, quickly leads to death. Around 60% of the patients with the postductal form have slight accompanying malformations. These are mostly aortic and mitral valve defects, occasionally also a small persisting ductus arteriosus. This form of stenosis of the aortic isthmus often remains undiscovered in infants, as it is much less likely to lead to a quickly progressing form of heart failure. Increasing left-heart hypertrophy and comparatively slower development of myocardial insufficiency come to the fore in these patients. In almost all cases, these patients develop a collateral circulation, which frequently lead to radiologically detectable rib lesions in the area of the affected hypertrophied intercostal arteries.

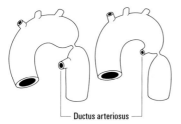

Ductus arteriosus

Figure 16.1: The aortic isthmus as the by far most frequent localization of an aortic coarctation (ca. 98 %).
Left side: Preductal type, stenosis located proximal to the ductus arteriosus (ligamentum arteriosum); frequently associated with right-to-left shunt).
Right side: Postductal type of aortic coarctation, stenosis located distal to the ductus arteriosus.

16.1.2.1 Atypical localizations of aortic coarctation

The various other localizations of aortic coarctation (aortic arch, descending aorta, suprarenal and interrenal abdominal aorta) are usually accompanied by arterial hypertension. The absence of increased arterial blood pressure values in infrarenal localizations of coarctation of the aorta underlines the probability of a pathogenic significance for the RAAS in the maintenance of hypertension in the other forms. In the differential diagnosis, these extremely rare congenital malformations of the aorta must be differentiated from acquired aortic changes, which may appear, for example, in the context of (mostly aortic) arteritis (Takayasu's disease; see also Figure 13.1).

16.1.3 Diagnosis

As a rule, the presence of a stenosis of the aortic isthmus in infancy is generally accompanied by pronounced clinical symptoms due to a progressively developing global heart failure. A typical cyanosis of the lower extremities develops already in newborns, due to the shunting of blood from the descending aorta through the pulmonary artery via the open ductus arteriosus. As has already been mentioned, this is generally accompanied by a preductal, multiple, and lengthy stenosis of the aortic vessel, as well as further severe accompanying malformations.

The diagnosis of a stenosis of the aortic isthmus after the first year of life is often made accidentally during a routine examination, because patients are often completely free of complaints during adolescence and early adulthood. Headaches, cold legs, low capacity for physical stress, tinnitus, visual impairment and nose bleeds are non-specific, hypertension-related symptoms, which are present in about 50% of affected patients. The leading clinical symptom of stenosis of the aortic isthmus is arterial hypertension in the upper body half with simultaneous low blood pressure conditions in the lower body region. A strong pulse in the arms and a barely perceptible or absent pulse in the feet are often noticed in the physical examination. With moderate aortic constriction, normotone blood pressure values can be measured in the arms under resting conditions. However, with physical exercise, these values increase inordinately in comparison to the pressure in the legs. Auscultatory examination reveals a late systolic murmur, whose maximum is projected left parasternally to the 2nd and 3rd intercostal space. In addition, systolic-diastolic vascular bruits can almost always be heard between the shoulder blades. Electrocardiographic examination produces mostly normal results during the early phases of the disease. Signs of left ventricular hypertrophy and occasionally non-specific conduction disorders, however, do appear with increasing duration and stress on the left ventricle. Left ventricular, hypertensive-related hypertrophy is also characteristic of the radiological picture of stenosis of the aortic isthmus. In addition, X-rays of the thorax often show costal lesions or erosions, which be accepted as radiological evidence of a collateral circulation.

Although the diagnosis of stenosis of the aortic isthmus can be made clinically (blood pressure measurement, auscultation), aortography should be performed in every case, at the latest before the initiation of specific therapeutic measures.

16.1.4 The therapy of stenosis of the aortic isthmus

Because the average life expectancy of patients with an untreated stenosis of the aortic isthmus is only 30−35 years due to worsening of heart failure and additional complications, corrective surgery should be performed in every case. The optimal time for operation is 9 years of age or less.

Dilatation of a stenosis of the aortic isthmus with the use of a balloon catheter has become technically possible over the past several years, both for children and adults. However, long-term observations have shown aneurysmatic changes in the aorta in the region of the dilatation site in some patients. These changes required surgical correction. Due to the limited experience, the value of balloon angioplasty can thus not be definitively evaluated in comparison to surgical correction of stenosis of the aortic isthmus at the present time.

Hypertension sometimes persists, even after the successful repair of the stenosis. While the pathogenic cause for this can be linked to residual stenosis in only a minority of patients, the cause remains unknown for the majority. Because the likelihood of persistent hypertension after correction increases relative to the length of the existing malformation, it is conceivable that the central blood pressure regulating mechanisms adapt themselves to the hypertension which has existed since earliest childhood. After correction, they may thus aim at a "false normalization" of the blood pressure within the hypertensive range.

Summary (Section 16.1)

- Congenital coarctation of the aorta is an infrequent, but potentially curable form of secondary hypertension.
- The region of the aortic isthmus (stenosis of the aortic isthmus) is by far the most common localization (98%) of congenital aortic coarctation.
- The leading clinical symptom of stenosis of the aortic isthmus diagnosed after the first year of life is arterial hypertension in the upper body half with simultaneous hypotension in the lower body region.
- An untreated stenosis of the aortic isthmus leads to progressive, hypertension-related heart failure with an average life expectancy of 30−35 years of age.
- The established therapy for all forms of aortic coarctation is operative correction of the stenosis. Balloon angioplasty is becoming increasingly significant as an alternative form of treatment.

16.2 Systolic cardiovascular hypertension

For a cardiac disease, an isolated increase in systolic arterial blood pressure is the consequence of a compensatory increase in stroke volume.

16.2.1 Hyperkinetic heart syndrome

In younger tachycardiac patients, the systolic hypertension resulting from increased stroke volume indicates the presence of hyperkinetic heart syndrome. The suspected cause of the increased sympathetic tone is an increased sensibility of the beta$_1$-adrenergic receptors to the normal or slightly increased release of endogenous catecholamines. An additional, inadequate increase in the heart rate and blood pressure is found with exercise stress. The consequence is a limited capacity for physical exercise. Patients with hyperkinetic heart syndrome show a normalization of blood pressure, tachycardia and defined capacity for bicycle/treadmill ergometric exercise test when under beta-receptor blockade drug therapy.

In the differential diagnosis, the possibility of hyperthyroidism, in particular, must be excluded.

16.2.2 Aortic valvular insufficiency

The increased amplitude of the blood pressure found in aortic valvular insufficiency is related to an increase in systolic and a decrease in diastolic blood pressure values. The cause of the increased amplitude of the blood pressure is an increased stroke volume, the sum of which is taken from the amount of blood actually ejected into the aorta and the amount regurgitated.

16.2.3 Sclerosis of the aorta (Windkessel hypertension)

The isolated systolic hypertension of the elderly is usually the expression of a decrease in the aortic Windkessel function, as a consequence of the increasing, arteriosclerosis-related loss of elasticity in the vessel wall. A reduction in arterial blood pressure is observed in diastole, resulting in a significantly increased amplitude of the blood pressure.

16.2.4 Severe bradycardia

Severe bradycardia is often accompanied by an increase in systolic blood pressure. This systolic hypertension is the consequence of a compensatory increase in stroke volume. Severe bradycardia are observed, for example, in 3rd degree atrioventricular blocks, which are characterized by complete atrial and ventricular dissociation. The resulting ventricular escape rhythm from the region of the AV node or from tertiary ventricular centers can be recognized with electrocardiography in the bundle branch block-like widening that is not associated to the P-waves.

16.2.5 Other cardiovascular diseases accompanied by systolic hypertension

Other, uncommon cardiovascular diseases accompanied by systolic hypertension are:

– patent ductus arteriosus,
– aorto-pulmonary window (hole in the septum between the aorta and pulmonary artery immediately after their exit from the heart),
– arteriovenous fistulas.

Summary (Section 16.2)

• The systolic hypertension present in cardiovascular forms of hypertension is conditioned by the frequently compensatorily increased stroke volume. In almost all forms there is a reduction in diastolic blood pressure.

• The most common causes of cardiovascular-related systolic hypertension are:

– hyperkinetic heart syndrome and
– increasing sclerosis of the aorta with loss of elasticity.

Literature (Chapter 16)

Cohen M, Fuster V, Steele PM, Driscoll D, McGoon DC. Coarctation of the aorta. Long-term follow-up and prediction of outcome after surgical correction. Circulation 1989; 80: 840–845.

Gillum RF, Teichholz LE, Herman MV, Gorlin R. The idiopathic hyperkinetic heart syndrome: clinical course and long-term prognosis. Am Heart J 1981; 102: 728–734.

Rocchini AP. Cardiovascular causes of systemic hypertension. Pediatr Clin N Am 1991; 40: 141–156.

Shaddy RE, Boucek MM, Sturtevant JE, Ruttenberg HD, Jaffe RB, Tani LY, Judd VE, Veasy LG, McGough EC, Orsmond GS. Comparision of angioplasty and surgery for unoperated coarctation of the aorta. Circulation 1993; 87: 793–799.

Stewart AB, Ahmed R, Travill CM, Newman CGH. Coarctation of the aorta: life and health 20–44 years after surgical repair. Br Heart J 1993; 69: 65–70.

17 Hypertension induced by medication or other substances/drug-induced hypertension

Although a large number of drugs can potentially induce and maintain arterial hypertension (Table 17.1 and, also, Table 29.2), the development of hypertension from these medications is in no way the rule and should be viewed as the exception. The diagnosis of hypertension caused by intake of medication or other substances (i. e. alcohol) is generally based on the patient history and a positive withdrawal trial for the substance in question.

In the following sections, a few medications and substances are presented in more detail, because, on the one hand, they are generally taken chronically and, on the other, they induce arterial hypertension with above-average frequency.

Table 17.1: Examples of drugs which may cause hypertension

Substance	Mechanism
Monoamine oxidase inhibitors	(tyramine related) Stimulation of sympathetic nervous system
Sympathomimetics − Nose drops (phenylephrine) − Broncholytics − Catecholamines	Stimulation of sympathetic nervous system
Tricyclic antidepressants (Imipramine and others)	Stimulation of sympathetic nervous system? (Inhibition of neuronal reuptake of norepinephrine)
Thyroid hormones	Thyroxine effect
Oral contraceptives	Sodium retention (?) Stimulation of renin angiotensin system (?)
Nonsteroidal anti-inflammatory agents (Phenylbutazone and others)	Sodium retention? Inhibition of prostaglandin synthesis
Carbenoxolone, licorice	Sodium retention
Glucocorticoids	Sodium retention (?), incresae of vascular reactivity to Ang II and norepinephrine
Cyclosporine	Stimulation of sympathetic nervous system? Sodium retention? Increased synthesis and release of endothelin (ET-1)?
Erythropoietin	Unknown

17.1 Oral contraceptives and post-menopausal hormone replacement therapy

17.1.1 Oral contraceptives (OCs)

The intake of oral contraceptives (OC) leads to a slight increase in blood pressure within the normal range in most women. In a few cases, however, arterial hypertension develops and is reversible with the discontinuation of the OC intake. It is possible that the incidence of OC-related hypertension was overestimated in the past, because the first generation of OCs contained a significantly higher amount of estrogen. Nonetheless, many premenopansal women do display a higher sensitivity to exogenously administered estrogen and they also develop arterial hypertension with the administration of the currently common OCs with low estrogen and progesterone content. Higher age, obesity, a low-grade renal insufficiency or genetic factors can represent additional predisposing factors for the development of hypertension under therapy with OCs. The question as to whether OC-induced hypertension should be interpreted as unmasked primary hypertension still can not be answered.

The pathogenesis of OC-induced hypertension has not been clearly explained. Increased sodium retention may play a role in the development of hypertension, as both estrogen and a portion of the synthetic progestagen contained in contraceptives (in contrast to the natriuretic effect of endogenous progesterones) have sodium-retentive properties.

An stimulation of the renin angiotensin aldosterone system (RAAS) is seen in more-or-less all patients who take OCs over a longer time period. This stimulation of the RAAS is the result of estrogen-related increases in the hepatic formation of angiotensinogen with its subsequent transformation into vasoactive Ang II. There is also a consequent stimulation of aldosterone release (secondary aldosteronism). The pathophysiological significance of RAAS activation for the development and maintenance of hypertension, however, has still not been clarified.

The diagnosis of OC hypertension results from the normalization of blood pressure after its discontinuation of administration. This normalization is observed after 1−3 months in most cases and over a longer time period in a few cases. If hypertension persists over a time period of more than 6 months after interrupting the administration of the "pill", this suggests the presence of a primary, renal or endocrine hypertension.

From a medical perspective, the development of hypertension with the administration of oral contraceptives demands the discontinuation of treatment in every case. For psycho-social reasons, however, such a discontinuation can be particularly difficult when no other possible forms of contraception offer a realistic alternative due to a lack of tolerance to or rejection of these methods by the woman or her partner. The same difficulty is encountered in patients with known hypertension who do not want to have children and for whom the intake of OCs alone can be expected to offer a reliable form of contraception for reasons already mentioned.

Although arterial hypertension represents a relative contraindication for the intake of OCs and, vice versa, OCs are to be discontinued on principle upon development of hypertension (see above), a blanket solution for difficult cases should definitely be rejected. As is so often the case, the decision of the physician here must be oriented on the individual case. In the process of deciding, however, one should confront the conceptual possibility that, in exceptional cases, the continuation of OCs despite mild hypertension may be the "lesser evil". Diuretics offer a first-line medication with antihypertensive effectiveness for the continuing intake of oral ovulation inhibitors, because they counteract the increased sodium retention.

Therapy with OCs is contraindicated in every case for patients who have pre-existing or are developing moderately or severe hypertension, upon the presence of additional cardiovascular risk factors and where hypertension-related end-organ damage exists.

17.1.2 Post-menopausal hormone replacement therapy (HRT)

The presence of arterial hypertension does not present a contraindication for the initiation of after menopause hormone replacement therapy (HRT), because the administration of low dosages of estrogen, in particular, is usually accompanied by a lowering of blood pressure and a beneficial effect on other cardiovascular risk factors. Regular blood pressure monitoring is still recommended, however, because the development of hypertension has been observed in individual post-menopausal women in extremely rare cases.

Due to an increased incidence of neoplasias of the cervix with therapy with estrogen alone, the administration of a combined (estrogen/progesterone) HRT is increasingly preferred (exception: history of hysterectomy). Although the blood pressure-lowering effect of estrogen may thus be eliminated or at least reduced by the additional administration of progesterone, there exist no contraindications for the combined HRT for patients with arterial hypertension.

Summary (Section 17.1)

- The intake of OCs can cause an arterial hypertension, which is generally reversible after discontinuation.

- A long-term administration of OCs must therefore be accompanied by regular blood pressure measurement.

- The diagnosis of OC-induced hypertension is justified when increased blood pressure returns to normal (ca. 3−6 months) after discontinuation of OC intake:

- Postmenopausal HRT does not normally increase blood pressure and is thus not contraindicated for patients with arterial hypertension.

17.2 Carbenoxolone- and licorice-induced hypertension (pseudoaldosteronism)

Heavy consumption of licorice and a drug therapy with carbenoxolone can induce hypokalemic hypertension, whereby the causative mineralocorticoid effect is triggered by the glycyrrhetinic acids contained in these substances. This results in a corresponding increase in sodium and water resorption in the distal tubules comparable to the effect of aldosterone. The diagnosis generally results from a carefully investigated patient history and the proof of a hypokalemic hypoaldosteronism with suppressed renin secretion. After the discontinuation of licorice or medication intake the blood pressure usually normalizes within a short period of time. Like the hypokalemia, the hormonal changes are also reversible.

If no carbenoxolone or licorice consumption can be detected when the constellation of laboratory results described above are found, an autonomous production of mineralocorticoid-effective precursors of steroid synthesis should be considered in the differential diagnosis (Section 14.4)

Summary (Section 17.2)

- The glycyrrhetinic acid contained in licorice and carbenoxolone is mineralocorticoid-effective and can induce hypokalemic hypertension.
- Every case of hypokalemic hypertension requires the exclusion (via patient history) of carbenoxolone or licorice consumption.
- In contrast to primary aldosteronism, the aldosterone secretion is suppressed.

17.3 Glucocorticoid therapy

In comparison to autonomous endogenous hypercortisolism (Section 14.5), hypertension under the exogenous administration of glucocorticoids is much less frequently observed. It is usually possible to control hypertension in patients who have received a kidney transplant through dosage reduction or through an alternating pattern of therapy days and therapy-free days. Low-dosed long-term therapy with glucocorticoids, such as is common to widely varied diseases, is not likely to trigger hypertension.

17.4 Erythropoietin

Recombinant human erythropoietin (EPO) is increasingly being used in the treatment of dialysis patients with renal anemia. Approximately $30-35\%$ of the patients on this therapy, however, develop an increase in peripheral vascular resistance with consecutive arterial hypertension. The pathogenesis of the development of hypertension can not be satisfactorily explained by an increase in the hemocrit or a direct vasoconstrictive effect of the EPO. Hypertension is less frequently observed with a slow increase of the hematocrit, possibly because there is sufficient time for processes of adjustment.

Hypertension under EPO therapy is conventionally treated with the usual antihypertensive effective medications. If no sufficient decrease in blood pressure can be achieved, the EPO dosage should be reduced or temporarily discontinued.

Summary (Section 17.4)

- Approximately one-third of the patients treated with erythropoetin (EPO) develop arterial hypertension of currently unclear genesis.
- The treatment of hypertension does not show any particularities. If no satisfactory control of blood pressure can be achieved with medications, the EPO dosage should be reduced or temporarily discontinued.

17.5 Cyclosporine

Cyclosporine has been therapeutically used for the suppression of endogenous immune response after organ transplantation since 1983. In addition, cyclosporine is used in the local and systemic treatment of various autoimmune diseases. Hypertension is relatively frequently associated with cyclosporine treatment. Approximately 50−70% of all transplant recipients and approximately 20% of patients who are treated with cyclosporine for other reasons develop hypertension. The suspected cause is an increased renal sodium retention, which is in turn the consequence of a constriction of the afferent arteriole with a decrease of the renal blood flow and the glomular filtration rate. The vascular constriction under cyclosporine is likely based on various mechanisms, such as an activation of the sympathetic nervous system, an increased formation and release of endothelin, an increased responsiveness of the renal vascular musculature to vasopressors, changes in the local prostaglandin production and a disturbed arteriolar production of nitric oxide (NO). While the arteriolar vasospasm is functional and thus generally reversible at the beginning of cyclosporine therapy, after some years morphological changes begin to set in, which in their further development are accompanied by nephrosclerosis. At this stage pathological changes are irreversible.

The therapeutic efforts in cyclosporine-associated hypertension are thus aimed at reducing the dosage of cyclosporine or at switching to a therapy with azathioprin. If it is not possible to do without the administration of cyclosporine, then calcium antagonists (dilation of the afferent arterioles), combined alpha/beta adrenergic blockers (labetalol) or centrally acting adrenergic alpha-blockers are recommended. It should be noted that calcium antagonists elevate the plasma level of cyclosporine. The sodium retention and the increased intravascular volume suppress renin secretion and thus may explain the poor effectiveness of ACE inhibitors in cyclosporine-induced hypertension.

Summary (Section 17.5)

- Cyclosporine induces intrarenal changes, which lead to sodium and water retention.
- These changes, which lead to hypertension in most patients, are initially reversible through dosage reduction or discontinuation of the cyclosporine therapy.

17.6 Alcohol

The relationship between the consumption of alcohol and hypertension has long been known. While acute alcohol consumption tends to have a blood pressure reducing effect, chronic alcohol consumption leads to an increase in the arterial blood pressure. It is estimated that alcohol is responsible for the increase in blood pressure in approximately 10% of the patients with hypertension. The pathogenesis of alcohol-induced hypertension is not known. Currently under discussion are a stimulation of the sympathetic nervous system, an increased secretion of glucocorticoids, an increased insulin resistance with reactively increased insulin secretion (hyperinsulinemia) and an increased cellular uptake of free calcium ions (with consecutive increase in the peripheral vascular resistance).

Discontinuation of alcohol consumption leads to a decrease in blood pressure and should thus be the first therapeutic measure for hypertensive patients with the corresponding history.

Summary (Section 17.6)

- Alcohol is possibly the most common cause of secondary hypertension.
- Discontinuation of alcohol consumption thus represents therapy of choice for chronic hypertension in many cases.

Literature (Chapter 17)

Abe H, Kawano Y, Kojima S, Ashida T, Kuramochi M, Matsuoka H, Omae T. Biphasic effects of repeated alcohol intake on 24-hour blood pressure in hypertensive patients. Circulation 1994; 89: 2626–2633.

Beilin LJ. Alcohol, hypertension and cardiovascular disease. J Hypertens 1995; 13: 939–942.
Bennett WM, Porter GA. Cyclosporine-associated hypertension. Am J Med 1988; 85: 131–132.

Bokemeyer D, Meyer-Lehnert H, Kramer HJ. Rolle von Endothelin bei den Ciclosporin-Nebenwirkungen Nephrotoxizität und arterielle Hypertonie. Dtsch med Wschr 1994; 119: 1706−1711.

Canadian Erythropoeitin Study Group. Effect of recombinant human erythropoeitin therapy on blood pressure in haemodialysis patients. Am J Nephrol 1991; 11: 23−26.

Driscoll DF, Pinson CW, Jenkins RL, Bistrian BR. Potential protective effects of frusemide against early renal injury in liver transplant patients receiving cyclosporin A. Critical Care Med 1989; 17: 1341−1343.

Farese Jr RV, Biglieri EG, Shackleton CHL, Irony I, Gomez-Fontes R. Licorice-induced hyper-mineralocorticoidism. N Engl J Med 1991; 325: 1223−1227.

Glim K, Isles CG, Hodsman GP, Lever AF, Robertson JWK. Malignant hypertension in women of childbearing age and its relation to the contraceptive pill. Br Med J 1987; 294: 1057−1059.

Malatino LS, Glen L, Wilson ESB. The effects of low-dose estrogen-progesteron oral contraceptives on blood pressure and the renin-angiotensin system. Curr Ther Res 1988; 43: 743−749.

Randin D, Vollenweider P, Tappy L, Jequier E, Nicod P, Scherrer U. Suppression of alcohol-induced hypertension by dexamethason. N Engl J Med 1995; 332: 1733−1737.

Sturrock NDC, Lang CC, Struthers AD. Cyclosporin induced hypertension precedes renal dysfunction and sodium retention in man. J Hypertens 1993; 11: 1209−1216.

Sturrock NDC, Lang CC, Coutie WJ, Struthers AD. Cyclosporin-induced renal vasoconstriction is augmented by frusemide and by angiotensin II in humans. J Hypertens 1995; 13: 987−991.

Victor RG, Hansen J. Alcohol and blood pressure − a drink a day... N Engl J Med 1995; 332: 1782−1783.

Walker BR, Edwards CRW. Licorice-induced hypertension and syndromes of apparent mineralocorticoid excess. Endocrinol Metab Clin N Am 1994; 23: 359−377.

Wing LMH, Tonkin AL. Drug-induced hypertension. In: Swales JD (ed). Textbook of Hypertension. Blackwell Scientific Publications, London 1994: 923−940.

Yamakado M, Umezu M, Negano M, Tagawa H. Mechanisms of hypertension induced by erythropoeitin in patients on hemodialysis. Clin Invest Med 1991; 14: 623−629.

18 Neurogenic hypertension

The term "neurogenic hypertension" refers to all chronic forms of hypertension, which are attributable to neurological diseases.

18.1 Sleep apnea syndrome

Sleep apnea syndrome is accompanied by arterial hypertension with above-average frequency.

Sleep apnea syndrome is defined as the appearance of at least five episodes of nocturnal interruption of breathing (apnea index > 5/h). The cessation of breathing is usually preceded by loud, irregular snoring. The sudden interruption of breathing, lasting up to 90 seconds, can lead to pronounced arterial hypoxemia. The cessation of breathing are terminated by arousal from sleep, of which the subject is often not conscious. A causal differentiation is made between a central (the lack of central activation of the muscle groups necessary for breathing), and obstructive (inspiratory obstruction of the upper respiratory tract by relaxation or inactivation of the muscle groups which keep the extrathoracic respiratory tract open) and a combined central/obstructive form of sleep apnea syndrome. The latter form is the most common one and is found in approximately 2−4% of all male and 1−2% of all female adults.

Patients with sleep apnea syndrome complain of extreme daytime fatigue, the likely consequence of the interruption of sleep, the shortening of the deep sleep phase and the reduction of the REM ("rapid eye movement") sleep. Correspondingly, the patients affected are approximately 2−3 times more likely to be involved in traffic accidents than normal persons. Patients with sleep apnea syndrome are more likely to acquire and also die from coronary heart disease or a stroke than the average population.

The intermittent, nocturnal increases in blood pressure during the apneic phases and immediately thereafter are most likely caused by activation of the sympathetic nervous system, triggered by repeated sleeping disturbances (with shortening of the deep sleep phase and the reduction of the REM sleep). However, it is unclear how these transient, nocturnal increases in blood pressure can lead to a lasting hypertension, which persists during the day. Obesity is to be discussed as a possible cause of the hypertension, as it is found in a majority of patients with sleep apnea syndrome and is also accompanied by arterial hypertension with above-average frequency.

The suspicion of a sleep apnea syndrome is justified in overweight, hypertensive patients with sleeping disorders and pronounced daytime fatigue for whom a third person report (e.g., spouse) shows loud and irregular snoring, broken by the cessation of breathing. In addition, if the physical examination reveals signs of a constriction of the upper respiratory tract, muscular disease, disorders and/or diseases of the sympathetic nervous system, targeted diagnostic measures are to be initiated (for example, a graduated program for the diagnosis of disturbances of the nocturnal respiratory and circulatory regulation has been put together by the German Pneumology Society). The final diagnosis of sleep apnea syndrome occurs with the help of polysomnography, which is costly in terms of methodology and personnel and which can only be conducted under hospitalized conditions.

General therapeutic measures for verified sleep apnea syndrome are weight reduction, restriction of alcohol consumption (alcohol can strengthen the obstruction through a relaxing effect of the pharyngeal musculature) and the avoidance of medications with a depressing effect on respiration (sleeping pills and sedatives, beta receptor blockers). The most successful therapy for apnea is nasal continuous positive airway pressure (nCPAP), which can lead to a normalization of arterial blood pressure.

Summary (Section 18.1)

- The sleep apnea syndrome is characterized by recurrent nocturnal cessation of breathing.
- Sleep disturbances, daytime fatigue, and irregular snoring, interrupted by cessation of breathing are the leading symptoms of sleep apnea syndrome.
- The combined central/obstructive form of apnea is the most common and affects 4% of male and 2% of female adults.
- Sleep apnea syndrome is accompanied by obesity and arterial hypertension with above-average frequency.
- Patients with sleep apnea syndrome are more likely to acquire and also die from coronary heart disease and/or stroke than the normal population.
- The diagnosis of sleep apnea syndrome is made with the use of polysomnography.
- The most successful therapy is nasal continuous positive airway pressure (nCPAP).

18.2 Other neurogenic causes of arterial hypertension

The following neurological diseases can also cause arterial hypertension:

- Increased intracranial pressure (e.g., as result of a tumor),
- Guillain-Barre syndrome,

− meningitis,

− encephalitis,

− quadriplegia.

These disorders are not given close attention in this book, because their therapy of choice (to the degree possible) represents a neurological or neurosurgical problem.

Their symptomatic drug treatment follows the usual therapeutic guidelines for blood pressure reduction.

Literature (Chapter 18)

Douglas NJ, Polo O. Pathogenesis of obstructive sleep apnoea/hypopnoea syndrome. Lancet 1994; 344: 653−655.

Dickinson CJ. Hypertension and central nervous system disease. In: Swales JD (ed). Textbook of Hypertension. Blackwell Scientific Publishing, Oxford 1994, 980−986.

Hla KM, Young TB, Bidwell T, Palta M, Skatrud JB, Dempsey J. Sleep apnea and hypertension. A population-based study. Ann Intern Med 1994; 120: 382−388.

Hoffstein V. Blood pressure, snoring, obesity, and nocturnal hypoxaemia. Lancet 1994; 344: 643−645.

Phillipson EA. Sleep apnea − a major public health problem. N Engl J Med 1993; 328: 1271−1273.

Polo O, Berthon-Jones M, Douglas NJ, Sullivan CE. Management of obstructive sleep apnoea/hypopnoea syndrome. Lancet 1994; 344: 656−660.

Wiemann J, Sanner B, Sturm A. Schlafapnoesyndrom. Dtsch med Wschr 1992; 117: 1928−1934.

Young T, Palta M, Dempsey J, Skatrud J, Weber S, Badr S. The occurence of sleep-disordered breathing among middle-aged adults. N Engl J Med 1993; 328: 1230−1235.

III Management

19 General therapeutic aspects of arterial hypertension

19.1 Fundamentals of treatment

Chronically elevated arterial blood pressure demands treatment. The goal of therapy is the reduction of the morbidity and mortality associated with high blood pressure while making as little use as possible of treatment associated with side-effects. To this end, most therapy guidelines recommend reducing blood pressure to a level below 140/90 mmHg (casual blood pressure measurement) or below 135/85 mmHg (continuous ambulatory blood pressure monitoring). To what extent a greater reduction in already normal blood pressure may lead to a further decrease in cardiovascular risk is still unknown. Retrospective evaluation of long-term studies in which the number of cardiac episodes in relation to diastolic blood pressure level was therapeutically reduced has yielded a J-shaped curve (Figure 19.1): A reduction in blood pressure to 90 mmHg during antihypertensive treatment reduced the frequency of ischemic heart disease, whereas reduction to diastolic blood pressure levels below 85 mmHg caused a renewed increase. The SHEP Study, among others, did not validate the J-curve hypothesis. This study primarily examined the effect of a medicinal treatment (ACE inhibitors) on morbidity and mortality in older patients with isolated systolic hypertension. In this study, the medicinal reduction of average diastolic blood pressure from 77 mmHg (starting point) to 67 mmHg (end point) was accompanied by a 25% reduction in cardioischemic episodes. Since a refutation or validation of the J-curve hypothesis or its associated therapeutic implications is currently impossible in the absence of appropriate prospective studies, it seems advisable not to reduce systolic blood pressure below 125 mmHg, or diastolic blood pressure below 85 mmHg. Particu-

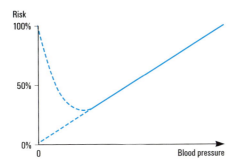

Figure 19.1: The "J-shaped curve"-theory: Relationship beween blood pressure and the risk of morbidity and mortality. (Adapted from Hannson L, Am J Hypertens 1988; 1: 414—420)

larly in older patients, a lowering of blood pressure below these values should be carried out only under the strictest observation of cardiac and (to the extent possible) cerebral functions.

Treatment methods for arterial hypertension can in principal be categorized as non-drug and drug therapy.

19.1.1 Deciding on the type and urgency of treatment

The type and urgency of therapeutic intervention must be determined individually in every case. It is nevertheless a rule of thumb that the lowering or normalizing of elevated arterial blood pressure should be brought about slowly. The attending physician should in any case refrain from switching modes of therapy too quickly, since their effectiveness frequently takes weeks (drug therapy) or months (changes in lifestyle or eating habits) to assess (see below).

In contrast, cases of moderate, severe or malignant hypertension (USA: Stages 2−4), always calls for a medicinal treatment whose effectiveness can be judged in the shortest time possible. Too dramatic a decrease in blood pressure should in any case be avoided because of the possibility of reduced cardiac and/or cerebral perfusion (Table 19.1). − The treatment of a hypertensive crisis is dealt with separately (Section 32.1).

Table 19.1:   Recommendations for diagnostic and therapeutic procedures in relation to the severity of hypertension*

Severity/stage	Diagnostic procedure	Therapeutic procedure
Mild:**		
140−180 mmHg (SBP) and/or 90−105 mmHg (DBP)	Basic (Chap. 7)	Procedure as shown in Table 19.2
Moderate to severe**		
≥180−209 mmHg (SBP) and/or ≥105−119 mmHg (DBP)	Extended, exclusion of secondary hypertension (Chap. 7)	Antihypertensive drug treatment, life-style modifications (Chap. 20−30)
Very severe:**		
≥210 mmHg (SBP) and/or ≥120 mmHg (DBP)	Extended exclusion of secondary hypertension (possibly under inpatient conditions) (Chap. 7 and 13−18)	Immediate start of drug-treatment (consider hospitalization) (Chap. 21−30)

  * Based on WHO/ISH- and JNC-V-classification (Tables 4.1a and 4.1b)
** USA: mild = stage 1−2; moderate to severe = stage 3; very severe = stage 4
SBP = systolic blood pressure
DBP = diastolic blood pressure

19.1.2 Therapeutic procedures for mild and borderline hypertension

According to the guidelines of the WHO (World Health Organization) and the ISH (International Society of Hypertension), elevated blood pressure values under 105 mmHg diastolic and/or 180 mmHg systolic (mild hypertension) – presuming the understanding and cooperation of the patient – should be treated primarily by non-drug therapies/lifestyle modifications (diet, weight loss, exercise; Chapter 20) and measured at brief intervals for at least three to six months (Figure 19.2; some guidelines – for example, those in the USA and Great Britain, among others – have proposed borderline values of < 100 mmHg and/or < 160 mmHg). If blood pressure does not normalize within this time, then – depending on the blood pressure level – the introduction of a medicinal antihypertensive therapy ought to be considered. Norms for the lower blood pressure value above which a medicinal therapy is recommended vary world-wide, however (Table 19.2). These differences mirror the current insecurity with respect to the benefits, risks and costs of medicinal therapy for diastolic blood pressure values of 90–99 mmHg and systolic blood pressure values of 140–159 mmHg (169 mmHg in New Zealand). Whereas in the United States, for example, drug therapy is recommended above a blood pressure reading of 140/90 mmHg and/or 150/95 mmHg (JNC V), the same recommendation is made in other countries only above a reading of 160/100 mmHg. The WHO and the ISH recommend drug therapy for mild hypertension when blood pressure values remain above 160/95 mmHg despite a six-month period of nonpharmacologic therapy and observation (Figure 19.2).

Table 19.2: International blood pressure threshold values for the initiation of antihypertensive drug therapy

Country/ Organization	DBP*	SBP*	Observation period	Threshold value with additional risk factors
	(mmHg)		(months)	(mmHg)
WHO/ISH**	95	160	3–6	140/90
Germany	95	160	3–6	
USA***	90	140	3–6	
	95	150	3–6	90
Canada	100			90
England	100	160	3–6	90
Australia	100	160	1	95
New Zealand+	100	170	6	90

```
 *    DBP  = diastolic blood pressure
      SBP  = systolic blood pressure
 **   WHO  = World Health Organization
      ISH  = International Society of Hypertension
***            Two different opinions are reflected for the USA in the JNC V
 +             See explanation in text
```

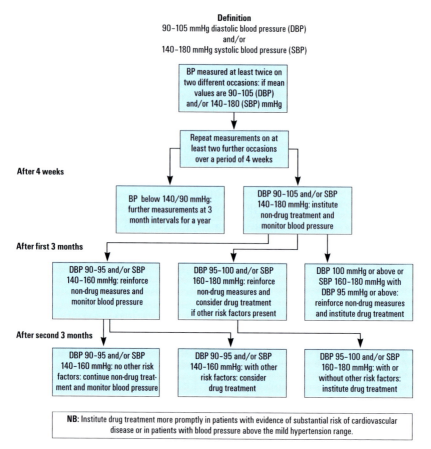

Figure 19.2: Definition and management of mild hypertension as recommended by the World Health Organization/International Society of Hypertension.
DBP, diastolic blood pressure; SBP, systolic blood pressure; BP, blood pressure.

For the attending physician, the practical consequence of this variation in recommendations is that diastolic blood pressure readings between 90−99 mmHg and systolic blood pressure readings between 140−159 mmHg become mere orientation values within whose limits the evaluation of the individual benefits and risks of a medicinal antihypertensive treatment are the doctor's to determine. The decision process, accordingly, should take account of the overall cardiovascular risk based on age, sex, weight, concomitant diseases (including hypertension-induced end-organ damages), lipid and carbohydrate metabolism, nicotine use, and both work and leisure activities (Table 19.3). The corresponding hypertension treatment guidelines from New Zealand do take account of such a concept, insofar as they recommend antihypertensive drug treatment only when it is estimated that a patient's absolute risk of developing a cardiovascular disease within ten years exceeds twenty percent. This excludes patients between 40 and 60 years of age with re-

Table 19.3: Coexisting conditions which influence the choice of therapy for patients with arterial hypertension

Lifestyle
  Occupational activity
    (e. g. sitting or physical labor, noise pollution, stress, shift-work, etc.)
  Leisure activity
    (a lot or a little physical activity, sport, etc.)

Risk factors

  Smoking
  Disorders of lipid metabolism
    (increased serum levels of total cholesterol and/or LDL; decrease in HDL)
  Carbohydrate metabolism disorders
    (Insulin resistance/Hyperinsulinemia, manifest diabetes mellitus)
  Increased fibrinogen level
  Overweight/truncal obesity
  Male gender
  Postmenopausal status
  Family medical history of early cardiovascular disease

Coexisting cardiovascular diseases/End organ damage

  Coronary artery disease
    with or without angina pectoris
    with or without proof of silent myocardial ischemia
  Myocardial infarction
  Condition following coronary revascularization (PTCA or bypass)
  Heart failure
  Left ventricular hypertrophy
  Peripheral arterial occlusive disease
  Hemodynamically relevant carotid stenoses
  Transient ischemic attack
  Apoplexy
  Familiar hyperlipidemia
  Renal diseases
  Retinal abnormalities

peated blood pressure measurements above 170/100 mmHg, for whom a medicinal therapy is recommended even where overall cardiovascular risk is lower than twenty percent (National Advisory Committee on Core Health and Disability Support Services, 1992). A decision which takes account of overall risk and possible side effects saves on cost as well, benefiting both the patient and the health care system and should therefore − despite all the practical difficulties it adds to a doctor's daily routine − be taken seriously.

Blood pressure self measurement ("home measurement") and/or ABPM (Figure 19.3) are useful in choosing an appropriate treatment since they can identify patients with "white coat" hypertension (Sections 2.3.1 and 2.3.2), and thereby obviate unnecessary treatment. They are less useful, however, in deciding whether or not to resort to medication in treating an already diagnosed mild hypertension.

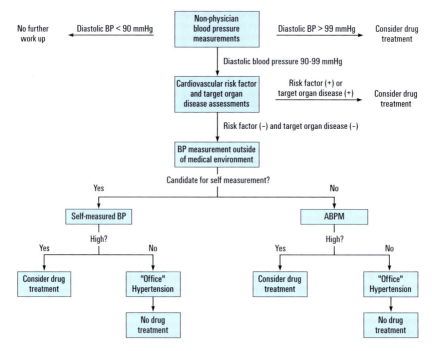

Figure 19.3: Diagnostic procedure including non-physician blood pressure measurements, home blood pressure measurement and ABPM (ambulatory blood pressure monitoring) in patients with mild hypertension and suspected white-coat hypertension.

19.2 General problems in long-term treatment / special problems in the treatment of hypertension

The most common cause of a "therapy resistant" hypertension is the patient's lack of cooperation or dependability (non-compliance) in carrying out the doctor's orders. When an antihypertensive therapeutic regime fails, the reason is frequently a pseudo-resistance indicative of a fundamental problem in the treatment of chronic illnesses. Since a patient's compliance with a therapeutic regime depends on, among other things, the subjective threat of pain, arterial hypertension, since it is mostly painless, must be considered a premier example of an illness whose clinical picture includes a priori a much higher risk of a patient's non-compliance with the demands of therapy.

19.3 Encouraging therapeutic compliance before beginning treatment

Once hypertension has been diagnosed and a decision reached to treat it, it is a good idea, for the reasons above, to draw up a plan for integrating not only the specifics of treatment, but the continuous care and advising of the patient as well. Only in this way can the risk of "pre-programmed" non-compliance be reduced. The introduction and implementation of the long-term treatment of arterial hypertension should therefore be administered according to the following principle rules:

1. Preliminary consultation with the doctor,

2. individualized treatment taking account of the patient's lifestyle,

3. integration of medicinal and non-medicinal therapy,

4. frequent blood pressure controls, at brief intervals and by scheduled appointment, during the first few months of treatment,

5. after satisfactory blood pressure reduction: routine measurement of blood pressure and other cardiovascular risk factors at intervals of 1−6 months,

6. patient participation in progress evaluation (blood pressure self-/home-measurement),

7. group therapy for hypertensive patients

19.3.1 Significance and content of the preliminary consultation

Since most patients experience no pain from arterial hypertension, they are scarcely willing to accept the importance of its treatment. Their understanding of and readiness for a lifetime of dietetic restrictions and medication depends to a considerable degree on the doctor's powers and tools of persuasion. These include not only an explanation of the damage expected to ensue from an untreated hypertension, but a thorough and careful discussion of the possible side-effects of medication. What the patient needs to understand before therapy begins can be summarized as follows:

− what blood pressure is;
− when and where normal or high blood pressure is anticipated;
− what damage can result from high blood pressure;
− how high blood pressure can be lowered;
− how and to what extent an effective antihypertensive therapy can prevent later damages;
− what restrictions and/or side-effects need to be taken into account;
− that treatment for hypertension normally lasts a lifetime and should not be discontinued on one's own authority.

Communicating this to the patient presumes, on the one hand, the doctor's thorough familiarity with the subject, since knowledge alone truly has the power to convince. On the other hand, it also presumes the doctor's sympathy, a large measure of which is necessary to get a feel for the patient's − often unspoken − reservations and fears. Finally, the doctor should speak clearly and understandably.

For most patients, treatment for hypertension means breaking from and frequently changing habits developed over a lifetime. The doctor's clear, open and thorough explanation will be a deciding factor in the patient's compliance or non-compliance.

19.3.2 Individualised treatment

The success and usefulness of any therapy correlate closely with the capabilities of the patient. Physical and mental ability, social circumstances and work environment must all be considered (see also Table 19.3). Rigid treatment guidelines defined solely by blood pressure values should therefore be avoided.

19.3.3 Follow-up examinations during initiation of antihypertensive treatment

Weight and blood pressure should be measured at weekly or biweekly intervals at the beginning of treatment, and in one to four month intervals once blood pressure has been successfully normalized. Additionally, where medication is involved, laboratory tests (serum lipids, potassium, creatinine, etc.) should follow. The results should be discussed with the patient. When patients mention no side effects – particularly at the outset of long-term medication – the doctor, out of respect for the patient, should inquire about them and put them into perspective.

Lastly, frequent check-ups offer the opportunity, through detailed consultation, to motivate the patient to remain true to the therapeutic regime. This appears initially quite important, since the patient experiences subjectively greater discomfort in this phase of antihypertensive treatment.

19.3.4 Follow-up examinations after blood pressure normalisation

Regular check-ups for blood pressure, body weight and various laboratory parameters remain important even after a successful therapeutically induced normalization of blood pressure. Appointments should therefore be scheduled for the patient in advance. These follow-up examinations should be treated as yet further opportunities for a thorough doctor-patient consultation, since a weakening of therapeutic resolve is often observed after blood pressure normalization.

19.3.5 Patient integration in the monitoring of therapy

The patient's integration in monitoring therapeutic progress is a further means to improve compliance. Blood pressure self/home measurement is recommended for this purpose, since it allows the patient to assess the effectiveness of treatment more frequently and in the comfort of his own home. Furthermore, documentation of the recorded measurements in a diary presents the attending physician with important additional information. Blood pressure self measurement is not recommended, however, for patients tending toward hypochondria.

19.3.6 Education and support groups for hypertensives

Another means of furthering compliance is the establishment of monthly "collective" office hours for hypertensive patients, a forum which would afford patients in the area the opportunity to better inform themselves, and to share experiences with others similarly afflicted. To date, such continuing education has unfortunately not been regularly included in treatment, although it would lead over time to a significantly greater patient insight and thus encourage greater therapeutic compliance.

Summary (Chapter 19)

- Firmly diagnosed arterial hypertension requires therapy the goal of which is the reduction of blood pressure to values below 140/90 mmHg.

- The urgency and scope of therapy, as well as the selection of available means of treatment, are determined by the patient's medical profile (overall cardiovascular risk, age, sex, concomitant diseases, hypertension-induced target-organ damage).

- The use of medication in controlling chronically elevated blood pressure whose highest measured values nonetheless remain lower than 95 and/or 160 mmHg is not compulsory according to the WHO and ISH.

- Where risk factors other than hypertension exist, or where end-organ damage is already observable, most national and international hypertension organizations recommend drug therapy above a blood pressure level of 140/90 mmHg.

- The absence of pain, the general necessity of life-long treatment and, where medication is involved, the potential occurrence of side-effects are factors which add to the risk of non-compliance from the very start of treatment.

- Before beginning treatment, an individualized mid- to long-term plan for encouraging patient compliance should be formulated.

Literature (Chapter 19)

Appel LJ, Stason WB. Ambulatory blood pressure monitoring and blood pressure self-measurement in the diagnosis and management of hypertension. Ann Intern Med 1993; 118: 867−882.

Alderman MH. Blood pressure management: individualized treatment based on absolute risk and the potential for benefit. Ann Intern Med 1993; 119: 329−335.

Cruickshank JM, Thorp JM, Zacharias FJ. Benefits and potential harm of lowering high blood pressure. Lancet 1987; i: 581−585.

Dahlf B, Lindholm LH, Hansson L, Schersten B, Ekbom T, Wester PO. Morbidity and mortality in the Swedish Trial in Old Patients with Hypertension (STOP-Hypertension). Lancet 1991; 338: 1281−1285.

Farnett L, Mulrow CD, Linn WD, Lucey CR, Tuley MR. The J-curve phenomenon and the treatment of hypertension. Is there a point beyond which pressure reduction is dangerous? JAMA 1991; 265: 489−495.

Ford GA, Asghar MN. Management of hypertension in the elderly: attitudes of general practioners and hospital physicians. Br J Clin Pharmacol 1995; 39: 465−469.

Guidelines Sub-Committee. 1993 guidelines for the management of mild hypertension: memorandum from a World Health Organization/International Society of Hypertension meeting. J Hypertension 1993; 11: 905−918.

Hansson L. What are we really achieving with long-term drug therapy? Am J Hypertens 1988; 1: 414−420.

Joint National Committee on Detection, Evaluation, and Treatment of High Blood Pressure. The Fifth Report of the Joint National Committee on Detection, Evaluation, and Treatment of High Blood Pressure (JNC V). Arch Intern Med 1993; 153: 154−183.

McVeigh GE, Flack J, Grimm R. Goals of antihypertensive therapy. Drugs 1995; 49: 161−175.

Phillips RA. The cardiologist's approach to evaluation and management of the patient with essential hypertension. Am Heart J 1993; 126: 548−666.

Rudd P. Partial compliance: implications for clinical practice. J Cardiovasc Pharmacol 1993; 22 (suppl A): 1−5.

SHEP Cooperative Research Group. Prevention of stroke by antihypertensive drug treatment in older persons with isolated hypertension. JAMA 1991; 265: 3255−3264.

Sever P, Beevers G, Bulpitt C, Lever A, Ramsay L, Reid J, Swales J. Management guidelines in essential hypertension: report of the second working party of the British Hypertension Society. Br Med J 1993; 306: 983−987.

Swales JD. Guidelines on guidelines. J Hypertens 1993; 11: 899−903.

Thürmer HL, Lund-Larsen PG, Tverdal A. Is blood pressure treatment as effective in a population setting as in controlled trials? Results from a prospective study. J Hypertens 1994; 12: 481−490.

Trenkwalder P, Ruland D, Stender M, Gebhard J, Trenkwalder C, Lydtin H, Hense HW. Prevalence, awareness, treatment and control of hypertension in a population over the age of 65 years: results from the Starnberg Study on Parkinsonism and Hypertension in the Elderly (STEPHY). J Hypertens 1994; 12: 709−716.

Weber MA, Laragh JH. Hypertension: steps forward and steps backward. Arch Intern Med 1993; 153: 149−152.

Zanchetti A. Guidelines for the management of hypertension: the World Health Organization/International Society of Hypertension view. J Hypertens 1995; 13 (suppl 2): 119−122.

20 Non-drug treatment of arterial hypertension

20.1 Indications and importance of general treatment

Whereas the usefulness of blood pressure reduction in achieving lower morbidity and mortality in more severe cases of hypertension has been demonstrated, it remains uncertain to what extent its value is negated in the treatment of milder hypertension by the side effects of medication. In at least two larger, controlled studies (Hypertension Detection and Follow-up Cooperative Group, HDFP, 1984; Multiple Risk Factor Intervention Trial, MRFIT, 1985) higher coronary morbidity and mortality were found in patients treated with antihypertensive medication than in untreated patients with borderline diastolic hypertension (90−94 mmHg). Furthermore these studies did not bear out the usefulness of medicinal intervention in cases where diastolic blood pressure values lay between 95 and 99 mmHg.

The potential risk involved in prescribing medication for hypertension is witnessed by the recommendation of all national and international professional societies to treat mild hypertension non-medicinally where no end-organ damage exists. Non-drug treatment in terms of life-style modifications is recommended moreover in all cases as an accompaniment and support to medication.

The most important non-pharmacological means to lower blood pressure are weight reduction in cases of obesity, reduction of salt intake and other dietary measures, reduction in consumption − or outright renunciation − of alcoholic beverages, and an increase in physical activity (Table 20.1).

Table 20.1: Relative effectiveness of non-pharmacological measures in hypertension

	Blood pressure reduction	Coronary protection
Weight control	+++	++
Alcohol reduction*	+++	+
Salt restriction	++	?
Moderate exercise**	++	++
Vegetarian-like diets***	+	++
Dietary fish	+	+++
Stopping smoking	−	+++

  * Reduction from 4−5 to 1−2 drinks per day
 ** Endurance sports, moderate exertion (age-adjusted heart rate, see Section 20.2.4)
*** Low-fat diet, fruits and vegetables
Adapted from Beilin LJ, J Hypertens, 1994; 12 (suppl 10): S 71−S 81

20.2 Specific non-drug therapies/life-style modifications

20.2.1 Weight reduction

There exists a positive, age-independent correlation between obesity and hypertension, so that the heavier the patient, the likelier the development of hypertension (see also Section 19.3.5). The risk of developing hypertension is more than three times greater for patients whose body weight is 20% or more above average. This direct relationship between obesity and hypertension has been confirmed by large epidemiological studies of both men and women all over the globe (see, for example, Chicago Heart Study, Figure 20.1). It has been further confirmed that obese patients with hypertension can significantly lower or even normalize their blood pressure by losing weight.

Since the blood pressure of chronically obese patients can only be reduced, if at all, by large doses of multiple medications, weight reduction has to be considered the first and foremost therapy. Daily caloric intake has to be kept unmistakably

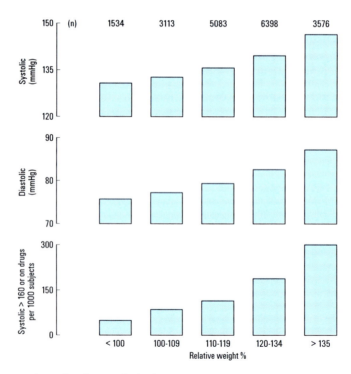

Figure 20.1: Relationship beween body fat (relative weight) and blood pressure or prevalence of hypertension in men aged 18–64 (data from the Chicago Heart Study; figure adapted from Beilin LJ, J Hypertens 1994; 12 (suppl 10): S71-S81)

lower than the common daily requirement. For example, to lose one kilogram of excess fat per week, a 7000 Kcal reduction in the normal weekly requirement is necessary. Since an elevated insulin level can be seen as a partial pathogenetic factor in obesity-related hypertension, a reduction in carbohydrate intake becomes an important part of reduced calorie diets. Weight reduction therefore represents a direct therapeutic approach to the treatment of obesity and hypertension. A multitude of tables with detailed information on the calories provided by specific foods are available for controlling the rate of weight loss. Virtually every magazine offers a diet plan, so guidelines abound. Naturally the weight loss plans available are so numerous, they can not be individually explored within the scope of this book. It is nevertheless important to point out that every diet should make ample allowance for water, vitamins and minerals. It is therefore advisable to counsel a patient prior to beginning a therapeutic weight loss program.

20.2.1.1 Definition of obesity

An adult's normal body weight can be determined either by use of the body mass index (BMI), or with the help of the "Broca" formula (known in German-speaking countries).

Body mass index:

Body mass index (BMI): Body weight (kg)/height (m)^2

Values over 25 kg/m^2 qualify as overweight.

"Broca" formula:

Normal weight: Body height (cm) -100 (kg)

Departures from the norm can be determined by the Broca-index:

Body weight (kg)/Normal weight (kg) $\times$ 100$-$100
Overweight: Body weight more than 10% $>$ normal weight
Obesity: Body weight more than 20% $>$ normal weight

Body fat distribution is also significant, since truncal obesity in particular is viewed as a cardiovascular risk factor.

20.2.2 Restriction of dietary sodium

The restricted use of table salt (sodium chloride) is one of the oldest, most widely employed means of lowering arterial blood pressure. Although a person's actual daily requirement for sodium chloride is only about 2$-$4 grams depending upon one's level of physical activity (hard physical labor with attendant greater perspiration may increase the need), in the western industrialized countries people consume an average of 8 to 15 grams of sodium chloride a day in their food. Epidemiological studies have accordingly demonstrated that a positive correlation exists be-

Table 20.2:   Food with low, medium and high sodium content

Food with low-sodium content*	Food with medium-sodium content*	Food with high-sodium content*
	Recommended for patients with hypertension?	
Yes**	Only in limited amounts	Generally no
Meat and sausages		
All fresh meats	Roast beef	All sausages
ground meat, tatar (without		Long-keeping sausage
additives)		Ham, raw or smoked
Fresh fowl		Pickled meat
Game		Meat and sausage salad
Fish		
All fresh fish	Bloater, smoked	Herring
	Mackerel, smoked	Eel, smoked
	Canned shrimp	Canned fish
	Canned tunafish	Fish salad
		Mock salmon
		Sardines
		Haddock
		Pollack, smoked
Fats, oils		
Diet margarine	Herbal butter	Mayonnaise
Unsalted fat		Bacon
Dairy products		
(Low-fat) milk	Fresh cheese	Edamer, gouda, tilsiter, roma-
Buttermilk	Swiss cheese	dur, limburger, camembert,
(Low-fat) yogurt		brie
Eggs		Sliced cheese
Bread, baked goods		
Flakes	Butter cookies	Rolls
Semolina	Rye bread	Pumpernickel
Noodles, spaghetti	Linseed bread	Cornflakes
Rice	Wheat and rye bread	Potato chips
Apple pie	White bread	Pretzels
Pie crust	Zwieback	
Shortbread		(Pretzel sticks, crackers)
Vegetables, salads, mush-		
rooms, potatoes		
All sorts of fresh or frozen	Canned vegatables	Mixed pickles
nuts (unsalted)	Vegetable juices (without so-	Olives, capers
	dium chloride)	Canned mushrooms
	Potato dumplings (raw or	Salted pickles
	half and half)	Sauerkraut
	Red beets	Salad dressings
		Salted nuts or almonds
Fruit		
All sorts		
Canned fruit		
Fruit juice		

Table 20.2: Continued

Food with low-sodium content*	Food with medium-sodium content*	Food with high-sodium content*
	Recommended for patients with hypertension?	
Yes**	Only in limited amounts	Generally no
Special products, packaged food Low-sodium or sodium-reduced foods		Canned soups Instant meals (frozen or canned) Instant sauces Packaged potato products
Herbs and spices All fresh, dried and frozen herbs (basil, mugwort, chervil, dill, oregano, estragon, garlic, cress, parsley, rosemary, cellary, thyme, lemon, onion) All pure spices (bay leaf, nutmeg, caraway, cloves, paprika, pepper, juniper, cinnamon) Salt-free curry, mustard, and tomato paste		Salt, salt mixtures, seasoned salts, curry, boullion, liquid seasonings, soup or meat extracts, packaged sauces, marinades, normal mustard, ketchup

* Low-sodium   < 120 mg sodium/100 g food = < 0.3 g sodium chloride/100 g food
  Medium-sodium: 120−400 mg sodium/100 g food = 0.3−1 g sodium chloride/100 g food
  High-sodium: > 400 mg sodium/100 g food = > 1 g sodium chloride/100 g food
** Recommended with regard to the sodium content. In some cases the content of cholesterol and saturated fatty acids must be considered.
Adapted from "German Hypertension Society". Kochsalz und Hochdruck (sodium chloride and hypertension) 2nd edition, 6/1993

tween daily salt intake and arterial blood pressure. From these studies it is obvious that populations with a very low sodium intake (< 75 mmol daily, e.g. native Indians in Brazil) display a significantly lower incidence of hypertension than for example the population of Japan, whose average consumption of sodium exceeds 300 mmol/day.

Various large and small placebo-controlled studies have ascertained that a reduction in sodium chloride intake in patients with primary hypertension can lead to as much as a 5 mmHg reduction in diastolic blood pressure. The blood pressure-reducing effect of a sodium-restricted diet is frequently greater in older patients, since the kidneys' ability to excrete sodium often diminishes with increased age. It has already been noted elsewhere (Section 9.3.3) that a reduction in salt intake results in a lowering of arterial blood pressure in only a minority of those affected by hypertension (so-called "salt sensitive" hypertension; ca. 30−40%). Since no sure indicators for the presence of salt sensitivity have yet been identified, extreme, in any event impractical reductions of salt intake to less than 1−2 g/day are in general not advisable, especially since smaller studies have noted a rise in cholesterol level and − at least where "salt-resistant patients" are concerned − a paradoxical, compensatory activation of the renin-angiotensin system is imaginable.

An individually suited salt intake of 2−4 grams (see above) would be ideal; however, because of the salt hidden in most food available today (bread, cheese, sausage, meat, etc.) it is all but impossible in day-to-day life. Moreover the sense of taste of the populations of the industrialized countries demands salt, so that adequate compliance is hardly to be expected. The currently valid recommendation to reduce daily salt intake to 5−6 grams (ca. 105 mmol sodium) is based therefore on the practicability of such a therapy. This recommendation is additionally valid for patients with primary hypertension, since a low-salt diet boosts the effectiveness of most antihypertensive drugs and is advantageous as well for salt-sensitive hypertension patients.

Preparation of food without salt, renunciation of the use of salt at the table, and conscious selection of low-sodium food are the most important measures to recommend to patients with primary hypertension. In addition to focused dietary counseling, doctors and/or their dietary assistants should provide detailed, geographically and culturally adapted tables with information on the amount of salt contained in various foods (see, for example, recommendations from the German Hypertension Society, 1993; Table 20.2).

Potassium-rich fare is furthermore recommended (e.g. fruit, vegetables, potatoes with their skins), since on the one hand digestion renders all food low in potassium, and on the other several studies have demonstrated that additional potassium has a blood pressure-lowering effect. The substitution of potassium chloride for sodium chloride is in principle possible and on therapeutic grounds absolutely desirable, but as regards taste, not generally accepted.

20.2.3 Limitation of alcohol consumption

There exists a positive correlation between the level of arterial blood pressure and the amount of alcohol consumed by patients with hypertension. Whereas this correlation is certain where daily alcohol intake exceeds 40 g (ca. one liter of beer or 0.3 to 0.4 liters of wine), the significance of lower daily consumption can not be so unambiguously interpreted. An increase in the proportion of high-density lipoproteins and an associated lowering of cardiovascular risk under conditions of a moderate alcohol intake of fewer than 30 g/day contradicts other studies which have found hypertension to prevail even in this range of consumption.

The reduction or cessation of the consumption of alcohol at levels above 40 g/day takes on the nature of a direct therapeutic approach to the treatment of arterial hypertension. Moreover the effectiveness of antihypertensive medication can be significantly improved by minimizing alcohol intake (see also Section 17.6).

20.2.4 Sports/physical activity

Regular participation in aerobic endurance sports can bring about a lowering of both the resting and exercising blood pressure. To achieve this, however, continuous exercise lasting more than 20 minutes at least three times a week is necessary. Exercise lasting less than 20 minutes has no apparent blood pressure-reducing effect.

The following mechanisms have been put forward as possible explanations of the blood pressure-reducing effect of duration training:

− lower heart rate and lower cardiac output,
− decrease in total peripheral resistance as a consequence of increased muscular metabolism,
− minimized response of vascular smooth musculature to norepinephrine and other vasoconstrictive stimuli,
− decrease in sympathetic activity with minimal release of catecholamines, and possibly
− increased vagal activity.

Sports involving isotonic exercise (e.g. running, cycling, cross-country skiing) are ideally suited for patients with hypertension. Sports that are primarily isometric but which induce momentary blood pressure peaks (contact sports, weight lifting, dashing etc.) are however particularly poorly suited for hypertensive patients with already diagnosed end-organ damage (Table 20.3).

The standard recommended exercise pulse can be determined by subtracting the patient's age from 180. Detailed, age-indexed values for running, cycling and

Table 20.3:   Suitability of various types of sports for hypertensive patients*

Suitability	Type of sport
Well-suited	− Endurance sports with isotonic stress (running, cycling, cross-country skiing, etc.) − Team sports with relatively low physical stress (volleyball, doubles tennis) − Golf
Suitable**	− Swimming − Alpine skiing − Games with minimum to moderate work load (ping-pong, tennis, etc.) Team sports with a moderate level of work load (field hockey, soccer)
Unsuited	− Competitive, high-performance sports − Track and field − Games with high stress levels (squash) − Team sports with high stress levels (ice hockey, basketball, etc.) − Combatant sports (boxing, karate, wrestling, etc.) − Power sports (weightlifting, body building, acrobatics) − Gymnastics

 * Adapted from Rost (1987)
** Depending on severity of hypertension and previous athletic activity

swimming are presented in Tables 20.4 a-c. Practically speaking, it is easier to judge by a patient's respiration, which should always allow for the possibility to speak while exercising.

Although one should not overestimate the antihypertensive benefit of regular physical exercise, it nevertheless represents a sensible addition to other therapeutic measures. Where patients faithfully participate in an endurance sport, one therefore witnesses an increase in HDL cholesterol level, and a decrease in total choles-

Table 20.4a−c: Maximal heart rate under physical training conditions adjusted to age and heart rate at rest. Recommendations for various endurance sports*

a) Running

Heart rate at rest (bpm)**	Age under 30	30−39	40−49	50−59	60−70	Over 70
Under 50	140	140	135	130	125	120
50−59	140	140	135	130	125	120
60−69	145	145	140	135	130	125
70−79	145	145	140	135	130	125
80−89	150	145	140	135	130	125
90−100	150	150	145	140	135	130
Over 100	155	150	145	145	140	130

b) Swimming

Heart rate at rest (bpm)**	Age under 30	30−39	40−49	50−59	60−70	Over 70
Under 50	130	130	125	120	115	110
50−59	130	130	125	120	115	110
60−69	135	135	130	125	120	115
70−79	135	135	130	125	120	115
80−89	140	135	130	125	120	115
90−100	140	140	135	130	125	120
Over 100	145	140	135	130	125	120

c) Cycling

Heart rate at rest (bpm)**	Age under 30	30−39	40−49	50−59	60−70	Over 70
Under 50	135	135	130	125	120	115
50−59	135	135	130	125	120	115
60−69	140	140	135	130	125	120
70−79	140	140	135	130	125	120
80−89	145	140	135	130	125	120
90−100	145	145	140	135	130	125
Over 100	150	145	140	140	135	125

* From Druckpunkt 2/1995 (modified)
** bpm = beats per minute

terol level, in LDL's, and in triglycerides, and an improvement of diabetic metabolic condition. Regular physical activity not only produces these benefits to the cardiovascular profile, but often fundamentally changes a patient's habits as well (quitting smoking and/or drinking, losing weight, etc.). These changes in turn make a not insignificant contribution to antihypertensive therapy.

All endurance training should be systematically planned. Whether or not the patient has fun from the very start of this — unaccustomed — exercise will be a determining factor in cooperation/compliance. Goals set too high from the outset and the stress frequently associated with them not only frustrate the patient, but are also physically harmful. As an example, the weeks-long, gradually accelerating running program displayed in Table 20.5 shows how physically inactive hypertension patients can slowly work their way into practicing an endurance sport.

Table 20.5:   Jogging program for hypertensive patients with no previous training*

Week	Intensity of training
1	10 min rapid walking
2	3 × 1 min jogging with 3 min walking intervals
3	3 × 2 min jogging with 3 min walking intervals
4	3 × 3 min jogging with 3 min walking intervals
5	3 × 4 min jogging with 3 min walking intervals
6	3 × 5 min jogging with 3 min walking intervals
7	3 × 6 min jogging with 3 min walking intervals
8	3 × 7 min jogging with 3 min walking intervals
9	3 × 8 min jogging with 3 min walking intervals
10	1 × 12 min jogging
after 11	Increase duration of jogging by ca. 1 min/week until ca. 20−30 min running is attained

* Acc. to Druckpunkt 2/1995 (modified)

20.2.5 Special diets

A vegetarian, potassium-rich diet encourages a lowering of the blood pressure. Opinions differ on whether or not this effect holds for omega-3 fatty acids containing fish oil. The incorporation of fish foods into reduced-fat diets leads nevertheless to a reduction of various cardiovascular risks. The often conjectured blood pressure-reducing effect of garlic has yet to be convincingly demonstrated.

20.2.6 The elimination of other cardiovascular risk factors

Diabetes mellitus, hyperinsulinemia, hypercholesteremia, and smoking are further decisive factors, apart from arterial hypertension, influencing cardiovascular risk. Optimization of carbohydrate metabolism for diabetics, weight reduction leading to the breakdown of insulin resistance in type IIb diabetics, and the resulting hyperinsulinemia, dietetic (or, if necessary, medicinal) normalization of elevated blood lipids, as well as the total cutting out of smoking are therefore integral components in the treatment of hypertension.

Summary (Chapter 20)

- Weight loss, reduction in or renunciation of alcoholic beverages, restricted salt intake and physical endurance training are all non-pharmacological measures that reduce blood pressure in at least a portion of patients with hypertension.

- Non-drug treatment should precede any other therapeutic measures in cases of mild hypertension (USA: stage 1), and should accompany primary drug-treatment in more severe cases of hypertension.

Literature (Chapter 20)

Anonymous. Sport-Anleitung für Selbst-Hilfe-gruppen. Druckpunkt 1995 (2): 27−29.

American College of Sports medicine. Physical activity, physical fitness and hypertension. Med Sci Sports Exerc 1993; 25: i-x.

Arroll B, Hill D, White G, Sharpe N, Beaglehole R. The effect of exercise episode duration on blood pressure. J Hypertens 1994; 12: 1413−1415.

Beilin LJ. Non-pharmacological management of hypertension: optimal strategies for reducing cardiovascular risk. J Hypertens 1994; 12 (suppl 10): S71−S81.

Cappuccio FP, MacGregor GA. Does potassium supplementation lower blood pressure? J Hypertens 1991; 9: 465−473.

Cutler JA, Follmann D, Elliott P, Suh IL. An overview of randomized trials of sodium restriction and blood pressure. Hypertension 1991; 17 (suppl I): I-27-I-33.

Deutsche Liga zur Bekämpfung des hohen Blutdruckes e.V. Deutsche Hypertonie Gesellschaft. Kochsalz und Hochdruck. Merkblatt, 1993.

Frost CD, Law MR, Wald NJ. By how much does dietary salt reduction lower blood pressure? II. Analysis of observational data within populations. Br Med J 1991; 302: 815−818.

Hoffmann G. Hypertension and sports. [in German] Dtsch Z Sportmed 1993; 44: 153−166.

Kenney WL. Parasympathetic control of resting heart rate: relationship to aerobic power. Med Sci Sports Exerc 1985; 17: 451−455.

Knapp HR, Fitzgerald GA. The antihypertensive effects of fish oil: a controlled study of polyunsaturated fatty acid supplements in essential hypertension. N Engl J Med 1989; 320: 1037−1043.

Krishna CC, Kapoor SC. Potassium depletion exacerbates essential hypertension. Ann Intern Med 1991; 115: 77−83.

Law MR, Frost CD, Wald NJ. By how much does dietary salt reduction lower blood pressure? I. Analysis of observational data among populations. Br Med J 1991; 302: 811−815.

Law MR, Frost CD, Wald NJ. By how much does dietary salt reduction lower blood pressure? III. Analysis of data from trials of salt reduction. Br Med J 1991; 302: 819−824.

Liebson PR, Grandits GA, Dianzumba S, Prineas RJ, Grimm RH, Neaton JD, Stamler J for the Treatment of Hypertension Study Research Group. Comparison of five antihypertensive monotherapies and placebo for change in left ventricular mass in patients receiving nutritional-hygienic therapy in the Treatment of Mild Hypertension Study (TOMHS). Circulation 1995; 91: 698−706.

Narkiewicz K, Maraglino G, Biasion T, Rossi G, Sanzuol F, Palatini P on behalf of the HARVEST Study Group (Italy). Interactive effect of cigarettes and coffee on daytime systolic blood pressure in patients with mild to moderate hypertension. J Hypertens 1995; 13: 965−970.

National High Blood Pressure Education Program Working Group. National High Blood Pressure Education Program Working Group

Report on Primary Prevention of Hypertension. Arch Intern Med 1993; 153: 186−208.

Mac Mahon S. Alcohol consumption and hypertension. Hypertension 1987; 9: 111−121.

Mann SJ, James GD, Wang RS, Pickering TG. Elevation of ambulatory systolic blood pressure in hypertensive smokers: a case-control study. JAMA 1991; 265: 2226−2228.

Paffenbarger RS, Hyde RT, Wing AL, Lee IM, Jung DL, Kampert JB. The association of changes in physical-activity level and other lifestyle characteristics with mortality among men. N Engl J Med 1993; 328: 538−545.

Palmer AJ, Fletcher AE, Bulpitt CJ, Beevers DG, Coles EC, Ledingham JGG, Petrie JC, Webster J, Dollery CT. Alcohol intake and cardiovascular mortality in hypertensive patients: report from the Department of Health Hypertension Care Computing Project. J Hypertens 1995; 13: 957−964.

Prichard BNC, Smith CCT, Ling KLE, Betteridge DJ. Fish oils and cardiovascular disease. Br Med J 1995; 31o: 819−820.

Silagy CA, Neil AW. A meta-analysis of the effect of garlic on blood pressure. J Hypertens 1994; 12: 463−468.

Somers VK, Conway J, Johnston J, Sleight P. Effects of endurance training on baroreflex sensitivity and blood pressure in borderline hypertension. Lancet 1991; 337: 1363−1368.

The Joint National Committee on Detection, Evaluation, and Treatment of High Blood Pressure. The Fifth Report of the Joint National Committee on Detection, Evaluation, and Treatment of High Blood Pressure (JNC V). Arch Intern Med 1993; 153: 154−183.

Van Dusseldorp M, Smith P, Lenders JWM, Thien T, Katan MB. Boiled coffee and blood pressure: a 14-week controlled trial. Hypertension 1991; 18: 607−613.

Victor RG, Hansen J. Alcohol and blood pressure − a drink a day... N Engl J Med 1995; 332: 1782−1783.

World Hypertension League. Nonpharmacological interventions as an adjunct to the pharmacological treatment of hypertension: a statement by WHL. J Hum Hypertens 1993; 7: 159−164.

21 Drug treatment of arterial hypertension

The introduction of a medicinal treatment for arterial hypertension is recommended when:

- Blood pressure values exceed 160 mmHg systolic and /or 95−100 mmHg diastolic, or
- no satisfactory blood pressure reduction can be achieved through non-drug treatment (including life-style modifications) after three to six months (ISH/WHO: < 160 mmHg systolic and/or < 95 mmHg diastolic; JNC V: < 140 mmHg systolic and/or < 90 mmHg diastolic), or
- hypertension-induced end-organ damage is already evident at blood pressure values over 140/90 mmHg, or
- other cardiovascular risk factors exist above blood pressure values of 140/90 mmHg (diabetes mellitus, hyperinsulinemia, hyperlipidemia etc.) (see Figure 19.2).

The goal of antihypertensive therapy is a reduction in mortality and morbidity. According to the guidelines of the ISH/WHO, the desired therapeutic "pressure norm" is

- < 140/90 mmHg for adults and older patients with diastolic and systolic hypertension,
- 120−130/80 mmHg for young patients with mild hypertension,
- 140 mmHg for patients with isolated systolic hypertension.

21.1 General guidelines for the drug treatment of arterial hypertension

To obtain the greatest possible patient compliance, the following points must be raised relative to any antihypertensive drug treatment:

- Effectiveness;
- number of side-effects (ideally none at all);
- when possible, monotherapy (maximum two doses per day);
- in the case of double or multiple combinations, uncomplicated prescription instructions;
- no aggravation of existing risk factors;
- no aggravation of possible related illnesses.

21.2 Beginning medication

The medicinal treatment of arterial hypertension can in principle be accomplished

- by monotherapy,
- by a free combination of two or more antihypertensive drugs,
- by a so-called "fixed" combination of two or more antihypertensive drugs.

As an introduction to the drug treatment of a confirmed mild to moderate hypertension (JNC V, USA: stages 1 and 2), the prescription of a single basic medication (a so-called "first-line" antihypertensive) is recommended virtually worldwide. The lowest possible dosage should be chosen first, although where no reduction in blood pressure is forthcoming but tolerance remains, the dose may be increased. Switching to another substance is another alternative. Where blood pressure reduction is still insufficient ($> 140/90$ mmHg), therapy should be expanded to include a second first-line antihypertensive drug from another pharmacological class and with a different mode of action.

In the event of severe or malignant hypertension (USA: Stages 3 and 4), adequate reduction of blood pressure is seldom achieved by a mere increase in the dosage of a single substance. More often than not it requires the prescription of at least two or more varied antihypertensives.

21.2.1 Basic ("first-line") medications for the treatment of primary arterial hypertension

All national and international guidelines for the treatment of hypertension have traditionally recommended beginning the long-term drug treatment of primary hypertension with monotherapy, using one of the recognized basic ("first-line") antihypertensive agents. The following conditions are imposed on first-line medications in the treatment of arterial hypertension:

1. A sufficient antihypertensive effect when used as monotherapy:
The proof that an antihypertensive administered as a monosubstance provides "adequate" blood pressure reduction stems from clinical studies performed mostly still as placebo-controlled ones during the development of a substance (phase II, or in particular phase III). Reduction of the diastolic blood pressure, whose so-called "trough" value (see Section 2.5) — before the next dosage and 24 hours after the last — should be at least 5 mmHg more pronounced, is the current primary evaluation criteria. The so-called "responder-rate", normally defined as a normalization (< 90 mmHg) and/or a reduction of diastolic blood pressure by more than 10 mmHg, lies between 40% and 60% for all substance classes confirmed as first-line medications. Higher responder rates result from studies which focus on more or less pre-selected patients (therefore on patients who are known to respond particularly well, therapeutically, to a particular class of substance).

2. Reduction of mortality and morbidity when used as monotherapy:
Medications are increasingly chosen for their ability to influence morbidity and mortality over the long-term. The treatment of cardiovascular risk factors − or in other words taking "surrogates" as end points − is in itself uninteresting if it does not take improvement in life expectancy and quality as its goal. This conclusion has to date only been drawn in the USA, in the 1993 JNC V Report. This report recommended only diuretics and beta-adrenergic blockers as first-line antihypertensives, since as of that time only these substance classes were proven to reduce mortality and morbidity.

3. A known safety profile based on the study of large numbers of patients
   over many years:
Data gathered in the course of clinical development on the safety of a substance is sufficient to certify it as a basic medication only when it involves a subsequent preparation ("me-too") of a single substance class already certified, with respect to its pharmacologically active properties and without a deviating safety profile, as a first-line therapy.

4. No negative influences on coexisting cardiovascular risk factors and/or
   diseases to be treated simultaneously:
Patients with high blood pressure often display other cardiovascular risk factors which first-line medications must not be allowed to aggravate lest they neutralize the anticipated long-term benefit of blood pressure reduction. The term "metabolic neutrality", used commonly in connection with carbohydrate, lipid and purine metabolism, summarizes this claim and represents a property that will be demanded of every new antihypertensive.

For the antihypertensive treatment of postmenopausal women (ca. 50% of all hypertensive patients), it will in future be demanded of a basic medication that it not aggravate the bone loss which occurs in this population when estrogen production stops. It must also be guaranteed that an antihypertensive certified as a first-line medication will not work against or outright counteract the osteoprotective effect of a simultaneous, long-term hormone replacement therapy ("osteoneutrality").

5. No reflex side-effects requiring suppression through the use
   of a second medication:
The treatment of hypertension with a monosubstance is only justified when it neither entails clinically relevant reflex side-effects nor demands the prescription of a second medication to suppress such side-effects (e.g. prescribing beta-blockers to compensate for a reflex tachycardia).

6. Once or twice daily administration:
The insistence that a first-line antihypertensive satisfactorily reduce blood pressure based on a dosage taken no more than twice a day is grounded on the acknowledgment that patient compliance decreases as the frequency of administration increases. The related assumption that it is better to take a given form of medication

once rather than twice a day is as yet unproved, although it is frequently advanced by the pharmaceutical industry as a sales argument.

Most national and international guidelines for the treatment of hypertension currently recommend five various substance classes as first-line medication for the treatment of primary hypertension (see also Section 21.3):

- Diuretics,
- beta-adrenergic blockers,
- (long-acting) calcium antagonists,
- angiotensin-converting enzyme (ACE) inhibitors, and
- alpha$_1$-adrenergic blockers.

Before the completion of appropriate long-term studies (e.g. the HOT Study, the ALLHAT-Study etc.), complete recognition of ACE inhibitors, calcium antagonists and alpha$_1$-blockers as basic antihypertensives proceeds from the assumption that these substance classes' demonstrated effectiveness in reducing blood pressure and their mostly favorable influence on other cardiovascular risk factors equate to a reduction in mortality and morbidity. Exceptions here are the USA, Canada and New Zealand, whose therapeutic guidelines recommend the initial use of diuretics and beta-blockers (see below).

21.2.1.1 Exceptional position of the JNC V

As noted above, the most recent recommendations of the US Joint National Committee on Detection, Evaluation and Treatment of High Blood Pressure (JNC V), last published in 1993, differ insofar as they name only diuretics and beta-blockers as preferred basic medications, since long-term hypertension studies had up to that time recorded a reduction in morbidity and mortality only for these substance classes.

The US recommendations have led to brisk discussion worldwide, and are not uncontested even in the USA (e.g. see American Journal of Hypertension 1994; 7: 857−885 and 1995; 8: 541−544), the more so as the previous US Report (JNC IV) had already named ACE inhibitors and calcium antagonists as basic medications. It should nonetheless be noted here that the JNC V, in contrast to many other therapy guidelines, took the trouble to ground its recommendations on actual, therapeutically-oriented, scientific fact. The preference given to diuretics and beta-blockers in the initial treatment of hypertension implies that a positive influence, for example, on cardiovascular risk factors − as demonstrated by ACE inhibitors, calcium antagonists and alpha-blockers − may be desirable in an antihypertensive, but nevertheless on the strictest scientific grounds is not as important as the supposed therapeutic goal, specifically the reduction of mortality and morbidity. Insofar as the authors of the JNC V in no way questioned, on the one hand, the value or significance of the newer antihypertensives as modern, individually adjustable treatments for hypertension, they tried, on the other hand, to establish clear scientific criteria against which the effectiveness of a basic medication could be measured. The merit of the JNC V is that it opposes the "watering down" of therapeutic goals: the supposed goal of treatment is neither the reduction of blood pressure nor the positive influencing of other cardiovascular risk factors (being nothing more than surrogates), but − see above − a reduction of the mortality and morbidity that result from chronically high arterial blood pressure. The JNC V authors also hardly doubt that the new antihypertensives will in all probability receive the same approbation already given to beta-blockers and diuretics. They moreover do not consider it "unethical" to prescribe an ACE inhibitor, a (long-acting) calcium antagonist or an alpha$_1$-blocker as an initial basic medication when the effectiveness and safety profile of one of these substance classes would fulfill a patient's individual needs.

21.2.2 Choosing a basic medication

The choice of a first-line medication should be made based on the particulars of the patient's individual profile (concomitant diseases, cardiovascular risk profile, physical activity, age, race, etc.) Therapeutic generalizations like those so often heard in the past (e.g. "beta-blockers for younger, calcium antagonists for older hypertension patients") break down under critical analysis and are increasingly exposed as unsuitable in practice.

The patient must be informed about the doctor's reasons for choosing one or another preparation, and, more importantly, must understand these reasons.

Monotherapy with one of the first-line drugs induces satisfactory blood pressure reduction in ca. 40% and 60% of all patients with mild to moderate hypertension (USA: stages 1 and 2), making the prescription of a second antihypertensive agent in many cases unnecessary. Since many of the available substances reach their optimum effectiveness only after two to five weeks, premature changes in preparation or rapid increases in dosage should be avoided.

21.2.4 Practical procedures in the event of a necessary expansion of therapy

In the event that an increase in the dose of a monosubstance brings about an increase of side-effects, a reduction in daily dosage is advisable, as is the earliest possible introduction of a second (and, if necessary, a third) antihypertensive-reinforcing medication in the lowest possible dose. The prescription of a second antihypertensive is also recommended in the event of unsatisfactory blood pressure reduction. A change in substance class is also an alternative, and is to be preferred when substance-typical, dose-unrelated side-effects occur (e.g. dry cough with ACE inhibitors, flushing or ankle edema with calcium antagonists, etc.)

Every change in therapy must be understandably explained to the patient. Too quick or too frequent changes in preparation are pharmacologically, and therefore therapeutically, not sensible. They rob the substance of any opportunity to reach optimum effectiveness (see above), and leave the patient feeling insecure, thus potentially further reducing therapeutic compliance.

21.3 National and international therapeutic guidelines for the drug treatment of arterial hypertension

21.3.1 International Society of Hypertension (ISH)/World Health Organisation (WHO)

The ISH/WHO guidelines recommend monotherapy using a preparation from among the recognized substance classes for the start of a medicinal treatment of mild hypertension. The list includes:

1. Diuretics,
2. beta-adrenergic blockers
3. ACE inhibitors, (long-acting) calcium antagonists, alpha$_1$-blockers.

The reduction in mortality and morbidity under long-term treatment forms the basis of ranking diuretics and beta-blockers higher in this list than other first-line antihypertensive drugs. However, the patient's overall profile is the most relevant criterion for choosing the initial antihypertensive substance class. The decision must be left to the doctor, and must not be liable to unalterable restrictions.

If the chosen monotherapy is ineffective, then a switch to another confirmed "first-line" substance class is recommended. In the event of marginal (therefore unsatisfactory = > 140/90 mmHg) blood pressure reduction through monotherapy, the treatment should be expanded to include a second basic medication from another substance class. The following examples are given:

- Diuretic plus beta-blocker,
- diuretic plus ACE inhibitor,
- diuretic plus alpha$_1$-blocker, or
- beta blocker plus alpha$_1$-blocker,
- beta blocker plus dihydropyridine calcium antagonist, or
- ACE inhibitor plus calcium antagonist.

Guidelines for the use of multiple combinations in the treatment of severe and/or therapy-resistant (for definition see Section 32.3) hypertension have not been provided by the WHO or the ISH to date.

21.3.2 Treatment algorithm of the Fifth Report of the Joint National Committee (JNC V), USA

The JNC V has published a treatment algorithm, which is depicted in Figure 21.1. Though it gives priority to diuretics and beta-blockers as first-line medications for use at the outset of treatment for hypertension (see section 21.3.1.1), the JNC V also emphasizes the patient's individual needs as an important criterion in the choice of a substance class, and so leaves the attending physician free to choose an ACE inhibitor, a calcium antagonist or an alpha$_1$-blocker.

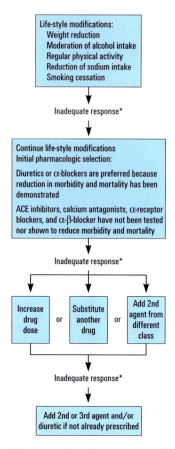

Figure 21.1: Treatment algorithm as suggested by the Joint National Committee on Detection, Evaluation, and Treatment of High Blood Pressure (JNC V). Asterisk (*) indicates that response means the patient achieved goal blood pressure or is making considerable progress toward this goal (from Arch Intern Med 1993; 153: 154−183)

21.3.3 Recommendations of the German Hypertension Society (10/1994)

If blood pressure can not be reduced below 140/90 mmHg through monotherapy with one of the basic medications (diuretics, beta blockers, calcium antagonists, ACE inhibitors, alpha$_1$-blockers), the recommendation of the German Hypertension Society, valid since October 1994, is to use combinations of two first-line medications, one of which should be either a diuretic or a calcium antagonist. Since beta blockers or ACE inhibitors are recommended as combination partners to calcium antagonists, diuretics, according to this schema, are best paired with beta blockers, calcium antagonists, ACE inhibitors and alpha$_1$-blockers. Combinations of a diuretic with reserpine, or of a diuretic with a central sympatholytic are also given as alternatives.

If none of these combinations proves sufficient, the prescription of an additional centrally acting sympatholytic or of some other combination of three is recommended (see Figure 21.2).

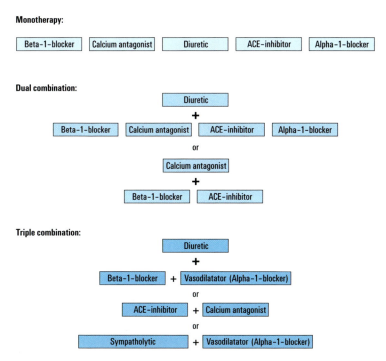

Figure 21.2: Recommendations of the "German Hypertension Society" for the mono- and combination treatment of arterial hypertension (10/1994)

21.4 Summary of the introduction to antihypertensive drug therapy

The basic guidelines for beginning medicinal treatment of primary hypertension can be summarized as follows:

Summary (Chapter 21)

- Antihypertensive drug therapy is indicated where
  1. diastolic blood pressure is $> 95-100$ mmHg and/or systolic blood pressure is $> 160-180$ mmHg,
  2. diastolic blood pressure is $> 90-95$ mmHg and/or systolic blood pressure is $> 140-160$ mmHg and where non-drug antihypertensive treatment/life-style modifications remain ineffective over a three- to six-month observation period,

3. blood pressure is $> 140/90$ mmHg and
   hypertension-induced target-organ damage or coexisting cardiovascular
   risk factors are present

- The therapeutic goal of antihypertensive therapy is the reduction of mortality
  and morbidity. The desired "target value" for the reduction of blood pressure is

  - $< 140/90$ mmHg for adult patients with diastolic and systolic hyperten-
    sion,
  - $120-130/80$ mmHg for young patients with mild hypertension
  - 140 mmHg for patients with isolated systolic hypertension.

- The available basic medications include

  - diuretics,
  - beta blockers and
  - ACE inhibitors, calcium antagonists and alpha$_1$-blockers.

  Up to 1995, a reduction in morbidity and mortality was observed only for
  diuretics and beta blockers.

- Before beginning drug treatment, a comprehensive discussion between doctor
  and patient is essential.

- In mild to moderate hypertension (USA: Stages 1 and 2), treatment should
  begin with a monotherapy with one of the first-line antihypertensives.

- First-line medication should be chosen based on the particulars of an individual patient's profile (concomitant diseases, additional risk factors, athletic
  activity, age, sex, race, etc.).

- The treatment of mild to moderate hypertension should begin with the lowest possible recommended dose (maximum twice a day).

- If no reduction in blood pressure is observed, treatment should be switched
  to another first-line substance class. In the event of marginal or unsatisfactory blood pressure reduction, the dosage can be increased as long as no side
  effects are noticed. If side effects occur after an increase in the dosage, the
  dosage can be reduced and the therapy expanded through the addition of a
  low dosage of a second first-line antihypertensive agent.

- The components of any combination therapy should be chosen from different
  substance classes. In the event of mild to moderate hypertension, the combination of first-line medications is recommended. In the event of severe hypertension, therapy should incorporate further substance classes (centrally-acting sympatholytics, direct vasodilators, etc.).

- Dosage increases, basic medication changes, or treatment expansion should
  be brought about slowly, since many medications reach their optimum effectiveness only after two to five weeks.

- Substance-class-specific, dosage-unrelated side-effects demand an immediate change of substance class. A change of preparations within a single substance class is pointless.

- Side effects and changes in therapy should be discussed with the patient.

- Indices of the effectiveness and safety of therapy (blood pressure, weight, and − according to medication − calcium, creatinine, uric acid, glucose, blood lipids) should be checked at regular intervals.

Literature (Chapter 21)

Alderman MH. Blood pressure management: individualized treatment based on absolute risk and the potential for benefit. Ann Intern Med 1993; 119: 329−335.

Boissel JP, Collet JP, Lion L, Ducruet T, Moleur P, Luciani J, Milon H, Madonna O, Gillet J, Gerini P, Dazord A, Haugh MC, and the OCAPI Study Group. A randomized comparison of the effect of four antihypertensive monotherapies on the subjecticve quality of life in previously untreated asymptomatic patients: field trial in general practice. J Hypertens 1995; 13: 1059−1067.

Brunner HR, Menard J, Waeber B, Burnier M, Biollaz J, Nussberger J, Bellet M. Treating the individual hypertensive patient: considerations on dose, sequential monotherapy and drug combinations. J Hypertens 1990; 8: 3−11.

Dahlöf B, Lindholm LH, Hansson L, Schersten B, Ekbom T, Wester PO. Morbidity and mortality in the Swedish trial in Old Patients with Hypertension (STOP-Hypertension). Lancet 1991; 338: 1281−1285.

Deutsche Liga zur Bekämpfung des hohen Blutdruckes e.V. Deutsche Hypertonie Gesellschaft. Empfehlungen zur Hochdruckbehandlung in der Praxis und zur Behandlung hypertensiver Notfälle. 11. Auflage, Oktober 1994.

Editorials on Government Guidelines. Am J Hypertens 1994; 7: 857−858.

Fenichel RR, Lipicky RJ. Combination products as first-line pharmacotherapy. Arch Intern Med 1994; 154: 1429−1430.

Gavras H, Gavras I. On the JNC V report. A different point of view. Am J Hypertens 1994; 7: 288−293.

Hjemdahl P, Wiklund IK. Quality of life on antihypertensive drug therapy: scientific end-point or marketing exercise? J Hypertens 1992; 10: 1437−1446.

Hoffmann G. Hypertonie und Sport. Z Sportmed 1993; 44: 153−166.

Jones JK, Gorkin L, Lian JF, Staffa JA, Fletcher AP. Discontinuation of and changes in treatment after start of new courses of antihypertensive drugs: s study of a United Kingdom population. Br Med J 1995; 311: 293−295.

Kaplan NM. Guidelines for the treatment of hypertension: an American view. J Hypertens 1995; 13 (suppl 2): S113-S117.

Materson BJ, Reda DJ, Cushman WC, Massie BM, Freis ED, Kochar MS, Hamburger RJ, Fye C, Lakshman R, Gottdiener J, Ramirez EA, Henderson WG. Single-drug therapy for hypertension in men. A comparison of six antihypertensive agents with placebo. N Engl J Med 1993; 328: 914−921.

McVeigh GE, Flack J, Grimm R. Goals of antihypertensive therapy. Drugs 1995; 49: 161−175.

Menard J. Oil and water? Economic advantage and biomedical progress do not mix well in a government guidelines committee. Am J Hypertens 1994; 7: 877−885.

Moser M. Comments on the American Journal of Hypertension editorials regarding the JNC V. Am J Hypertens 1995; 8: 542−544.

Oparil S. Antihypertensive therapy − efficacy and quality of life. N Engl J Med 1993; 328: 959−961.

Phillips RA. The cardiologist's approach to evaluation and management of the patient with essential hypertension. Am Heart J 1993; 126: 648−666.

Saito T, Sugiyama Y, Inagaki Y. Hemodynamic effects of antihypertensive agents: a comparison of diuretics, beta-blockers, calcium antagonists, and angiotensin converting enzyme inhibitors. Curr Therap Res 1992; 52: 863−877.

Sever P, Beevers G, Bulpitt C, Lever A, Ramsay L, Reid J, Swales J. Management guidelines in essential hypertension: report of the second working party of the British Hypertension Society. Br Med J 1993; 306: 983−987.

SHEP Cooperative Research Group: Prevention of stroke by antihypertensive drug treatment in older persons with isolated systolic hypertension. JAMA 1991; 265: 3255−3264.

Swales JD. Guidelines for treating hypertension: improved care or retarded progress? Am J Hapertens 1994; 7: 873−876.

Swales JD. Pharmacological treatment of hypertension. Lancet 1994; 344: 380−385.

The HOT Study Group: The hypertension optimal treatment study (HOT Study). Blood Pressure 1993; 2: 62−68.

The Joint National Committee on Detection, Evaluation, and Treatment of High Blood Pressure. The Fifth Report of the Joint National Committee on Detection, Evaluation, and Treatment of High Blood Pressure (JNC V). Arch Intern Med 1993; 153: 154−183.

Tobian L, Brunner HR, Cohn JN, Gavras H, Laragh JH, Materson BJ, Weber MA. Modern strategies to prevent coronary sequelae and stroke in hypertensive patients differ from the JNC V consensus guidelines. Am J Hypertens 1994; 7: 859−872.

Weber MA, Laragh JH. Hypertension: steps forward and steps backward. Arch Intern Med 1993; 153: 149−152.

WHO/ISH Guidelines Subcommittee. 1993 Guidelines for the management of mild hypertension: memorandum from a WHO/ISH meeting. J Hypertens 1993; 11: 905−918.

22 Specific drug treatment of hypertension

A considerable number of pharmacologically different medications for the treatment of arterial hypertension have been registered worldwide. As a result of multiple offerings of many monosubstances and the multitude of fixed combination preparations the supply of antihypertensive medications is becoming more and more difficult to keep track of. This supply brings with it an increasing complexity, which makes it ever more difficult, especially for the non-specialized physician, to make a proper choice in the individual case.

However, on the basis of the pharmacological mode of action, it is possible to divide most of the available antihypertensives into a few classes of substances (see also Table 22.1, next page):

- diuretics (Chapter 23),
- sympatholytics (Chapter 24),
- vasodilators (Chapter 25),
- calcium antagonists (Chapter 26),
- inhibitors of the renin-angiotensin-system (Chapter 27), and
- other antihypertensive acting substances (Chapter 28).

Tab. 22.1: Classification of antihypertensive drugs according to mode of action

---

1. **Diuretics**

a) Thiazides and related sulfonamides
b) Loop diuretics
c) Potassium-sparing diuretics
   - Aldosterone antagonists
   - Other potassium-sparing diuretics

2. **Sympatholytics**

a) Sympatholytics with primarily central action sites

   - Alpha-methyldopa
   - Imidazoline receptor agonists
   - Guanfacine

b) Sympatholytics with central and peripheral action sites

   - Reserpine
   - Urapidil
   - Indoramin

c) Sympatholytics with primarily peripheral action sites

   - Alpha-receptor blockers
   - Beta-receptor blockers
   - Combined beta-/alpha-receptor blockers

3. **Calcium antagonists**

   - Phenylalkylamines (verapamil type)
   - 1,4-dihydropyridines (nifedipine type)
   - Benzodiazepines (diltiazem type)
   - Others

4. **Inhibitors of the renin-angiotensin system**

   - Renin inhibitors
   - Angiotensin-converting enzyme (ACE) inhibitors
   - Angiotensin II receptor antagonists

5. **Vasodilators**

   - Hydralazine/Dihydralazine
   - Minoxodil
   - Sodium nitroprusside
   - Diazoxide

6. **Miscellaneous antihypertensive substances**

---

23 Diuretics

Diuretics are amongst the oldest medications in the treatment of hypertension and are considered first-line antihypertensives in most countries. Along with beta-adrenergic blockers they are the only class of antihypertensive substances for which there is proof of a reduction in morbidity and mortality under long-term therapy.

23.1 Mode of action and classification of diuretics

The common basic principle of all diuretics is the inhibition of the sodium and water reabsorption in the nephron, which occurs to a varying degree in the individual segments. About 60 to 70% of the glomerularly filtered sodium chloride and the free water are reabsorbed in the proximal tubule. The resorption occurs almost isoosmotically. While the sodium reabsorption continues in the ascending limb of the loop of Henle, water absorption can not be detected here. The tubular fluid therefore becomes increasingly hypertonic and the renal medulla hypotonic, so that — with continued sodium chloride absorption — water reabsorption may occur in the distal portions of the tubule. For the most part free water is then absorbed in the collecting tubule. The reabsorption of sodium chloride in the terminal segment of the nephron is then only slightly pronounced.

On the basis of their chemical structure and the resultant varying sites of action in the nephron (Figure 23.1; Table 23.1), diuretics can be categorized in various classes of substances:

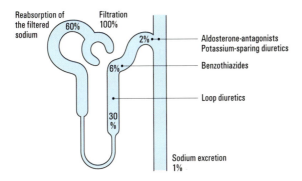

Figure 23.1: Diuretics' renal site of action

Table 23.1:   Profile of action for diuretics

Substance	Mechanism of action	Site of action	Instensity of action*	Duration of action (hr)
Thiazides	Inhibition of the Na$^+$-reabsorption	Distal tubule	++	18–72
Loop diuretics	Inhibition of the Na$^+$-reabsorption	Thick ascending limb of Henle's loop	+++	ca. 6
Aldosterone antagonists	Competitive inhibi-tion of aldosterone	Late distal tubule and collecting duet	+	up to 96
Other potassium-sparing diuretics	Blockade of Na$^+$ channels	Late distal tubule and collecting duct	+	8–24

* + weak;   ++ moderate;   +++ strong

1. Thiazide diuretics and related sulfonamides,
2. loop diuretics,
3. potassium-sparing diuretics (aldosterone antagonists and other potassium-sparing diuretics).

Osmotically active diuretics and carbonic anhydrase inhibitors are not used in the treatment of hypertension.

The administration of diuretics increases the secretion of sodium, free water and − with the exception of potassium-sparing diuretics − of potassium. Therefore, at the beginning of treatment, the diuretics cause a reduction in the extracellular and plasma volumes, whereby the venous return and therefore the cardiac output are reduced. The slight decrease of blood pressure observed during this phase causes a reflex increase in the peripheral vascular resistance, which however, again decreases during long-term diuretic treatment. Although the cardiac output has already normalized in this phase, a slight negative sodium and water balance persists under chronic treatment with diuretics. This serves to explain the diuretic-induced activation of the renin-angiotensin system with the resultant constellation of a secondary aldosteronism.

The antihypertensive pathomechanism of long-term diuretic treatment still remains completely unexplained. It does, however, appear certain that the decrease in peripheral vascular resistance can be viewed as at least partially causal for the decrease in blood pressure under chronic diuretic therapy. A direct relaxing effect of the diuretics on vascular smooth muscle can, however, be excluded. It is rather assumed that the renal effect with the increase in natriuresis is secondary to altered sodium and calcium ion distribution and therefore to reduced vascular muscular tone in the arterial resistance vessels. Another cause for the antihypertensive long-term effect of diuretics in patients with primary hypertension under discussion is a reduced cardiovascular response to catecholamines. A volume depletion as a potential pathomechanism of the chronic drop in blood pressure is quite unlikely, because the reduction of the extracellular volume under long-term diuretic treatment is at best discrete in the dosages normally applied in the treatment of hypertension.

23.2 Thiazide diuretics and related sulfonamides

Chlorthalidone, indapamide, metolazone, and xipamide are related to the thiazides, despite structural differences and are therefore discussed concurrently.

23.2.1 Mode of action, therapeutic application

Thiazide diuretics (benzothiazides, chlorothiazides, hydrochlorothiazides, etc.) and related substances (see above) inhibit the resorption of sodium and chloride ions in the early distal tubule. This then also results in a reduced uptake of potassium, so that the monotherapies with representatives of this class of substances are often accompanied by hypokalemia.

Seventy percent of the maximum antihypertensive effect is attained with dosages as low as 25 mg hydrochlorothiazide, 500 mg chlorothiazide and 25 mg chlorthalidone. To reach the full antihypertensive potential of these substances requires dosages 4 times as high. This relatively small increase in the therapeutic efficacy comes at the cost of a considerably higher and more pronounced rate of side effects (hypokalemia, hyperuricemia, reduced glucose tolerance). It is also possible that the metabolic changes attributed to the diuretics (increase in the triglycerides and cholesterol) are also a dose-dependent phenomenon, which could be avoided by lower, but therapeutically reasonable dosages. An increase in the blood lipids represents an additional cardiovascular risk and would offset the favorable effect of the normalization of the blood pressure. On the basis of the current state of medical knowledge, it is therefore recommendable that the blood lipids of patients under chronic diuretic therapy be routinely monitored in 6- to-12 month intervals.

As a result of the negative correlation between the antihypertensive efficacy of the thiazide diuretics and the reabsorption of sodium chloride, it is necessary that the patient be put on a low-sodium diet. Only in this manner can an (side-effect increasing, see above) increase in the dosage be avoided.

Antihypertensive therapy with diuretics should began at a low dosage. Due to the fact that the antihypertensive effect of the diuretics can only be assessed after a period of three to four weeks, it is not recommended that the substance be changed too early. If there is, however, a lack of or unsatisfactory response, it is recommended to avoid significantly increasing the dosage, due to the only slight increase in the efficacy and the danger of increased side effects (recommended dosages in the treatment of hypertension are for example, 12.5−25 mg hydrochlorothiazide, 15−25 mg chlorthalidone or 2.5 mg indapamide).

Instead, the early administration of a suitable second antihypertensive (ACE-inhibitor, beta blocker) should be considered, because an additive antihypertensive effect can be expected – with a constant, low-level of side effects. Good antihypertensive efficacy has also been reported for extremely low dosages of hydrochlorothiazide in combination with low dosages of other antihypertensives (6.25 mg hydrochlorothiazide/2.5 mg bisoprolol or 6.25 mg hydrochlorothiazide/3.75 mg moexipril).

Due to the fact that the pharmacological effects of thiazides are dependent on a functioning tubular secretion, their therapeutic efficacy is reduced with increasing renal insufficiency. The administration of thiazide diuretics is generally ineffectual with serum creatinine concentrations of more than 2.0 mg/dl and connected with a proportional increase in the rate of side effects with accumulation. The additional administration of a thiazide is certainly justified in cases of chronic renal insufficiency and therapeutic resistance to loop diuretics, and frequently leads to therapeutic success.

Osteoprotective effects of diuretics, suspected for years, have recently been shown in a randomized, placebo-controlled study with chlorthalidone in postmenopausal women with isolated systolic hypertension (Figure 23.2).

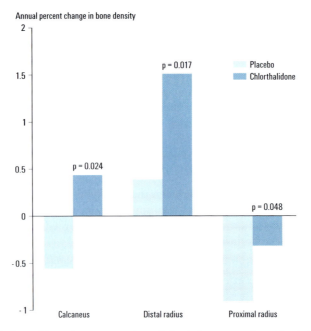

Figure 23.2: Annual bone loss rates at three skeletal sites comparing chlorthalidone use (12.5 mg-25 mg/d) with placebo in postmenopausal women with systolic hypertension participating in the SHEP-study (Systolic Hypertension in the Elderly Program). (From Wasnich RD et al., Osteoporosis Int 1995; 5: 247–251)

23.2.2 Side effects

The most important side effect of long-term diuretic therapy with thiazide diuretics and related substances is, as mentioned above, hypokalemia, which can lead to severe arrhythmia in patients with previous cardiac damage. Furthermore, the reinforcing effect of a diuretically-induced hypokalemia on glycoside therapy should be noted.

An increased calcium resorption under treatment with thiazides with simultaneous immobilization always leads to clinically relevant hypercalcemia. In addition, there have been repeated reports of impaired glucose tolerance or insulin resistance (see Section 9.3.4 for the clinical relevance of insulin resistance/hyperinsulemia as cardiovascular risk factors) under long-term treatment. For that reason it is recommended that the serum glucose be monitored after commencing therapy. In patients with disturbed glucose metabolism or manifest diabetes mellitus thiazide diuretics can lead to a further deterioration of the metabolic state, so that their administration can only be recommended in exceptional cases in this patient group (see also Section 31.5.1).

The probable dosage dependence of the LDL and the triglyceride increase and the usually asymptomatic course of the uric acid increase was dealt with above.

Impotence was observed more frequently with the long-term application of thiazide diuretics in comparison to other antihypertensives.

23.3 Loop diuretics

23.3.1 Mode of action, therapeutic use

Loop diuretics are a chemically heterogeneous group of substances whose mode of action is based on the inhibition of sodium chloride reabsorption ($Na^+/Cl^-/K^+$-cotransport system) in the ascending limb of the loop of Henle. This inhibition occurs primarily from the lumen of the tubule, so that the hypertonic state of the renal medulla in these portions is canceled and the passive water reabsorption from the collecting tubules is impaired. While the antihypertensive efficacy of the loop diuretics exhibits a comparably flat dosis-effect curve to that of the thiazides, the diuretic effect of the loop diuretics is dose dependent and marked by a peaked dosis-effect curve. As a result of this considerably more pronounced diuresis and saluresis, compared to thiazides, as well as the therapeutic effect even in the case of impaired renal function, loop diuretics are administered in the long-term treatment of high blood pressure, especially in the presence of impaired kidney function with hypervolemia and hypernatremia. The intravenous application of furosemide in combination with other fast-acting antihypertensives has proven itself to be especially valuable as a first-aid medication in the treatment of hypertensive crises (Section 32.1). It should, however, be noted in such emergency situations that the application of a high-dosed diuretic in patients with normal or reduced plasma volumes may show no effect or even lead to an increase in the hypertensive status, due to the increased activation of the renin-angiotensin-system as a result of the additional loss of fluid, and the resultant increased formation of angiotensin II "fixes" the vasoconstriction already present.

The use of furosemide as a monotherapy in the long-term treatment of uncomplicated hypertension is less common, because a weaker antihypertensive effect without any metabolic advantage is observed in comparison to thiazide diuretics.

Torasemide, piretanide, bumetanide, ethacrynic acid, etozoline and muzolimine are other loop diuretics, which are basically suited for long-term treatment, but vary in the degree to which they are accepted and licensed throughout the world.

23.3.2 Side effects

The range of the metabolic side effects is basically the same as that of thiazides (hypokalemia, hyperuricemia, hyperglycemia, hyperlipidemia). These side effects have not been observed with low-dosed therapy with torasemide (2.5−5.0 mg/ day). A possible hearing impairment may occur with long-term treatment with loop diuretics. This is most probably attributable to a change in the composition of the otic fluid.

In contrast to the thiazide diuretics, calcium excretion is actually promoted by the loop diuretics and therefore can be used in the treatment of hypercalcemic syndromes.

23.4 Potassium-sparing diuretics

Potassium-sparing diuretics are:

− aldosterone antagonists (spironolactone) and
− other substances such as amiloride and triamterene.

23.4.1   Aldosterone antagonists

23.4.1.1 Mode of action, therapeutic use

Aldosterone, secreted by the adrenal cortex, causes an exchange of sodium and potassium ions and protons in the distal tubule. As a result, there is increased sodium, chloride and water retention on the one hand and increased potassium and hydrogen excretion on the other hand. Spironolactone and related substances inhibit aldosterone competitively at the specific receptors in the distal tubule so that the physiological effect of aldosterone is canceled. The resultant natriuresis and diuresis occurs without the accompanying increase of the potassium excretion.

The amount of sodium and water excretion and the antihypertensive efficacy of spironolactone is dependent on the amount of endogenous aldosterone secretion. The therapeutic administration of spironolactone is especially recommended in most forms of hyperaldosteronism (primary aldosteronism, secondary hyperaldosteronism with heart failure, cirrhosis of the liver, etc.). As a combination, spironolactone increases the antihypertensive effect of benzothiazides and loop diuretics and compensates the loss of potassium which frequently occurs with these medications.

23.4.1.2 Side effects

The administration of aldosterone antagonists in patients with impaired renal function should − if at all − only take place with great caution, due to the fact that the reduced capability of the damaged kidney to excrete potassium may lead to dangerous hyperkalemia.

Side effects such as gynecomastia and impotence in men or amenorrhea, loss of libido and hirsutism in women, which have been observed, for the most part, in higher dosages (> 100 mg/day), occasionally require the discontinuation of therapy.

23.4.2   Other potassium-sparing diuretics

23.4.2.1 Mode of action, therapeutic use

In contrast to spironolactone, triamterene and amiloride do not interfere with aldosterone binding. These diuretics do not inhibit sodium cotransport, but rather block the sodium channels located in the distal tubule and the collecting duct. By reducing the influx of the depolarizing sodium the transepithelial potential difference of the tubular cells is decreased so that a reduced potassium secretion results in the tubular lumen. As the inhibition of the total sodium reabsorption is not very pronounced, the diuretic effect of the potassium-sparing is only relatively weak. The same is true for the reduction in blood pressure, which is only minimal at best with monotherapy. Triamterene and amiloride are therefore suited as combination partners with benzothiazides, whose induced potassium loss is then balanced.

23.4.2.2 Side effects

Disturbances of the gastrointestinal motor functions have been observed. The most important potential side effect of potassium-sparing diuretics is however an occasional hyperkalemia, which occurs under long-term therapy. Triamterene and amiloride should therefore not be used in patients with impaired renal function or in combination with an aldosterone antagonist or an ACE-inhibitor.

Summary (Chapter 23)

- Diuretics are inexpensive drugs which have proven themselves effective in the long-term treatment of hypertension.

- Diuretics are known as first-line antihypertensives; along with beta blockers they are the only class of antihypertensive drugs which have been proven to reduce morbidity and mortality.

- The most important side effect of thiazide and loop diuretics is hypokalemia. An unfavorable effect has been observed on uric acid, lipid, and carbohydrate metabolism, especially under high dosages.

- The most important side effect of aldosterone antagonists and the other potassium-sparing diuretics is hyperkalemia. Their administration is therefore contraindicated in impaired renal function.

- Due to the side effects described, diuretics should be dosed as low as possible in the long-term treatment of hypertension. The antihypertensive efficacy — in contrast to diuresis — is hardly increased by higher dosages (flat dose-effect curve).

Literature (Chapter 23)

Carlsen JE, Kober L, Torp-Pederson L, Johansen P. Relation between dose of bendrofluazide, antihypertensive effect, and adverse biochemical effects. Br Med J 1990; 300: 975−978.

Cauley JA, Cummings SR, Seeley DG, Black D, Browner W, Kuller LH, Nevitt MC. Effects of thiazide diuretic therapy on bone mass, fractures, and falls. Ann Intern Med 1993; 118: 666−673.

Dahlöf B, Lindholm LH, Hansson L, Schersten B, Ekbom T, Wester PO. Morbidity and mortality in the Swedish trial in Old Patients with Hypertension (STOP-Hypertension). Lancet 1991; 338: 1281−1285.

Dirks JH, Sutton RAL (eds.). Diuretics: physiology, pharmacology and clinical use. WB Saunders, Philadelphia, 1986.

Hampton JR. Comparative efficacy of diuretics: benefit versus risk: results of clinical trials. Europ Heart J 1992; 13 (Suppl G): 85−91.

Harper R, Ennis CN, Sheridan B, Atkinson AB, Johnston GD, Bell PM. Effects of low dose versus conventional dose thiazide diuretic on insulin action in essential hypertension. Br Med J 1994; 309: 226−230.

Hoes AW, Grobbee DE, Peet TM, Lubsen J. Do non-potassium-sparing diuretics increase the risk of sudden cardiac death in hypertensive patients? Recent evidence. Drugs 1994; 47: 711−733.

Holzgreve H. Where now the diuretics in antihypertensive treatment? Europ Heart J 1992; 13 (Suppl G): 104−108.

Knauf H, Mutschler E. Diuretic effectiveness of hydrochlorothiazide and furosemide alone and in combination in chronic renal failure. J Cardiovasc Pharmacol 1995; 26: 394−400.

Mc Veigh G, Galloway D, Johnston D. The case for low dose diuretics in hypertension: comparison of low and conventional doses of cyclopenthiazide. Br Med J 1988; 297: 95−98.

Moser M. Diuretics and cardiovascular risk factors. Europ Heart J 1992; 13 (Suppl G): 72−80.

Moser M. Effect of diuretics on morbidity and mortality in the treatment of hypertension. Cardiology 1994; 84 (suppl 2): 27−35.

MRC Working Party. Medical Research Council trial of treatment of hypertension in older adults: principal results. Br Med J 1985; 304: 405−412.

Neaton JD, Grimm RH Jr, Prineas RJ, Stamler J, Grandits GA, Elmer PJ, Cutler JA, Flack JM, Schoenberger JA, McDonald R, Lewis CE, Liebson PR. Treatment of mild hypertension study (TOMHS): final results. JAMA 1993; 270: 713−724.

Prevention of stroke by antihypertensive drug treatment in older persons with isolated systolic hypertension. Final results of the Systolic Hypertension in the Elederly Program (SHEP). JAMA 1991; 265: 3255−3264.

Ramsay LE, Yeo WW, Jackson PR. Metabolic effects of diuretics. Cardiology 1994; 84 (suppl 2): 48−56

Siscovick DS, Raghunathan TE, Psaty BM, Koepsell TD, Wicklund KG, Lin X, Cobb L, Rautaharju PM, Copass MK, Wagner EH. Diuretic therapy for hypertension and the risk of primary cardiac arrest. N Engl J Med 1994; 330: 1852−1857.

Schmieder RE, Rockstroh JK. Efficacy and tolerance of low-dose loop diuretics in hypertension. Cardiology 1994; 84 (suppl 2): 36−42.

Storstein L. Diuretics, arrhythmias and silent myocardial ischaemia in hypertensive patients. Europ Heart J 1992; 13 (Suppl G): 81−84.

Wasnich RD, Davis JW, He YF, Petrovich H, Ross PD. A randomized, double-masked, placebo-controlled trial of chlorthalidone and bone loss in elderly women. Osteoporosis Int 1995; 5: 247−251.

24 Sympatholytic (antiadrenergic) agents

The causal interweaving of the sympathetic nervous system in the, to date, unexplained pathogenesis of primary hypertension takes the development of pharmacological substances into account whose antihypertensive effect results from a reduction in sympathetic tone. As a result of their direct interference with the sympathetic nervous system, these substances are summarized in the following as sympatholytics. A distinction is made between medications with primarily central sites of action (alpha-methyldopa, I_1-imidazoline-receptor agonists, guanfacine), with primarily peripheral sites of action (alpha$_1$ and beta-adrenergic receptor blockers) and those acting both peripherally and centrally (reserpine, urapidil).

24.1 Primarily centrally-acting sympatholytics

24.1.1 Alpha-methyldopa

24.1.1.1 Mode of action, therapeutic use

The blood-pressure reducing effect of alpha-methyldopa is obtained by acting on the brain stem where it is first of all absorbed by noradrenergic neurons and then forms the "false neurotransmitter" methylnorepinephrine. The methylnorepinephrine released stimulates central alpha$_2$-receptors and leads to a peripheral reduction of the sympathicotone. As a result there is a decrease in the peripheral vascular resistance. Heart rate and cardiac output remain for the most part constant. A reduction in the renal blood flow and the glomerular filtration rate is not observed following the administration of alpha-methyldopa. This is why this substance has long been used as the therapy of choice in hypertensives with impaired renal function. Due to an increase in the plasma volume, a combination therapy of methyldopa and a diuretic is recommended.

Alpha-methyldopa is initially dosed at 250 mg 1−2 times per day; with the maximum recommended dose of 2 g daily, the rate of side effects increases noticeably. Though duration of action is up to 24 hours, it is generally divided into two applications to obtain a satisfactory reduction in blood pressure throughout the day.

Although alpha-methyldopa has a good antihypertensive efficacy, it is no longer recommended as basic treatment as a result of the frequency of side effects.

24.1.1.2 Side effects

The most important side effect is the initial sedation occurring in 60% of the patients treated and persistent sedation in 20−30%. Fatigue, poor concentration and forgetfulness as well as dryness of the mouth and nasal congestion were frequently observed with long-term treatment with alpha-methyldopa (10−75%). The remaining spectrum of side effects includes depressive mood, dizziness, dyspnea, orthostatic dysregulation and increased tendency towards diarrhea.

24.1.2 Imidazoline receptor agonists

The discovery of imidazoline receptors (I_1 and I_2) and especially their importance for the centrally controlled regulation of the blood pressure has led to a new understanding of the antihypertensive mechanism of action of a number of centrally acting substances. Correspondingly it was possible to demonstrate that the antihypertensive effect of clonidine is not − as had long been suspected − the result of a stimulation of central alpha$_2$-receptors, but rather caused by an activation of I_1-imadazoline receptors.

Imadoziline receptors, however, bind not only imidazoline derivatives, but structurally similar molecules such as oxazolines (e.g. rilmenidine) or guanidine derivatives (e.g. guanethidine, guanfacine).

All agents of this class of substances lead to the reduction in hypertensive-related, left ventricular cardiac hypertrophy; an influence on the lipid and carbohydrate metabolism has not been observed under long-term therapy.

24.1.2.1 Clonidine

Mode of action, therapeutic use:

Clonidine is an imidazoline derivative. Until recently it was suspected that the hypertensive effect of clonidine was based on a stimulation of centrally located alpha$_2$-receptors in the medulla oblongata. It has been subsequently demonstrated that the antihypertensive effect of clonidine occurs either for the most part or exclusively via the I_1-imidazoline receptors, which are located in the ventrolateral portion of the medulla oblongata (rostral ventrolateral medulla). The resulting decrease in sympathetic tone leads to a relaxation of the peripheral vascular musculature, a drop in the heart rate and a decreased cardiac output. The result is a drop in the blood pressure which commences about 30 minutes after oral administration of clonidine, reaches its peak after about 3 hours and may last for as long as 24 hours.

Clonidine has a slight affinity to the imidazoline receptors (30%) and a high affinity to the alpha$_2$-receptors (70%). This might explain the side effects such as sedation and dryness of the mouth which have been observed under clonidine treatment and are probably the result of activation of the alpha$_2$-receptors. Since these side effects are dose-dependent, clonidine should not be dosed higher than 0.075 mg twice a day at the beginning. Intramuscular and intravenous administration of clonidine causes a considerably quicker or immediate decrease, injecting too quickly may however, cause an undesired, temporary increase of the arterial blood pressure. These forms of administration should, however, be reserved for hypertensive crises (Section 32.1).

Side effects:

Many patients describe the dryness of the mouth in particular as being very disturbing. By reducing the dose, it is often possible to avoid these concomitant events, whereby the possible decrease in antihypertensive effect may make it necessary to administer an additional antihypertensive. Diuretics, calcium antagonists, ACE inhibitors and dihydralazine are well suited for combination therapy in such cases.

Abrupt discontinuation of chronic clonidine treatment can precipitate a hypertensive crisis (rebound phenomenon) which can best be combated by intravenous administration of clonidine or labetalol (combined beta/alpha$_1$-receptor blocker).

Clonidine can "unmask" a clinically unmanifested sick sinus syndrome and thereby induce life-threatening bradycardia. Clonidine is contraindicated in patients with known sick sinus syndrome.

24.1.2.2 Moxonidine

Mode of action, therapeutic use:

With moxonidine (and rilmenidine, see below), a conscious attempt was made to develop a central antihypertensive with the highest possible affinity to the I$_1$-imidazoline receptor. Accordingly, moxonidine demonstrated a considerably higher selectivity for the I$_1$-imidazoline receptors located in the RVLM (rostral ventrolateral medulla). The affinity to the alpha$_2$-receptors is, in contrast, considerably lover. Since I$_1$-imidazoline receptors have also been identified in the adrenal medulla and the kidney, it is conceivable that the antihypertensive effect of the imidazoline receptor agonists occurs via peripheral mechanisms. Thus stimulation of these binding sites inhibits the release of renin and the reabsorption of sodium by the kidney and possibly the release of catecholamines from the adrenal medulla.

Placebo-controlled studies and active-controlled comparative studies have demonstrated that moxonidine has a comparable blood-pressure reducing efficacy to that of other antihypertensives. The recommended initial dose in patients with mild to moderate hypertension (USA: Stage 1 and 2) is 0.2 mg, the maximum recommended daily dose 0.6 mg. Dose increases should occur in three week intervals, in case the blood pressure has not decreased sufficiently.

Side effects:

Side effects like dryness of the mouth and sedation by a stimulation of central alpha$_2$-receptors have been observed less frequently under moxonidine than under clonidine. Should these results also be confirmed in larger patient populations in clinical routine, it would indicate a clinical relevance for the high affinity to the

I_1-imidazoline receptor and considerably lower affinity to the alpha$_2$-receptor. Rebound hypertension following the abrupt discontinuation of moxonidine has not been reported so far.

24.1.2.3 Rilmenidine

The mode of action, therapeutic application and side effects profile for rilmenidine do not essentially differ from those of moxonidine. The selectivity for the I_1-imidazoline receptor is, however, somewhat less. This has not been determined to be of clinical relevance.

The recommended initial dose of 1 mg/day can be doubled (1 mg b.i.d), if the antihypertensive effect is not satisfactory.

24.1.3   Guanfacine

24.1.3.1 Mode of action, therapeutic use

The substance guanfacine is similar to clonidine, with a considerably higher affinity to central alpha$_2$-receptors. To what extent the antihypertensive effect is determined by the stimulation of these receptors is not clear. An activation of I_1-imidazoline receptors in the RVLM is also a possible explanation for the blood-pressure reducing mechanism of action (see above), although the binding of guanfacine to these structures is only very weak.

24.1.3.2 Side effects

The side effects that can be expected are about the same as those of clonidine; dryness of the mouth and sedation appear somewhat less frequently and in the studies reported to date could be completely avoided by a dose reduction to 2 mg/day or less. The danger of a rebound phenomenon after discontinuation of a long-term treatment with guanfacine may also exist with this substance, even if there have only been a few reports dealing with this problem to date.

24.2   Sympatholytics with central and peripheral sites of action

24.2.1   Reserpine

24.2.1.1 Mode of action, therapeutic use

Norepinephrine, which is stored in the neuronal vesicles, is released by exocytosis into the synaptic gap during the transmission of sympathetic impulses, whereby a certain portion of this transmitter substance is subsequently taken up by the neuron and stored in specific vesicles.

Reserpine lowers the norepinephrine content of the central and peripheral neurons in that it inhibits the active transport of norepinephrine into storage vesicles. Furthermore, reserpine inhibits the transport of dopamine, a precursor of norepinephrine, into the vesicles. A consequence of the resulting transmitter depletion is a reduction in peripheral vascular resistance. Due to the strong binding of reserpine to the vesicle, the effect is only canceled by the resynthesis of adrenergic vesicles. For that reason reserpine's antihypertensive effect continues for several weeks even after the discontinuation of the substance. The reduced sympathetic tone leads to a predominance of vagal tone, which can cause a decrease in cardiac output, due to a drop in the heart rate.

Reserpine was, in 1953, the first agent approved for the long-term treatment of high blood pressure. Due to its poor control, the nonspecific effect on the sympathetic nervous system and the resultant − especially with high dosages − side effects, reserpine is no longer recommended as basic medication.

24.2.1.2 Side effects

Weariness, sedation, depressive mood and increased dreaming are reserpine's known side effects. The predominance of parasympathetic influences causes an increased production of gastric juices, which can, amongst other things, cause stomach ulcers.

The side effects are dose-dependent and observed considerably less often in the dosages recommended today (max. 0.5 mg/day).

Reserpine is available primarily in combination preparations, whereby benzothiazide diuretics and vasodilators have proven to be good partners.

24.2.2   Urapidil

24.2.2.1 Mode of action, therapeutic use

Urapidil is a substance with central and peripheral sites of action. On the one hand it has been proven to stimulate central serotonine receptors (5-hydroxy-tryptophan$_{1A}$-(5-HT$_{1A}$-) receptors) with consequent reduction of the sympathetic tone, on the other hand it inhibits the peripheral alpha$_1$-receptors. Urapidil's antihypertensive effect is attributable to the resulting decrease in the peripheral vascular resistance. A reflex increase in the heart rate should not be expected.

Long-term treatment with urapidil is initiated with 30 mg twice daily; a maximum daily dose of 180 mg should not be exceeded. Urapidil is available for intravenous administration for the treatment of hypertensive crises.

24.2.2.2 Side effects

Side effects described to date are dizziness, nausea and headache, in rare cases weariness, orthostatic dysregulation, dryness of the mouth and allergic skin reactions.

24.2.3   Indoramin

24.2.3.1 Mode of action, therapeutic use

Indoramin is another hybrid substance whose mechanism of action is, on the one hand (primarily) based on the blockade of peripheral alpha$_1$-receptors and in addition is possibly due to stimulation of medullary 5-HT$_{1A}$ receptors. The recommended dose is $25-200$ mg/day. Diuretics and beta-adrenergic receptor blockers are suitable combination partners. Indoramin is licensed in Germany.

24.2.3.2 Side effects

Side effects are sedation, fatigue, dryness of the mouth and ejaculation disturbances.

Summary (Sections 24.1 and 24.2)

- Sympatholytics with primarily or partially central sites of action have proven to be effective in reducing blood pressure.

- The most important side effects of these substances are sedation, fatigue and dryness of the mouth. Due to the dose dependence of these events, long-term treatment should only be conducted in low dosages.

- Lipid and carbohydrate metabolism are not affected.

- Hypertensive-related hypertrophy of the heart is reduced with long-term therapy.

- Combination with a second antihypertensive (e.g. diuretics) is recommended at an early date should the reduction in blood pressure be unsatisfactory.

- The abrupt discontinuation of long-term treatment with clonidine or guanfacine can precipitate a hypertensive crisis (rebound hypertension).

- Long-term experience with broad application in clinical routine will show to what extent the favorable side effect profile demonstrated by the new selective imidazoline receptor agonists to date truly exceed that of other centrally acting sympatholytics.

24.3 Primarily peripherally-acting sympatholytics

24.3.1 Alpha adrenergic receptor blockers

The alpha-receptor blockers currently available can be divided into non-selective and (alpha$_1$-) selective substances.

24.3.1.1 Non-selective alpha adrenergic receptor blockers

Phentolamine, phenoxybenzamine:

Mode of action, therapeutic use and side effects

Non-selective alpha-receptor blockers such as phentolamine and phenoxybenzamine are used in the treatment of pheochromocytomas (Section 34.4). Both substances block postsynaptic alpha$_1$-receptors in vascular smooth muscle as well as presynaptic (central) alpha$_2$-receptors. While the blocking effect of phentolamine is reversible and only of a short duration, phenoxybenzamine is accompanied by a covalent, irreversible binding to the receptors. In contrast to phentolamine, which has a short duration of action and is used almost exclusively in the acute treatment of hypertensive crises with pheochromocytoma, phenoxybenzamine demonstrates a long period of action. Phenoxybenzamine serves as a preoperative treatment and long-term treatment of non-operable pheochromocytomas (Section 34.4). Phenoxybenzamine and phentolamine have not been able to establish themselves in the treatment of primary hypertension due to pronounced orthostatic dysregulation, weariness and dizziness and a strong (reflex) tachycardia.

Urapidil, indoramin:

Urapidil and indoramin are hybrid substances whose blood pressure reducing effects are transmitted on the one hand by a blockade of peripheral alpha$_1$-receptors and, on the other hand, by a stimulation of central serotonine receptors (Sections 24.2.2 and 24.2.3).

24.3.1.2 Selective alpha$_1$-adrenergic receptor blockers

The selective alpha$_1$-receptor blockers recommended for the treatment of arterial hypertension have recently been classified as first-line medication by most professional societies, because, beside their proven antihypertensive efficacy and safety, they favorably influence other cardiovascular risk factors. An increase in HDL cholesterol and a drop in LDL and total cholesterol and triglycerides is observed with the administration of an alpha$_1$-receptor blocker. The metabolic state of patients with diabetes mellitus is not impaired; in overweight, normoglycemic hypertensive patients an improvement in insulin sensitivity was seen after the administration of prazosin and doxazosin. As with all modern antihypertensives, long-term therapy with selective alpha$_1$-receptors leads to a regression of left ventricular hypertrophy.

Therapeutic benefits from the consequences of a selective alpha$_1$-receptor blockade have also been attained for the symptomatic treatment of obstructive, benign prostatic hypertrophy. Elderly male hypertensives in particular could additionally benefit from this.

Prazosin:

Mode of action, therapeutic use

Prazosin was introduced as a nonspecific vasodilator for the treatment of arterial hypertension in the mid-seventies. Only later was it discovered that the antihypertensive effect is the result of a selective blockade of postsynaptic alpha$_1$-receptors. The related competitive inhibition of norepinephrine in vascular smooth muscle causes a dilation of the peripheral resistance vessels so that a reduction in arterial blood pressure results. Despite this vasodilatation a slight reflex tachycardia is observed. This phenomenon is attributed to the lack of influence on the presynaptic alpha$_2$-receptors.

The cardiac output, renal circulation and the glomerular filtration rate do not demonstrate any significant change under long-term treatment with prazosin.

As severe orthostatic reactions may occur initially, therapy with prazosin must be introduced slowly. An initial dose of 0.5 mg is recommended. This can then be increased to a maximum daily dose of 12 mg in the following days, depending on therapeutic response. In most cases it will be necessary to divide the dose into two or three dosages daily, because the plasma half-life of prazosin is 2–3 hours.

Diuretics reinforce the antihypertensive effect of prazosin and in the case of unsatisfactory reaction to the monotherapy are well-suited as are beta-receptor blockers for combination therapy.

Side effects

The most important and relatively frequently occurring side effects are the initial orthostatic complaints, which may occur along with headache, nausea, vomiting and palpitations. These complaints are, however, only of a temporary nature and generally do not require a dose reduction. Occasional side effects are rashes, polyarthritis, incontinence, priapism, headache, dryness of the mouth, nasal congestion and depressive mood.

Doxazosin, terazosin:

Mode of action, therapeutic application and the side effect profile of these newer alpha$_1$-receptor blockers are for the most part the same as those of prazosin. The only difference is the duration of action of these substances, which allows for the once-daily administration. Excessive hypotensive reactions at the beginning of treatment are apparently seen more seldom than with prazosin. Nevertheless, the danger of a pronounced hypotension with doxazosin or terazosin can not be excluded.

Summary (Section 24.3.1)

- The non-selective alpha-receptor blockers phentolamine and phenoxybenzamine are reserved for the treatment of hypertension with pheochromocytoma.
- Selective alpha$_1$-receptor blockers such as prazosin, doxazosin and terazosin are safe and effective antihypertensives, which, in the meantime, have been recognized in most countries as first-line drugs for the long-term treatment of primary hypertension.

- Selective alpha$_1$-receptor blockers have a favorable or neutral effect on the lipid and carbohydrate metabolism; left ventricular cardiac hypertrophy is reduced with long-term treatment.

- The most important side effect is the orthostatic hypotension, especially at the beginning of treatment, which therefore should be introduced slowly.

- Diuretics and beta-receptor blockers are recommended as combination therapy should the individual antihypertensive effect be insufficient.

24.3.2 Beta-adrenergic receptor blockers

Beta-adrenergic receptor blockers are recognized throughout the world as first line therapy for the treatment of primary hypertension. Together with diuretics they were until 1996 the only substance classes for which corresponding long-term studies had proven that they lead to a reduction in the increased incidence of mortality and morbidity in patients with primary hypertension (see Chapters 21 and 23). Beta-receptor blockers were first used for the treatment of coronary artery disease. Only in the mid-60s was their blood-pressure reducing effect and their benefit for the treatment of arterial hypertension discovered.

24.3.2.1 Mode of action, therapeutic use

The pharmacological effect of beta-receptor blockers is based on a competitive inhibition (blockade) of the sympathomimetic-acting neurotransmitters norepinephrine and epinephrine on the cellular beta-receptors of the specific target organ (Table 24.1). There is a positive correlation between the sympathetic activity and the beta-receptor blocker's intensity of effect. Despite more than 20 years of clinical experience in the treatment of arterial hypertension, the precise mechanism of action for blood-pressure reduction is still unclear. With the acute administration of a beta-receptor blocker there is first of all a decrease in cardiac output and an increase in peripheral vascular resistance; with long-term therapy the cardiac output again approaches, but does not reach, the initial values. The increased vascular resistance normalizes, for the most part, with the chronic administration of beta-receptor blockers. If, and in what manner, the humoral changes (increased plasma levels of epinephrine and norepinephrine, suppressed plasma-renin activity) play a role in triggering the blood-pressure reduction observed with the administration of beta blockers, is also unclear.

The maximum antihypertensive efficacy is generally attained after two to four weeks of treatment.

The differentiation between beta$_1$ and beta$_2$ receptors based on the various functional effects of norepinephrine and epinephrine led to the development of (rela-

Table 24.1:   Organ-specific effects of beta-receptor blockers

Target organ	Receptor class	Effect of the receptor blockade
Heart	Beta$_1$	Reduction in contractility Reduction in heart rate Slowing of sino-atrial rhythm and prolongation of the atrioventricular conduction Decreased excitability of the myocardium
Kidneys	Beta$_1$	Inhibition of renin release
Bronchi	Beta$_2$	Constriction
Smooth muscle tissue		
− Uterus	Beta$_2$	Constriction
− Intestines	Beta$_1$	Constriction
− Vasculature	Beta$_1$	Constriction of the coronary arteries
	Beta$_2$	Constriction
Skeletal muscles	Beta$_2$	Inhibition of glycogenolysis
Fat tissue (FT)		
− Subcutaneous FT, "white" fat cells	Beta$_{1/2/3}$*	Inhibition of lipolysis, retention of fat in fat cells
− Visceral FT, "brown" fat cells (thermogenesis)	Beta$_3$*	Thermogenetic inhibition; induction of obesity(?)
Pancreas	Beta$_2$	Inhibition of insulin secretion
Eyes		
− Intra-occular pressure	Beta$_1$	Decrease
− Lacrimal secretion	Beta$_2$	Decrease
Hormone release		
− Renin	Beta$_{1>2}$	Inhibition
− Insulin	Beta$_2$	Inhibition
− Glucagon	Beta$_2$	Inhibition

* Theoretical considerations based on knowledge of beta$_3$ receptor stimulation

tively) beta$_1$-selective ("cardioselective") receptor blockers and non-selective beta-receptor blockers (Table 24.2).

A further differentiating characteristic of the beta-receptor blockers is a sympathomimetic "residual activity" (intrinsic sympathomimetic activity − ISA) of some of the members of this class of substances, which is based on the similarity of their molecular structure with that of sympathomimetics and causes only a slight drop in resting heart rate and resting cardiac output (Table 24.2). Beta blockers with vasodilating or alpha receptor-blocking properties are dealt with in Section 24.3.3.

The organ-specific effects of beta-receptor blockers are summarized, as are the typical substance properties and dosages of numerous preparations, in Tables 24.1 and 24.3.

Table 24.2:   Classification of beta-receptor blockers according to cardioselectivity

Selectivity	ISA		Vasodilatory/ alpha-receptor blocking properties
	No	Yes	
Non-selective	Bupranolol	Alprenolol	Amusolol
	Carazolol	Bopindolol	Bucindolol
	Madolol	Bunitrolol	Carvedilol
	Metipranolol	Carteolol	Labetalol
	Propanolol	Mepindolol	Nipradilol
	Sotalol	Oxprenolol	
	Timolol	Penbutolol	
	Pindolol		
Selective	Atenolol	Acebutolol	Arotinolol
	Betaxolol	Celiprolol	Bevantolol
	Bisoprolol		
	Metoprolol		

ISA = intrinsic sympathomimetic activity

Beta-receptor blockers as monotherapy − like other first-line antihypertensives − sufficiently lower blood pressure in about 40−60% of the patients with mild to moderate hypertension (USA: Stages 1 and 2). In cases of insufficient therapeutic response, in principle any basic medication is suitable as a combination partner; for pharmacodynamic reasons the additional administration of a diuretic, a calcium antagonist of the dihydropyridine-(nifedipine-)-type or a selective alpha$_1$-receptor antagonist are especially favorable (see Chapter 30).

24.3.2.2 Side effects

The non-specific side effects common to therapy with other antihypertensives are − especially at the beginning − also observed with the use of beta-receptor blockers: headache, dizziness, fatigue, gastrointestinal complaints, impotence, symptomatic hypotension, etc.

Specific side effects are for the most part based on the inhibitory influence on the beta$_2$-receptors.

Arterial vascular system

Vasoconstriction induced in the areas of vascular smooth muscle, especially of peripheral arteries explains the feeling of "cold extremities"; in patients with Raynaud's phenomenon or a peripheral arterial occlusive disease, the reduced peripheral blood supply often leads to a deterioration in symptoms and the objective disease picture.

Bronchial system

In patients with bronchial asthma a blockade of the beta-receptors of smooth bronchial muscle may cause acute bronchial spasm. Although this danger is re-

Table 24.3: Pharmacological properties and recommended dosages of beta-receptor blockers

Substance	Tradename (examples in Germany)	Beta$_1$-selectivity*	Lipophilicity	ISA**	Bioavailability (%)	Normal daily dose (mg)
Acebutalol	Prent, Sectral	+	+	+	40–60	2 × 400–800
Atenolol	Tenormin	+	–	–	50	25–100
Alprenolol	Aptin	–	+	+	1–15	200–400
Betaxolol	Kerlone	+	–	–	80–90	10–20
Bunitrolol	Stresson	–		+	13–44	20–40
Bupranolol	betadrenol	–		–	>10	100–600
Carazolol	Conducton	–		–	>10	18–30
Carteolol	Endak, Cartrol	–	–	+	90	2,5–10 (20)
Celiprolol	Selectol, Corliprol	+	–	+	50–70	200–400
Mepindolol	Corindolan	–		+	>95	4–10
Metipranolol	Disorat	–	+	–	50	20–60
Metoprolol	Beloc; Lopresor	+	–	–	50	50–200
Nadolol	Solgol	–	–	–	20–34	60–120
Oxprenolol	Trasicor	–	+	+	24–60	40–160
Penbutolol	Betapressin, Levatol	–	+	+	>95	40
Pindolol	Visken	–	+	+	85	15–30
Propranolol	Dociton, Inderal	–	+	–	30	120–320
Sotalol	Sotalex, Betapace	–	–	–	70	80–160
Timolol	Temserin, Blocadren	–	+	–	75	10–60

* Relative selectivity;   ** Intrinsic sympathomimetic activity

duced under the administration of beta$_1$-selective substances, it is generally recommended to avoid treatment with beta blockers in such patients and in cases of concurrent hypertension to perform therapy with another class of antihypertensive substances. Therapy with beta blockers is also not recommended in patients with chronic obstructive lung diseases, since shortness of breath may increasingly occur.

Exercise tolerance

The reduction in exercise tolerance occurs independent of selectivity or ISA, so that therapy with beta-receptor blockers in patients who pursue sports is not ideal.

Cardiac conduction system

Beta-receptor blockers should not be given in cases of pronounced bradycardia, with atrioventricular (AV) blocks or with sick sinus syndrome (SSS).

It is generally not advised to combine therapy with a centrally active sympatholytic (e.g. clonidine), because the additive effect may precipitate bradycardia, or in extreme cases − asystolia (demasking of an SSS). Furthermore, there are doubts about the combined administration of beta-receptor blockers and calcium antagonists which delay the AV-conduction (verapamil, diltiazem). In known cases of AV blocks the combination is already contraindicated.

Heart failure

Therapy with beta-receptor blockers may lead to an acute decompensation in patients with pre-existing heart failure. Nevertheless, a general contraindication to heart failure, as has been advocated for many years, can, due to new information, no longer be universally made. For one, the benefit of beta-blockers in the secondary prophylaxis of patients who have suffered myocardial infarction (equivalent to a loss of ventricular muscular mass with, as a rule, reduced cardiac strength, as a rule at least equivalent to heart failure of NYHA classification I to II) has been proven. Beyond that patients with moderate to severe heart failure (NYHA stage III to IV) and insufficient response to preexisting therapy appear to profit from an additional low-dose administration of a non-selective beta-receptor blocker (about 40% of beta receptors in insufficient myocardium are beta-receptors) with vasodilatory properties. The proof of an actual reduction in mortality and morbidity in this patient population has thus far only been made for carvedilol as add-on therapy. The results of future studies with metropolol (BEST study), carvedilol (CHOICE study) and bucindolol must be evaluated before we can pass final judgment on the therapeutic value of a pharmacological beta-receptor blockade in the treatment of moderate to severe heart failure.

Metabolism

The influence on carbohydrate metabolism has been known for some time and affects both patients with diabetes mellitus as well as healthy individuals. While insulin resistance and − in comparison to untreated patients considerably more frequently − a manifest diabetes could develop under long-term treatment with beta-receptor blockers, there is an additional hazard of hypoglycemia in known diabetics. Since the counterregulation under hypoglycemic conditions, especially in insulin-dependent (and frequently low-glucagon) diabetics, is primarily determined by epinephrine, a blockade of the beta adrenergic receptors causes, a delay in metabolic normalization or a re-increase of the glucose.

The influence of the beta-receptor blockers on the distribution of the blood lipids depends on the class of the substance; with non-selective beta-receptor blockers without ISA there is an increase in triglycerides and a decrease in the HDL-cholesterol. The LDL-cholesterol does not change significantly. The lipid metabolism is hardly influenced, if at all, by selective substances with ISA or those with additional vasodilatory/alpha-receptor blocking properties (Table 24.2).

In evaluating this metabolic influence with the administration of non-selective beta-receptor blockers without ISA it must be kept in mind that a reduction in cardiovascular risk with long-term therapy has been proven with these substances, while the proof of any clinical relevance in the minimal lipid changes does not yet exist.

CNS

The most frequent central-nervous system side effects which have been reported with beta-receptor blockers are sleeplessness, depressive mood and nightmares.

Rebound hypertension

Long-term therapy with beta blockers should always be slowly tapered; a sudden release of the adrenergic receptors, which have been blocked for a long period of time should be avoided, because the receptors exhibit an increased sensitivity and the increased concentrations of catecholamines can set off a sympathetic overreaction (hypertension, tachycardia). Increased cardiac oxygen demand may lead to acute ischemia, especially in patients with concomitant heart disease.

Summary (Section 24.3.2)

- Beta-receptor blockers are recognized as a first line therapy for the treatment of arterial hypertension throughout the world; increased mortality and morbidity in hypertensive patients are reduced with long-term therapy.

- Beta-receptor blockers are a heterogeneous class of substances, which can be differentiated from each other by pharmacological properties such as relative cardiac (beta$_1$-) selectivity, an intrinsic sympathomimetic activity (ISA) and an additional (vasodilating) influence on the alpha$_1$-receptors.

- The therapeutic response rate in mild to moderate hypertension is 40 to 60%; the maximum antihypertensive effect is to be expected after two to four weeks.

- Diuretics, dihydropyridine calcium antagonists and selective alpha$_1$-receptor blockers are favorable combination partners in cases of unsatisfactory blood pressure response.

- As with all antihypertensives, non-specific side effects should be expected, especially at the beginning of treatment (headache, nausea, fatigue, etc.)

- In cases of heart failure, manifest, particularly insulin-dependent diabetes mellitus, peripheral arterial occlusive disease, obstructive pulmonary diseases and athletic patients, therapy with beta-receptor blockers should be carefully considered.

- Bradycardia and AV blocks (especially with elderly patients) and the presence of sick sinus syndrome are contraindications.

24.3.3 Beta adrenergic receptor blockers with additional pharmacological properties (hybrid substances)

The following table represents a summary of beta-receptor blockers which additionally have one or more vasodilatory, pharmacological modes of action available (so-called hybrids or pseudohybrids) (Table 24.4).

Table 24.4: Beta-receptor blockers with an additional vasodilator component*

Substance	Pharmacodynamic profile	
	Beta-receptor Selectivity	Vasodilator component
Amosulalol	$Beta_1$ and $beta_2$	$Alpha_1$-receptor blockade
Arotinolol	$Beta_1 > beta_2$	$Alpha_1$ and $alpha_2$-receptor blockade
Carvedilol	$Beta_1$ and $beta_2$	$Alpha_1$-receptor blockade
Labetalol	$Beta_1$ and $beta_2$	$Alpha_1$-receptor blockade
Bevantolol	$Beta_1 > beta_2$	"Direct" vasodilatation?
BW-A575C	$Beta_1$ and $beta_2$	ACE inhibition
Celiprolol	$Beta_1 \gg beta_2$	$Beta_2$-receptor agonism and "direct" vasodilatation
Nipradilol	$Beta_1$ and $beta_2$	"Direct" vasodilatation via cGMP

* Modified acc. to van Zwieten PA, 1993

24.3.3.1 Combined beta- and alpha$_1$-receptor blockers

Labetalol:

Mode of action, therapeutic use

The antihypertensive effect of labetalol is based on a non-selective beta-receptor blockade and a selective blockade of the postsynaptic alpha$_1$-receptors. As a beta-receptor blocker labetalol is considerably weaker than propanolol and as an alpha blocker weaker than prazosin. The beta-blocking effect of labetalol is about 3 to 7 times stronger than the alpha-blocking effect.

Under chronic long-term therapy with labetalol there is a reduction in both the resting and exercise heart rate, the peripheral vascular resistance, the myocardial contractility and the cardiac output.

The oral administration of labetalol should begin with low dosages (100 mg twice-daily); the maximum dosage is 800 mg/day. There have been repeated reports of increased sensitivity to the substance with increasing age. Orally and parenterally, labetalol is indicated for the treatment of hypertensive crisis. Due to a slight expansion of the plasma volume with labetalol, diuretics are suitable combination partners when blood pressure has been insufficiently decreased. It should, however, be noted that orthostatic decreases in blood pressure may occur more frequently.

Side effects

The most frequent side effect, complaints of which are most frequently heard at the beginning of therapy, is orthostatic hypotension. These complaints are considerably more frequent with concomitant therapy with diuretics or vasodilators.

Other, less frequent side effects are headache, nausea, nasal congestion, gastrointestinal disorders and rashes.

Since rare cases of liver cell damage have been reported with the use of labetalol, patients with a history of liver disorders should be subjected to particularly careful monitoring of the liver function.

An influence on the lipid metabolism — in accordance with the selective $alpha_1$-receptor blockers — has not been reported.

The contraindications for other beta-receptor blocking substances should also be considered to be binding for labetalol.

Carvedilol:

Carvedilol is another substance, which, along with its primarily inhibitive (non-selective) effect on the beta-adrenergic receptors, exhibits vasodilatory properties that are based on the additional blockade of peripheral $alpha_1$-receptors. Furthermore, carvedilol has been said to have calcium antagonistic properties which also possibly contribute to the substance's antihypertensive effect.

A further therapeutic application of carvedilol is to be expected as add-on therapy in patients with moderate to severe heart failure not sufficiently responding to preexisting standard therapeutic regimens.

Summary (Section 24.3.3)

- Beta-receptor blockers with additional blocking effects on peripheral alpha$_1$-adrenergic receptors are suitable for the initial treatment of hypertension.

- The side effects profile is for the most part the same as that of other beta-receptor blockers; an influence on the lipid metabolism, however, has not been observed ("metabolically neutral").

- Oral and intravenous administration of labetalol is suitable for the primary treatment of a hypertensive crisis.

Literature (Chapter 24)

Bengtsson C, Blohme G, Lapidus L, Lissner L, Lundgren H. Diabetes incidence in users and non-users of antihypertensive drugs in relation to serum insulin, glucose tolerance and degree of adiposity: a 12-year prospective study of women in Gothenburg, Sweden. J Intern Med 1992; 231: 583–588.

Bousquet P, Feldman J, Schwartz J. Central cardiovascular effects of alpha-adrenergic drugs: differences between catecholamines and imidazolines. J Pharmacol Exp Ther 1984; 230: 232–236.

Bousquet P, Feldman J, Tibirica E, Bricca G, Greney H, Dontenwill M, Stutzmann J, Belcourt A. Imidazoline receptors. A new concept in central regulation of the arterial blood pressure. Am J Hypertens 1992; 5: 47S–50S.

Brown MJ. To beta block or better block? Beta-1-selectivity rarely matters in clinical practice despite the hype. Br Med J 1995; 311: 701–702.

Bristow MR, O'Conell JB, Gilbert EM, French WJ, Letherman G, Kantrowitz NE, Orie J, Smucker J, Smuckker ML, Marshall G, Kelly P, Peitchman D, Anderson JL, for the Bucindolol Investigators. Dose-response of chronic beta-blocker treatment in heart failure from either idiopathic dilated or ischemic cardiomyopathy. Circulation 1994; 89: 1632–1642.

Chatterjee K. Potential use of third-generation beta-blockers in heart failure. J Cardiovasc Pharmacol 1989; 14 (Suppl. 7): S22–S27.

Chadda K, Goldstein S, Byington R, Curb J. Effect of propanolol after acute myocardial infarction in patients with congestive heart failure. Circulation 1986; 73: 503–510.

Chrisp P, Faulds D. Moxonidine. A review of its pharmacology, and therapeutic use in essential hypertension. Drugs 1992; 44: 993–1012.

Cruikshank JM. Beta-blockers: primary and secondary prevention. J Cardiovasc Pharmacol 1992; 20 (suppl. 11): S55–S69.

Giacobino JP. Beta-3-adrenoreceptor: an update. Eur J Endocrinol 1995; 132: 377–385.

Dahlöf B, Lindholm LH, Hansson L, Schersten B, Ekbom T, Wester PO. Morbidity and mortality in the Swedish trial in Old Patients with Hypertension (STOP-Hypertension). Lancet 1991; 338: 1281–1285.

Dominiak P. Moxonidin, ein neues Antisympathotonikum mit neuem Angriffspunkt? Herz/Kreisl 1994; 26: 419–424.

Fulton B, Wagstaff AJ, Sorkin EM. Doxazosin. An update of its pharamcology and therapeutic applications in hypertension and benign prostatic hyperplasia. Drugs 1995; 49: 295–320.

Hansson L. The place of beta-blockers in the treatment of hypertension in 1993. Clin Exper Hypertens 1993; 15: 1257–1262.

Haxhiu MA, Dreshaj I, Schäfer SG, Ernsberger P. Selective antihypertensive action of moxonidine is mediated mainly by I$_1$-imidazoline receptors in the rostral ventrolateral medulla. J Cardiovasc Pharmacol 1994; 24 (suppl. 1): S1–S8.

Laurent S, Safar M. Rilmenidine: a novel approach to first-line treatment of hypertension. Am J Hypertens 1992; 5: 99S–105S.

Lithell H. Metabolic effects of antihypertensive drugs interacting with the sympathetic nervous system. Eur Heart J 1992; 13 (suppl A): 53–57.

Lund-Johansen P, Hjermann I, Iversen BM, Thaulow E. Selective alpha-1 inhibitors: first- or second-line antihypertensive agents? Cardiology 1993; 83: 150–159.

Molderings GJ, Göthert M, Christen O, Schäfer SG. Imidazolrezeptoren und Blutdruckregulation. Hohe Rezeptorselektivität von Moxonidin. Dtsch med Wschr 1993; 118: 953−958.

MRC Working Party. Medical Research Council trial of treatment of hypertension in older adults: principal results. Br Med J 1985; 304: 405−412.

Persson H, Erhardt L. Beta receptor antagonists in the treatment of heart failure. Cardiovasc Drugs Ther 1991; 5: 589−604.

Prevention of stroke by antihypertensive drug treatment in older persons with isolated systolic hapertension. Final results of the Systolic Hypertension in the Elderly Program (SHEP). JAMA 1991; 265: 3255−3264.

Stimpel M, Wambach G. Therapie des Phäochromozytoms. Dtsch med Wschr 1987; 112: 1426−1427.

The BEST Steering Committee. Design of the Beta-Blocker Evaluation Survival Trial (BEST). Am J Cardiol 1995; 75: 1220−1223.

Van Zwieten PA. An overview of the pharmacodynamic properties and therapeutic potential of combined alpha- and beta-adrenoceptor antagonists. Drugs 1993; 45: 509−517.

Van Zwieten, Chalmers JP. Different types of centrally acting antihypertensives and their targets in the central nervous system. Cardiovasc Drugs Ther 1994; 8: 787−799.

Wikstrand J. Beta-blockers and cardioprotection − is there any good news from the recent trials? J Clin Pharmacol Ther 1987; 12: 347−350.

Wikstrand J, Warnold I, Olsson G, Tuomiletho J, Elmfeldt D, Berglund G. Primary prevention with metropolol in patients with hypertension. Mortality results from the MAPHY study. JAMA 1988; 259: 1976−1982.

25 Direct vasodilators

The category of direct vasodilators consists of substances which exert their anti-hypertensive effect by direct action on the peripheral vascular musculature. A differentiation is made between these antihypertensives, which are heterogeneous with regard to their chemical structure and their mode of action, and substance classes, which indirectly inhibit vasoconstrictive influences via other defined mechanisms of action (alpha-receptor blockers, Chapter 24, calcium antagonists, Chapter 26, inhibitors of the renin-angiotensin-system, Chapter 27) and thereby also cause a blood-pressure lowering vasodilation. It is now known that several vasodilators induce their effect on the vascular smooth muscle by opening ATP-(adenosine triphosphate) sensitive potassium channels (e.g., minoxidil, diazoxide). Other potassium channel openers (pinacidil, nicorandil, chromakalim, etc.) are currently in clinical development. As has been the case with all previously established, direct vasodilatory substances, however, both the RAAS and the sympathetic nervous system are activated as a reflex. Reflex tachycardia and palpitations as well as sodium and water retention caused by the activated RAAS have to be compensated by an additional medication (beta-receptor blockers, diuretics).

Vasodilators can be divided into those medications used for the long-term treatment (dihydralazine and minoxidil) and those used for acute treatment (sodium nitroprusside) of hypertension.

25.1   Vasodilators for the long-term treatment of hypertension

25.1.1   Hydralazine/ dihydralazine

25.1.1.1 Mode of action, therapeutic use

Hydralazine was introduced in the treatment of arterial hypertension in the early 1950s, making it one of the antihypertensives which has been available longest.

(Di-)Hydralazine causes a direct dilation of the vascular smooth musculature through a mechanism of action which has not yet been explained. The associated reduction in the vascular resistance causes the drop in the arterial blood pressure.

Long-term oral therapy with (di-)hydralazine is initiated with a daily dose of between 25 and 50 mg, generally divided into at least two separate administrations. The recommended maximum dose of 150 mg per day should not be administered over an extended time period, since the likelihood of lupus erythematosus is increased at a daily dose of 100 mg. Today, (di-)hydralazine is generally only administered in cases of severe or therapy resistant hypertension as an add-on therapy to preexisting antihypertensive multiple therapy.

In the rare cases where (di-)hydralazine is to be applied as a primary antihypertensive, a parallel therapy with a beta-receptor blocker and a diuretic should be included in order to compensate the occurrence of reflexive counterregulation (see above).

The intravenous administration of (di-)dihydralazine is limited to emergency situations. The intravenous administration of (di-)hydralazine has proven effective in lowering blood pressure in the face of threatening eclampsia (see Section 33.3.3).

25.1.1.2 Side effects

Side effects which frequently appear with (di-)hydralazine include headaches, tachycardia, palpitations and sweating. The risk of a hydralazine-induced lupus erythematosus has already been mentioned.

Due to reflex tachycardia associated with (di-)hydralazine administration, angina pectoris attacks or myocardial infarction may be triggered in patients with coronary artery disease or limited coronary reserve with hypertensive heart disease. Therapy with (di-)hydralazine should therefore be excluded for these patients.

In contrast to most other antihypertensives, no regression of the left ventricular hypertrophy has been observed under (di-)hydralazine administration.

25.1.2   Minoxidil

25.1.2.1 Mode of action, therapeutic use

Minoxidil causes a blood pressure reduction lasting up to 24 hours as the result of a very pronounced dilatation of the arterial vascular smooth musculature that is mediated by the activation of ATP-sensitive potassium channels.

Because the antihypertensive quality of minoxidil is very strong, the initial daily dosage should be very low (5 mg). The daily dosage of minoxidil can be raised to 50 mg, as necessary. Even the lowest dosage levels require the additional administration of a beta-receptor blocker and a diuretic, as minoxidil administration can lead to dangerous reflex tachycardia and significant sodium and water retention. The use of minoxidil is only recommended for the treatment of severe hypertension, which can not be controlled by other antihypertensives alone.

25.1.2.2 Side effects

The most common side effects are tachycardia, fluid retention with and without edema formation, as well as increased, generalized hair growth (especially problematic for women).

Minoxidil is contraindicated in the presence of coronary artery disease.

25.2   Vasodilators for the acute treatment of hypertension

25.2.1   Sodium nitroprusside

25.2.1.1 Mode of action, therapeutic use

Sodium nitroprusside is applied intravenously and causes a decrease of the blood pressure within a few seconds via mechanisms, which appear to correspond to those of the endogenous vasodilator nitric oxide formed in the endothelial cells (NO; formerly termed as "endothelial derived relaxing factor", EDRF). Nitroprusside dilates both arterial and venous vessels, so that, on the one hand, venous return to the heart is decreased (decrease in cardiac output and stroke volume, increase in heart rate) and, on the other, a reflex constriction of the arterial vascular bed is prevented.

Nitroprusside can be well regulated, so that an excessive drop in blood pressure can be counteracted within a few seconds by the interruption of the infusion.

Therapy with nitroprusside is reserved for hypertensive emergencies (see Section 32.1) and may only be performed where intensive care monitoring capabilities exist, so that possible hypotension can be counteracted immediately.

25.2.1.2 Side effects

Life threatening situations can arise from the release of cyanide at very high infusion doses of sodium nitroprusside.

25.2.2 Diazoxide

Diazoxide is, like minoxidil, a potassium channel opener, whose intravenous administration leads to a massive dilatation of the arterioles. The therapeutic use of diazoxide in arterial hypertension is currently still reserved for hypertensive emergency situations.

Diazoxide is contraindicated in coronary artery disease, pulmonary edema and suspected aortal aneurysm.

Diazoxide has a diabetogenic effect through a direct inhibition of insulin secretion. This property is used therapeutically in combination with thiazide diuretics as a conservative measure for bridging over the preoperative preparation in cases of organically caused hyperinsulinism (benign or malignant insulinoma). Where the condition is inoperable, this combination is also used for long-term treatment.

Summary (Chapter 25)

- Direct vasodilators are chemically and pharmacologically heterogeneous substances, whose effects are either mediated by activating membranous potassium channels of the vascular smooth muscle (e.g., minoxidil, diazoxide) or by mechanisms that have still not been entirely explained (e.g., (di-)hydralazine).

- Direct vasodilators reflexively trigger sodium retention and tachycardia, which — especially with long-term treatment — require the additional administration of a diuretic and a beta-receptor blocker.

- As a result, direct vasodilators are not recommended for the initial treatment of arterial hypertension despite good antihypertensive effectiveness.

- Today direct vasodilators are only to be administered as an add-on therapy to preexisting therapy of severe hypertension, in cases of therapy resistant hypertension ((di-)hydralazine, minoxidil) or in the acute treatment of a hypertensive emergency under intensive care conditions (sodium nitroprusside).

Literature (Chapter 25)

Cook NS. The pharmacology of potassium channels and their therapeutic potential. Trends Pharmacol Sci 1988; 9: 21–28.

Richer C, Pratz J, Mulder P, Mondot S, Giudicelli JF, Cavero I. Cardiovascular and biological effects of K+ channel openers: a class of drugs with vasorelaxant and cardioprotective properties. Life Sci 1990; 47: 1693–1705.

Koch-Weser J. Drug therapy — hydralazine. N Engl J Med 1976; 295: 320–323.

Pettinger WA. Minoxidil in the treatment of severe hypertension. N Engl J Med 1980; 303: 922–926.

Vidrio H. Interaction with pyridoxal as a possible mechanism of hydralazine hypotension. J Cardiovasc Pharmacol 1990; 15: 150–156.

26 Calcium antagonists

26.1 Classification, definition

The calcium antagonists represent a chemically heterogeneous substance class, whose common characteristic is the inhibition of the influx of calcium ions through specific membranous channels ("L-type" calcium channels) of excitable cells. Only selective calcium antagonists with a high affinity for the calcium channels of the L-type have thus far been developed for the treatment of arterial hypertension. They can be differentiated into the following three types based on their varied chemical structures, different binding sites on the calcium channel and an − at least partially − varying spectrum of effect (for the individual substances see Table 26.1):

− Phenylalkylamine derivatives ("verapamil type"),
− 1.4-dihydropyridine derivatives ("nifedipine type") and
− benzothiazepine derivatives ("diltiazem type").

A differentiation is to be made between these selective calcium antagonists, which bind to defined sites on the L-type calcium channel, and other substances, which either inhibit the influx of calcium ions into the cells in an nonselective fashion or through binding to different calcium channels or which influence the regulation of intracellular calcium storage. In addition to the above-mentioned, selective calcium antagonists, the International Union of Pharmacology (IUPHAR; 1994) differentiates the following additional types:

− Substances that interfere with yet-to-be-defined sites of the L-type channel,
− substances which selectively interact with other voltage-dependent, calcium selective channels (of the T-, N- and P-type),
− non-selective calcium channel modulators,
− substances which bind to other calcium-selective channels (calcium-releasing channels on the sarcoplasmic reticulum, receptor-operated calcium channels).

It remains to be seen whether the term proposed by the IUPHAR, "calcium channel modulators", will replace the expression "calcium antagonists" coined by A. Fleckenstein and applied worldwide.

26.2 Mode of action, therapeutic use

Calcium ions play a decisive role as second messengers in the regulation of the vascular smooth musculature. They do so by activating the enzyme decisive for the contraction of the muscle cells (i. e. the actin-myosin interaction), myosin light

Table 26.1: Classification and overview of specific calcium antagonists

Substance class	Agent (Generic name)	Daily dosage (in mg)	Side effects
Arylalkylamine-derivatives, "verapamil-type"	Amipamil** Gallopamil* Tiapamil* Verapamil Verapamil retard	$3 \times \ 40-120$ $1-2 \times 120-240$	Constipation, slowing of AV-conduction, bradykardia, headache, gingiva hyperplasia
Dihydropyridine-derivatives, "nifedipine-type"	Amlodipine Felodipine Isradipine Lacidipine* Nicardipine Nifedipine Nifedipine retard Nifedipine GITS Nilvadipine Nimodipine* Nisoldipine Nitrendipine	$1 \times 2.5-10$ $1 \times 5-20$ $2 \times 1.25-10$ $3 \times 20-40$ $3 \times 10-20$ $2-3 \times 20$ $1 \times 30-90$ $1 \times 8-16$ $2 \times 5-10$ $1-2 \times 10-20$	Ankle edema, facial flushing, (reflex-) tachycardia, headache, gingiva hyperplasia, hypotension, provocation of angina
Benzothiazepine-derivatives, "diltiazem-type"	Diltiazem Diltiazem, retard bzw. sustained release Diltiazem, extended release	$3 \times \ 30-120$ $2 \times \ 90-180$ $1 \times 180-360$	Headache, slowing of AV-conduction, bradykardia, gingiva hyperplasia

 * not approved as an antihypertensive agent
** in clinical development (1996)
AV   = atrio ventricular
GITS = gastrointestinal therapeutic system

chain kinase (MLCK). Cellular calcium homeostasis is essentially maintained through the following functional structures under physiological conditions:

— Voltage-dependent, specific calcium channels,
— receptor-operated, specific calcium channels,
— Na^+/Ca^{2+} exchangers (activity regulated by the membrane-based Na^+/K^+-ATPase).

The calcium ions entering the cells are absorbed and stored intracellularly (sarcoplasmic reticulum, mitochondria, etc.) and released according to need. Excess intracellular calcium ions can be transported out of the cell into the extracellular space by the Na^+/Ca^{2+} exchanger, which essentially works bi-directionally.

An increase in intracellular, free calcium ions in the arterial vasculature is associated with vasoconstriction. Accordingly, in numerous studies an increased intracellular calcium concentration was shown in patients with primary hypertension, which indicates an imbalance in the mechanisms involved in cellular calcium regulation. The suspected cause, at least in a portion of the patients with primary hypertension, is the release of a natriuretic hormone (digitalis-like factor, ouabain-like substance), which inhibits the membrane-based Na^+/K^+-ATPase (see also Section 9.3.6.4). The resulting increase in intracellular sodium ions with simultaneous decrease in potassium ions leads to a lowering of the membrane resting potential and consequently to an increased influx of calcium ions through voltage-operated calcium channels. Furthermore, the activity of the Na^+/Ca^{2+} exchange system may increase. In the process of reducing the increased intracellular sodium concentration this exchange system would bring even more calcium into the cell in exchange.

The calcium antagonists introduced for the treatment of arterial hypertension inhibit the transmembranous influx of calcium through voltage-operated channels by lowering the probability of their opening. The influencing of the calcium channels is dependent on the height of the membrane potential and leads to a reduced availability of free intracellular calcium ions. This, in turn, results in a decrease in muscle tone in the area of the arterial resistance vessels and a subsequent lowering of the blood pressure. The antihypertensive effectiveness of the calcium antagonists increases with rising levels of the initial blood pressure.

Calcium antagonists lower blood pressure irrespective of differences in age, sex or race. Their effectiveness has been shown for all degrees of severity of primary hypertension. The sublingual administration of nifedipine has proven effective in the treatment of hypertensive emergencies (see Section 32.1). In addition, calcium antagonists have been used successfully against a few forms of secondary hypertension (pheochromocytoma, primary aldosteronism, etc., see Sections 34.4 and 34.5, respectively). Calcium antagonists with long-lasting activity (once-daily administration) are therefore recommended in most countries as first-line antihypertensives.

The following additional effects of the calcium antagonists have been postulated or have been proven in corresponding studies:

− Anti-arteriosclerotic effect (has only been convincingly shown in animal experiments),
− renal protection (the results have varied to date),
− diuresis and natriuresis (particularly under dihydropyridines),
− reduction of left ventricular hypertrophy,
− anti-anginal effects, and
− "metabolic neutrality".

The results of the ALLHAT ("Antihypertensive and Lipid Lowering Treatment to Prevent Heart Attack Trial")-study and other presently ongoing studies will show, whether a reduction of increased mortality and morbidity associated with untreated hypertension can be expected under long-term treatment with calcium antagonists (Table 26.2).

Trial	Agents	Hypothesis	Projected no. of patients	Primary end point	Comments
Hypertension					
HOT	Felodipine at 5 and 10 mg doses plus ACE-I, BB, or D	Test the effects of DBP lowering to ≤90, ≤85, or ≤80 mmHg	18000	CV events	DBP shows only a small difference between groups (87±7, 85±8, and 83±8 mmHg at 3 months). This small contrast could limit the ability to show differences.
STOP	D vs ACE-I vs calcium antagonists	Effects of three classes of agents with the same BP target	6600	Major CV events	Adequate power to detect ≥25% difference between classes of agents, which may be unrealistically optimistic.
ALLHAT	D vs amlodipine vs lisinopril vs doxazosin	Relative effects of classes of agents with the same BP target	40000	CHD	High power to detect a 16% relative risk difference between arms.
INSIGHT	Nifedipine GITS vs amiloride and hydrochlorothiazide	Relative effects of two classes of agents	6600	CV events	May not have adequate power to detect plausible differences.
EURO-SYST	Nitrendipine + enalapril or hydrochlorothiazide	Impact of Ca^{2+} antagonist-based treatment vs placebo	3000	Strokes	
Heart failure					
V-HEFT-3	Felodipine vs standard treatment	Effect of a direct vasodilator or when added to ACE-I, dig, and D	600	Ex tolerance, LV function, and quality of life	Only moderate power to assess clinical outcomes.
PRAISE-2	Amlodipine vs placebo	Effects in patients without CHD	1800	Mortality and morbidity	
MACH-1	Mabefradil vs placebo	NYHA class II to IV and using ACE-I, dig, or D	2000	Mortality	

HOT indicates Hypertension Optimal Treatment; ACE-I, angiotensin-converting enzyme inhibitor; BB, β-blocker; D, diuretic; CV, cardiovascular; DBP, diastolic blood pressure; STOP, Swedish Trial in Old Patients with Hypertension; ALLHAT, Antihypertensive and Lipid Lowering Heart Prevention Trial; BP, blood pressure; CHD, coronary heart disease; INSIGHT, International Nifedipine Study, Intervention as a Goal in Hypertension Treatment; GITS, Gastrointestinal Therapeutic System; EURO-SYST, European Study of Systolic Hypertension; V-HEFT, Veterans Heart Failure Trial; dig, digoxin; PRAISE, Prospective Randomized Amlodipine Survival Evaluation; MACH-1, Mortality Assessment in Congestive Heart Failure; and NYHA, New York Heart Association. From Yusuf S; Circulation 1995; 92: 1079−1082.

26.3 Side effects

While the presently marketed dihydropyridine derivatives act in therapeutic doses almost exclusively on the peripheral vascular musculature, the administration of calcium antagonists of the verapamil and diltiazem types can, in addition, have a delaying effect on conduction in the atrioventricular node. Combination with a beta-receptor blocker or a centrally acting antiadrenergic substance increases this effect and can trigger high-grade atrioventricular blocks or asystole in patients with previous cardiac damage. Constipation occurs relatively frequently with the administration of verapamil and related substances.

Reflective stimulation of the sympathetic nervous system with resulting increases of pulse, tremor, palpitations, sweating and flush symptoms may occur with the administration of short-acting dihydropyridines. For that reason it is not recommended to give short-acting calcium antagonists to patients with concomitant, severe coronary heart disease – especially with instable angina pectoris or following a recent myocardial infarction – because the reactive sympathetic activation may cause acute ischemia. Instead, calcium antagonists which have a long period of action, or are offered in formulations which guarantee a slow release of the active ingredient, should be given preference (e.g. GITS, gastrointestinal therapeutic systems).

Indications of an increased cardiovascular risk with hypertensive patients who were treated with short-acting calcium antagonists (increase of the absolute risk compared to diuretics of 0.6%) are based on a retrospective, methodologically controversial case controlled study (Psaty et al., 1995). The publication of such analyses serve better to upset than to the benefit of either patients or attending physicians. On the other hand, they point out the lack of prospectively obtained data on mortality and morbidity under long-term treatment with the new antihypertensive substances in general and the calcium antagonists in particular.

Peripheral edema is observed relatively frequently following the intake of dihydropyridines and more frequently in women than in men.

The development of hyperplasia of the gingiva is a very rare side effect which occurs with the intake of calcium antagonists.

Summary (Chapter 26)

- Calcium antagonists inhibit the transmembranous influx of calcium through the L-type calcium channels.

- All selective calcium antagonists cause a decrease in muscle tone in the peripheral arterial musculature.

- Calcium antagonists of the verapamil and diltiazem types also delay conduction in the atrioventricular node. Their administration is thus contraindicated given a simultaneous presence of atrioventricular blocks, sick sinus syndrome and pronounced bradycardia.

- Long-acting calcium antagonists are recognized as first-line antihypertensives in most countries (exception: USA) and can be used as monotherapy in long-term treatment of primary hypertension. A reduction in the morbidity or mortality has, however, not yet been proven.

- Where the decrease in blood pressure is insufficient, dihydropyridine-type calcium antagonists can be combined with beta-receptor blockers, ACE inhibitors, diuretics and imidazoline agonists (e.g., clondine, moxonidine). The additional administration of beta-receptor blockers and imidazoline agonists with calcium antagonists of the verapamil and diltiazem types should be avoided, especially in elderly patients.

- Calcium antagonists do not cause any negative changes in metabolism and cause a regression of left ventricular hypertrophy.

- Long-acting calcium antagonists are recommended for the treatment of hypertension and concomitant coronary artery disease (CAD); however, short-acting substances of the dihydropyridine class should not be administered to hypertensive patients with coexisting severe CAD.

- The most common side effects of dihydropyridines are the development of peripheral edema and flushing, while the administration of calcium antagonists of the verapamil type cause obstipation. Initial headaches occur relatively frequently with all calcium antagonists.

Literature (Chapter 26)

Annonymus. Are calcium blockers safe for first-line therapy? The Genesis Report, June 1995: 14–21.

Borchard U. Kalziumantagonisten. Perspektiven für die 90er Jahre. Walter de Gruyter, Berlin-New York 1993, 1–122.

Chobanian AV. Can antihypertensive drugs reduce atherosclerosis and its clinical complications? Am J Hypertens 1994; 7: 119S–125S.

Dahlöf B, Lindholm LH, Hansson L, Schersten B, Ekbom T, Wester PO. Morbidity and mortality in the Swedish trial in Old Patients with Hypertension (STOP-Hypertension). Lancet 1991; 338: 1281–1285.

Fleckenstein A, Tritthard H, Fleckenstein B, Herbst A, Grün G: A new group of competetive Ca-antagonists (Iproveratril, D 600, Prenylamine) with highly potent inhibitory effects on excitation-contraction coupling in mammalian myocardium. Pflügers Arch Ges Physiol 1969; 307: 25.

Groth H, Stimpel M, Stricker M, Greminger P, Vetter W. Hypertensiver Notfall und schwere-

Hypertonie: Erfahrungen mit Nifedipin. Schweiz Rundschau Med 1985; 74: 491–495.

Henry PD, Bentley KI. Suppression of atherosclerosis in cholesterol-fed rabbits treated with nifedipine. J Clin Invest 1981; 68: 1366–1369.

Lijnen P. Once-daily antihypertensive treatment with calcium antagonists. Drugs Today 1995; 31: 283–292.

Mimran A, Ribstein J. Angiotensin-converting enzyme inhibitors versus calcium antagonists in the progression of renal diseases. Am J Hypertens 1994; 7: 73S–81S.

Opie LH. Clinical use of calcium channel antagonist drugs. 2nd ed. Kluwer Academic Publishers Boston-Dordrecht-London 1990, 1–326.

Opie LH, Messerli FH. Nifedipine and mortality. Grave defects in the dossier. Circulation 1995; 92: 1068–1073.

Psaty BM, Heckbert SR, Koepsell TD, Siscovick DS, Raghunathan TE, Weiss NS, Rosendaal FR, Lemaitre RN, Smith NL, Wahl PW, Wagner EH, Furberg CD. The risk of myocardial infarction associated with antihypertensive drug therapies. JAMA 1995; 274: 620−625.

Steele RM, Schuna AA, Schreiber RT. Calcium antagonist-induced gingival hyperplasia. Ann Intern Med 1994; 120: 663−664.

Stimpel M, Ivens K, Wambach G, Kaufmann W. Are calcium antagonists helpful in the management of primary aldosteronism? J Cardio-vasc Pharmacol 1988; 12 (Suppl. 6): S131−S134.

Yusuf S. Calcium anatgonists in coronary artery disease and hypertension. Time for reevaluation? Circulation 1995; 92: 1079−1082.

27 Inhibitors of the renin-angiotensin system

27.1 The renin-angiotensin system

The renin-angiotensin system (RAS) plays an important role in the regulation of arterial blood pressure. The enzyme renin is formed largely in the cells of the juxtaglomerular apparatus of the kidneys from the inactive precursors pre-pro-renin and pro-renin. It is released by a number of stimuli (hypotension, hyponatremia, hypovolemia, sympathetic activity, etc.). By cleavage of ten amino acids, renin converts the glycoprotein angiotensinogen to the decapeptide angiotensin I (Ang I). The systemically circulating Ang I is converted to the biologically active octapeptide angiotensin II (Ang II). This occurs particularly during passage through the lungs and almost entirely by the non-specific angiotensin converting enzyme (ACE), which is localized on the surface of endothelial cells. Although ACE also circulates systemically, it is apparently only involved in the conversion of Ang I to Ang II to a slight degree. − Ang II suppresses renin formation and release, so that a negative feedback mechanism exists, which controls the formation of Ang II. − In recent years, the discovery of components of the RAS in various organ systems, in particular, prompted the hypothesis that Ang II is not only a circulating, systemically active hormone, but that, as a locally formed hormone, it also performs autocrine or paracrine functions. The functional relationships between locally formed Ang II and the systemic regulation of the RAS have not yet been clarified.

The significance of an alternative formation of Ang II from Ang I, which is mediated by a specific chymase and which has been shown in the human heart, also remains unclear.

27.1.1 Angiotensin II

As the actual effective substance of the RAS, Ang II increases arterial vascular resistance through direct vasoconstriction and thus causes an increase in blood pressure. This effect is increased by an additional stimulation of catecholamine release from the adrenal medulla as well as an increase in the vascular sensitivity to catecholamines. Ang II also stimulates sodium reabsorption, on the one hand, through direct renal mechanisms and, on the other, indirectly through the increased release of aldosterone from the adrenal cortex, a hormone which also causes sodium retention. − As a whole, all the differing effects of Ang II serve to maintain arterial blood pressure in situations with extracellular volume depletion.

Trophic effects have also been detected for Ang II. Among others, it was shown that locally formed Ang II is probably decisively involved in the development of pressure-related, hypertrophic adjustment processes of the arterial vascular wall and of the myocardium. Locally formed Ang II also seems to play a role in the development of ateriosclerotic changes and to be involved in the process of wound healing.

In the kidneys Ang II causes a constriction of the efferent arterioles with a consequent increase in blood pressure in the preceding glomeruli. It is supposed that this Ang II effect contributes, at least partially, to the pathogenesis of progressively developing glomerular damage in untreated arterial hypertension.

Experimental data indicates that Ang II might also be involved in the regulation of bone turnover by stimulating bone resorption and/or the activity of the osteoclasts.

The effects of Ang II on target organs are transmitted via specific receptors, which can be differentiated based on structure and function into the AT_1 and AT_2 receptors. Most effects associated with Ang II, like vasoconstriction, renal effects, stimulation of the aldosterone and catecholamine release and mitogenic effects, are evidently consequences of an activation of the AT_1 receptors (the existence of the AT_{1A}, AT_{1B} and AT_{1C} isoforms in rat and mice has not yet been shown in humans). $-$ The (clinical) relevance of AT_2 receptors is less clear. They have only been shown in higher concentrations in embryonic tissue. AT_2 receptors are only expressed to a slight degree in the adult organism. They may possibly mediate antiproliferative effects.

27.1.2 Angiotensin-(1−7), Angiotensin-(3−8) and Angiotensin III

Recent studies have shown that Ang I is not only converted into Ang II, but that it is also a substrate for the enzymatic transformation into the vasodilatory heptapeptide Ang-(1−7). The cleavage of the residual amino acid takes place through various tissue-based endopeptidases, which have only been shown in larger concentrations in the brain, kidneys and vascular endothelium. The physiological role of Ang-(1−7), like that of other, some only recently identified, degradation products (Ang III and IV), remains, however, largely unclear.

27.1.3 Kallikrein kinin system

The ACE is not specific for the enzymatic conversion of Ang I to Ang II. It also interferes with the kallikrein kinin system, which is also vasoactive. Referred to here as kininase II, it causes the breakdown of the strongly vasodilatory bradykinin to inactive fragments.

27.2 Inhibition of the renin-angiotensin system

The RAS participates as an important factor in the development and maintenance of the elevated blood pressure in a large number of patients with primary hypertension. In various renal forms of hypertension the RAS is undoubtedly the "driving

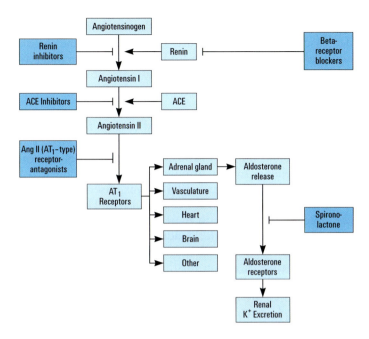

Figure 27.1: The renin angiotensin system and potential sites to block the system
ACE   = angiotensin converting enzyme
AngII = angiotensin II
AT_1 = angiotensin II type 1 receptor

force" and pathogenetically responsible for the elevation of the arterial blood pressure. Therefore, it is not surprising that the pharmacological inhibition of the RAS has proven itself as an effective principle of therapy in the treatment of hypertension.

The RAS inhibitors currently available or in development can be divided into the following substance classes based on their specific modes of action:

– Renin inhibitors,
– angiotensin I converting enzyme inhibitors (ACE inhibitors) and
– angiotensin II receptor antagonists.

Beta-receptor blockers interfere with the RAS by inhibiting the release of renin from the cells of the juxtaglomerular apparatus. However, because this is only one of several suspected antihypertensive mechanisms of action for the beta-receptor blockers, this substance class is not considered a specific inhibitor of the RAS (Chapter 24)(see also Figure 27.1).

27.2.1   Renin inhibitors

27.2.1.1 Mode of action, therapeutic use

The transformation of angiotensinogen to Ang I is prevented by the direct inhibition of renin. Ang I is a necessary substrate for the formation of Ang II and the resulting decrease in Ang II formation leads, on the one hand, to vasodilation and a subsequent decrease of the blood pressure. On the other hand, however, it also leads to a pronounced compensatory increase in renin secretion (negative feedback mechanism, see Section 27.1). To achieve a long-term inhibition of the RAS the substances in question must show a high affinity to the enzyme and reach the circulation in sufficient concentrations.

The orally applicable renin inhibitors synthesized to date have, in particular, not fulfilled the requirement of sufficient plasma concentration, as they consistently show a low to very low bioavailability. Thus, in clinical studies on healthy volunteers and patients with primary hypertension, a consistent re-increase of Ang I and Ang II to concentrations above the starting levels was observed after an initial and significant drop in the plasma levels had been achieved. There have been no placebo-controlled studies on patients with hypertension which have shown a long-lasting decrease in blood pressure with the administration of an oral renin inhibitor. It thus remains to be seen to what degree specific renin inhibition will be further pursued as a principle of action for the treatment of arterial hypertension due to the difficulties mentioned. Remikiren (Ro 42−5892), zankiren (A-72517) and enalkiren (A-64662, i.v.) are examples of renin inhibitors which are currently in clinical development (phase II) or whose development has already been terminated.

27.2.3   Angiotensin I converting enzyme (ACE) inhibitors

27.2.3.1 Classification of and differences between the ACE inhibitors

The currently available ACE inhibitors (Table 27.1) can be classified according to the following criteria:

Table 27.1:   Properties of various ACE inhibitors

Substance	Zinc ligand	Prodrug	Elimination	Daily dose (mg)	Dosage (x/day)
Alacepril	S	yes	renal	25−75	1
Benazepril	C	yes	renal	10−40	1
Captopril	S	no	renal	12.5−75	1−2
Cilazapril	C	yes	renal	2.5−5	1
Enalapril	C	yes	renal	5−40	1
Fosinopril	P	yes	renal + hapatic	10−20	1
Lisinopril	C	no	renal	5−40	1
Moexipril	C	yes	renal + hepatic	7.5−30	1
Perindopril	C	yes	renal + hepatic	1−16	1
Quinapril	C	yes	renal + hepatic	5−80	1
Ramipril	C	yes	renal	1.25−10	1
Spirapril	C	yes	hepatic + renal	12.5−50	1
Trandolapril	C	yes	renal + hepatic	2−4	1
Zofenopril	S	yes	renal + hepatic	30−60	1

C = Carboxyl; P = Phosphoryl; S = Sulfhydril

- chemical structure of the zinc ligands or the ACE binding sites (differentiations are made between by ACE inhibitors with sulfhydryl-, carboxyl- and phosphoryl-ligands),
- non-prodrug and prodrug forms (some ACE inhibitors are first transformed into the active metabolites in the liver),
- elimination (renal, renal-hepatic),
- duration of effect (clinical: single or multiple administrations),
- lipophilia (is said to be equivalent to a high affinity to local tissue RAS, e.g., in the heart, brain, vascular walls, etc.),
- affinity to the kallikrein kinin system.

Efficacy and/or safety advantages for individual ACE inhibitors have repeatedly been postulated based on these possibilities for differentiation. It has not been shown, however, that these differences are of significant clinical relevance.

27.2.3.2 Mode of action, therapeutic use

ACE inhibitors inhibit the ACE both systemically and locally in various tissues (heart, kidneys, adrenal glands, vessel wall, brain, etc.). Thus they also inhibit the conversion of Ang I to Ang II. The decreased formation of Ang II causes a decrease in the vasoconstriction mediated by Ang II and an inhibition in renal sodium and water reabsorption. Because ACE is identical to kininase II, which is responsible for the degradation of bradykinin, the inactivation of the vasodilatory bradykinin is also inhibited. ACE inhibitors thus cause the following hormonal changes:

- Increase in renin secretion,
- increase in Ang I,
- decrease in the activity of ACE or kininase II,
- decrease in Ang II,
- decrease in aldosterone secretion and
- increase in bradykinin.

The antihypertensive effect of ACE inhibitors is attributed above all to the decreased formation of Ang II, whereby the magnitude of the reduction in blood pressure is to a large degree dependent on the activity of the RAS. Salt reduction and/or the additional administration of a diuretic thus increase the antihypertensive effect of ACE inhibitors. Because a reduction in the blood pressure is also observed in patients with an only slightly activated RAS, it can be assumed that the antihypertensive effect of ACE inhibitors is not only achieved through an inhibition of the systemic RAS, but possibly also the consequence of an inhibition of local tissue RAS. It is also conceivable that the reduced degradation of bradykinin and the subsequent synthesis of vasodilatory prostaglandins and nitric oxide might also contribute to the dilatation of the resistance vessels and thus to the antihypertensive effectiveness of ACE inhibitors. Comparable to other antihypertensives, a sufficient reduction in blood pressure was achieved under monotherapy with ACE inhibitors for approximately 40—60% of patients with mild or moderate hypertension (USA: Stages 1 and 2). In cases of insufficient blood-pressure reduction, an increase in dosage or the additional administration of a second antihypertensive agent should first take place after 3–4 weeks, as the maximal effect of the ACE inhibitors can not be expected before this time. Diuretics and calcium antagonists are particularly well-suited as combination partners, as they provide a pharmacologically verifiable increase of the antihypertensive effect of ACE inhibitors by activating the RAS.

Despite blood-pressure reduction, heart rate, cardiac output and stroke volume remain unchanged under treatment with ACE inhibitors for patients with primary hypertension.

ACE inhibitors are acknowledged nearly worldwide as first line therapy for the treatment of primary hypertension. Their antihypertensive effectiveness does not show any dependence on age, however, it appears to be weaker among a portion of black African-American patients with hypertension (low-renin hypertension). ACE inhibitors are, however, also effective with this population in combination with a diuretic. The same is true for forms of hypertension with suppressed RAS (e.g., primary aldosteronism).

Additional effects of the ACE inhibitors:

Further additional effects have been shown for ACE inhibitors or are assumed based on preliminary and, in part, experimental data:

- No negative influence on lipid metabolism,
- increase in insulin sensitivity/reduction of hyperinsulinemia (studies with a small number of patients),
- improvement in proteinuria in patients with primary hypertension and diabetes mellitus ("renal protection", possibly mediated by dilatation of the vas efferens with a reduction in the intraglomular pressure),
- regression of left ventricular hypertrophy,
- delayed development or worsening of left ventricular dysfunction at the start of ACE inhibitor therapy at the earliest 1–2 days after a myocardial infarction and,
- related to this (SAVE Study, AIRE Study), prolonged survival time and reduction in cardiac mortality and morbidity,
- improvement in mortality and morbidity related to heart failure (V-HeFT II Study, SOLVD Study, SMILE Study),
- improvement in the compliance of arterial vessels in hypertensive patients/prevention of remodelling processes (experimental studies on a limited number of patients),
- improvement in cognitive functions (preliminary animal experimental investigations) and
- inhibition of osteoclastic-caused bone resorption (in vitro experiments).

The influence of long-term therapy with ACE inhibitors, as compared to other antihypertensive substance classes, on the increased mortality and morbidity of patients with primary hypertension has been one of the endpoints of the STOP Hypertension 2 Study, which has included approximately 6,600 patients (70–84 years of age) (see also Table 26.2).

27.2.3.3 Side effects

ACE inhibitors are considered to be effective antihypertensives with a favorable safety profile. The serious side effects witnessed in the first years after the introduction of captopril (e.g. acute renal failure etc.) were primarily a consequence of very high doses. The dosages recommended today are significantly lower.

A typical side effect for all ACE inhibitors, which is not dependent on dosage, is dry cough. It appears in around 4−20% of the patients treated and often necessitates a switch to another substance class. The reduced breakdown of bradykinin is the suspected, but not proved cause of this.

The appearance of angioneurotic edema under ACE inhibitor administration is infrequent and almost always appears within the first few hours or days of treatment (exceptions to this have already been described). It is usually associated with a swelling of the lips, tongue and other parts of the face. It can become life-threatening if parts of the upper respiratory passage are obstructed by the swelling and acute respiratory distress results. The development of angioneurotic edema demands the immediate withdrawal of ACE inhibitor treatment and the switch to another antihypertensive substance class.

Hypotensive blood-pressure reactions are observed particularly at the beginning of treatment with ACE inhibitors (first-dose hypotension). Particular attention should be paid to patients with an activated RAS (salt depletion, preexisting diuretic treatment). These patients should be monitored for a few hours in a hospital or at the physician's practice after the first administration of the ACE inhibitor. If this is not possible, it is recommended to stop the treatment with diuretics before the first administration of the ACE inhibitor.

For patients with bilateral renal artery stenoses or with renal artery stenosis in a solitary functioning kidney, ACE inhibitors may only be administered in exceptional cases and strict medical supervision.

Other typical, though rare, side effects are non-allergically related, maculopapular rash and a worsening of renal function.

Pregnancy, nursing and a known hypersensitivity to the respective ACE inhibitor are all considered contraindications.

Therapy with an ACE inhibitor should always begin with the lowest recommended dosage. A further reduction of dosage necessary for patients with reduced renal function. These precautionary measures should also be thoroughly considered when using ACE inhibitors with renal-hepatic elimination.

27.2.4   Angiotensin II (Ang II-) receptor antagonists

27.2.4.1 Classification of and differences between Ang II receptor antagonists

Studies were conducted already in the 1970s to inhibit the RAS through a pharmacological blockade of the Ang II receptors. Of the substances synthesized at that time, saralasin became the most widely recognized. However, the clinical development of this substance was stopped because it showed qualities which were partially agonistic to Ang II and because its peptide-like structure made it suited only for parenteral administration.

The renewed interest in developing Ang II receptor antagonists was tied to the discovery in the early 1980s that some non-peptide-like molecules with an uncomplicated chemical structure (benzyl-substituted imidazole) show Ang II antagonistic properties (Furokawa, 1982).

There are several (AT$_1$-receptor) specific Ang II antagonists now in preclinical and/or clinical development. These new, orally applied substances are largely Ang II receptor antagonists with high affinity to the AT$_1$ receptor (e.g., losartan, valsartan, candesartan, etc.). These substances should be differentiated from AT$_2$ selective Ang II receptor antagonists (prototype: PD 123319), which have only been used in experimental investigations.

As the first Ang II receptor antagonist to be so acknowledged, losartan was approved in early 1995 in the USA and several European countries for the treatment of primary hypertension.

27.2.4.1 Mode of action, therapeutic use

The clinical experiences that have been gathered with regard to the Ang II receptor antagonists only relate to the use of AT$_1$ selective substances. These are prodrugs, which are metabolized after their intestinal absorption. In most cases, the metabolite has a significantly higher affinity to the receptor than does the prodrug (for example, EXP3174 is the active metabolite of losartan) and is thus primarily responsible for the effects achieved. The feedback process, which begins after the administration of an Ang II receptor antagonist, causes an increased release of renin and, subsequently, an increase in Ang II concentration. Due to the increased formation of Ang II, which is displaced from the receptor, a more marked stimulation of the AT$_2$ receptor can be assumed, the functional role of which has not been clarified for the human organism.

The hemodynamic effects after administration of Ang II receptor antagonists largely correspond to the changes induced by ACE inhibitors and are explained by the displacement of Ang II from the AT$_1$ receptor (see above).

Additional effects, which have been observed after the administration of Ang II receptor antagonists, are

− no negative effect on metabolic parameters,
− a reduction in left ventricular hypertrophy,
− a reduction in proteinuria in patients with hypertension and
− an improvement in the hemodynamic and hormonal parameters in patients with left ventricular dysfunction.

It must, however, be emphasized that these data are to be considered preliminary, since they are based on studies with a very limited number of patients and volunteers from clinical development studies.

A once-daily administration of losartan in patients with mild to moderate primary hypertension causes a blood-pressure reduction, which has been evaluated as satisfactory by the medical authorities and thus led to the approval for this indication. Losartan can be combined with a diuretic or a calcium antagonist if monotherapy causes an unsatisfactory blood-pressure reduction. The maximal antihypertensive effect is to be expected after approximately 3−6 weeks.

All of the precautionary measures required for ACE inhibitors also apply to losartan.

27.2.4.2 Side effects

Due to the minimal clinical experience with Ang II receptor antagonists, only a limited evaluation of the safety profile of this substance class is possible. In principle, however, it should correspond to that of the ACE inhibitors.

The lack of influence that Ang II receptor antagonists have on the kallikrein kinin system may explain the significantly lower incidence of dry cough, when compared to ACE inhibitors. Whether the development of angioneurotic edema will also be observed less frequently due to the unaffected breakdown of bradykinin, can only be judged after broader and sufficiently long clinical use.

Summary (Chapter 27)

- The renin angiotensin system (RAS) plays an important role in blood pressure regulation. As a local system it is involved in trophic adaptation processes of various tissues.

- Inhibition of the RAS is a sensible principle of effect for the treatment of arterial hypertension and possibly for its associated end-organ damage, as well.

- Substance classes have been developed for the specific, pharmacological inhibition of the RAS. They target different segments of the RAS: renin inhibitors, angiotensin I converting enzyme inhibitors (ACE inhibitors) and angiotensin II receptor antagonists.

- The effectiveness of the renin inhibitors synthesized to date has been limited by a compensatory increase in renin secretion with poor bioavailability.

- The effectiveness and safety of ACE inhibitors have been supported by worldwide use on a large number of patients. This substance class is recognized in most countries as first line therapy for the treatment of primary hypertension.

- The antihypertensive effectiveness of the ACE inhibitors is weaker among a portion of black African-American patients with hypertension (low-renin hypertension).

- The combination with a diuretic or a calcium antagonist is recommended, if blood pressure does not respond sufficiently to a monotherapy with an ACE inhibitor.

- There has not yet been proof of a reduction in mortality and morbidity under long-term therapy with ACE inhibitors in patients with hypertension.

- Further positive effects of ACE inhibitors are the reduction in left ventricular hypertrophy, "metabolic neutrality", improvement in proteinuria and the improvement in mortality and morbidity related to heart failure and myocardial infarction ("secondary prevention").

- The most important side effects that can occur with ACE inhibitors are dry cough, angioneurotic edema, non-allergic rash, neutropenia, "first dose" hypotension and headache.

- Because ACE inhibitors are eliminated either renally or renal-hepatically, the physician should always consider the necessity of dosage reduction when treating patients with impaired renal function.

- Clinical experience with Ang II receptor antagonists has been very limited. As the first substance of this class, losartan was launched for the treatment of arterial hypertension in 1995.

- The efficacy and safety profile of Ang II receptor antagonists is expected to largely correspond to that of the ACE inhibitors. The missing inhibition of the breakdown of bradykinin may explain the lower incidence of dry cough, when compared to ACE inhibitors.

Literature (Chapter 27)

Albaladejo P, Bouaziz H, Duriez M, Gohlke P, Levy BI, Safar M. Angiotensin converting enzyme inhibition prevents the increase in aortic collagen in rats. Hypertension 1994; 23: 74−82.

Ambrosioni E, Borghi C, Magnani B for the Survival of Myocardial Infarction Long-Term Evaluation (SMILE) Study Investigators. The effect of the angiotensin-converting-enzyme inhibitor zofenopril on mortality and morbidity after anterior myocardial infarction. N Engl J Med 1995; 332: 80−85.

Arakawa K, Brunner HR. Angiotensin II receptor antagonists: can they go beyond angiotensin converting enzyme inhibitors? J Hypertens 1994; 12 (suppl 9): S1−S38.

Bönner G, Rahn KH (eds.). ACE-Hemmer-Handbuch, 2. Aufl. Schattauer Verlag, Stuttgart-New York 1994.

Cody RJ. The clinical potential of renin inhibitors and angiotensin antagonists. Drugs 1994; 47: 586−598.

Cohn JN, Johnson G, Ziesche S, Cobb F, Francis G, Tristani F, Smith R, Dunkman B, Loeb H, Wong M, Bhat G, Goldman S, Fletcher RD, Doherty J, Hughes CV, Carson P, Cintron G, Shabetai R, Haaken-son C. A comparison of enalapril with hydralazine-isosorbide dinitrate in the treatment of chronic congestive heart failure. N Engl J Med 1991; 325: 303−310.

Crozier I, Ikram H, Awan N, Cleland J, Stephen N, Dickstein K, Frey M, Young J, Klinger G, Makris L, Rucinska E for the Losartan Hemodynamic Study Group. Losartan in heart failure. Hemodynamic effects and tolerability. Circulation 1995; 91: 691−697.

Flamenbaum W. A comparison of the efficacy and safety of a beta-blocker, a calcium channel blocker, and a converting enzyme inhibitor in hypertensive blacks. Arch Intern Med 1990; 150: 1707−1713.

Fletcher AE, Palmer AJ, Bulpitt CJ. Cough with angiotensin converting enzyme inhibitors: how much of a problem? J Hypertens 1994; 12 (suppl 2): S43−S47.

Goldberg AI, Dunlay MC, Sweet CS. Safety and tolerability of losartan potassium, an angiotensin II receptor antagonist, compared with hydrochlorothiazide, atenolol, felodipine ER, and angiotensin-converting enzyme inhibitors for the treatment of systemic hypertension. Am J Cardiol 1995; 75: 793−795.

Hansson L. Update on STOP-Hypertension. Am J Hypertens 1995; 8: 26A.

Hoyer J, Schulte KL, Lenz T. Clinical pharmacokinetics of angiotensin converting enzyme (ACE) inhibitors in renal failure. Clin Pharmacokinet 1993; 24: 230−254.

Ichiki T, Labosky PA, Shiota C, Okuyama S, Imagawa Y, Fogo A, Niimura F, Ichikawa I, Hogan BLM, Inagami T. Effects on blood pressure and exploratory behaviour of mice lacking angiotensin II type-2 receptor. Nature 1995; 377: 748−750.

Israili ZH, Hall WD. Cough and angioneurotic edema associated with angiotensin-converting enzyme inhibitor therapy. A review of the literature and pathophysiology. Ann Intern Med 1992; 117: 234−242.

Johnston CI. Angiotensin receptor antagonists: focus on losartan. Lancet 1995; 346: 1403−1407.

Kleinert HD. Renin inhibition. Cardiovasc Drugs Ther 1995; 9: 645−655.

Lewis EJ, Hunsicker LC, Bain RP, Rohde RD. The effect of angiotensin-converting-enzyme inhibition on diabetic nephropathy. N Engl J Med 1993; 329: 1456−1462.

Menard J. Anthology of the renin-angiotensin system: a one hundred reference approach to angiotensin II antagonists. J Hypertens 1993; 11 (suppl 3): S3−S11.

Opie LH. Angiotensin converting enzyme inhibitors. Scientific basis for clinical use. Wiley-Liss, Author's Publishing House, New York 1992.

Parish RC, Miller LJ. Adverse effects of angiotensin converting enzyme (ACE) inhibitors. An update. Drug Safety 1992; 7: 14−31.

Pfeffer MA, Lamas CA, Vaughan DE, Parisi AF, Braunwald E. Effect of captopril on progressive ventricular dilatation after anterior myocardial infarction. N Engl J Med 1988; 319: 80−86.

Saunders E, Weir MR, Kong BW, Hollifield J, Gray J, Vertes V, Sowers JR, Zemel MB, Curry C, Schoenberger J, Wright JT, Kirkendall W, Conradi EC, Jenkins P, McLean B, Massie B, Berenson G, Flamenbaum W. A comparison of the efficacy and safety of a beta-blocker, a calcium channel blocker, and a converting enzyme inhibitor in hypertensive blacks. Arch Intern Med 1990; 150: 1707−1713.

Saunders E, Weir MR, Kong BW, Hollifield J, Gray J, Vertes V, Sowers JR, Zemel MB, Curry C, Schoenberger J, Wright JT, Kirkendall W, Conradi EC, Jenkins P, Mc Lean B, Massie B, Berenson G, Shotan A, Widerhorn J, Hurst A, Elkayam U. Risks of angiotensin-converting enzyme inhibition during pregnancy: experimental and clinical evidence, potential mechanisms, and recommendations for use. Am J Med 1994; 96: 451−456.

Stimpel M, Bonn R, Koch B, Dickstein K. Pharmacology and clinical use of the new ACE-inhibitor moexipril. Cardiovasc Drug Rev 1995; 13: 211−229.

Timmermans PBMWM, Wong PC, Chiu AT, Herblin WF, Benfield P, Carini DJ, Lee RJ, Wexler RR, Saye JAM, Smith RD. Angiotensin II receptors and angiotensin II receptor antagonists. Pharmacol Rev 1993; 45: 205−251.

The Acute Infarction Ramipril Efficacy (AIRE) Study Investigators. Effect of ramipril on mortality and morbidity of survivors of acute myocardial infarction with clinical evidence of heart failure. Lancet 1993; 342: 821−828.

The SOLVD Investigators. Effect of enalapril on survival in patients with reduced left ventricular ejection fractions and congestive heart failure. N Engl J Med 1987; 325: 293−302.

The SOLVD Investigators. Effect of enalapril on mortality in the development of heart failure in asymptomatic patients with reduced left ventricular ejection fractions. N Engl J Med 1992; 327: 685−691.

Van den Meiracker AH, Man in 't Veld AJ, Admiraal PJJ, van Eck HJR, Boomsma F, Derkx FHM, Schalekamp MADH. Partial escape of angiotensin converting enzyme (ACE) inhibition during prolonged ACE inhibitor treatment: does it exist and does it affect the antihypertensive response? J Hypertens 1992; 10: 803−812.

Weber MA, Neutel JM, Essinger I, Glassman HN, Boger RS, Luther R. Assessment of renin dependency of hypertension with a dipeptide renin inhibitor. Circulation 1990; 81: 1768−1774.

Weber MA, Byyny RL, Pratt H, Faison EP, Snavely DB, Goldberg AI, Nelson EB. Blood pressure effects of the angiotensin II receptor blocker, losartan. Arch Intern Med 1995; 155: 405−411.

28 Other drugs with antihypertensive efficacy

Serotonin antagonists and agonists:

5-hydroxytryptophan$_2$ (5-HT$_2$) antagonists

The vasoconstrictive properties of serotonin (5-hydroxytryptophan), a tissue hormone which appears physiologically in, among other sites, the intestine, brain and platelets, are mediated largely via 5-HT$_2$ receptors (large arteries, precapillary resistance vessels). Despite the normal or rather reduced level of serotonin in the plasma, with primary hypertension, it is thought that blocking the 5-HT$_2$ receptors causes vasodilatation of the precapillary resistance vessels. This gives it a pharmacological mechanism of action suitable for blood-pressure reduction in arterial hypertension. Corresponding investigations with the highly selective 5-HT$_2$ receptor antagonist ritanserin, however, showed no blood-pressure reducing effect, so that this mode of action is no longer being pursued in the development of antihypertensive substances.

The antihypertensive effect of ketanserin, a hybrid substance with a low affinity for the 5-HT$_2$ receptor, is perhaps most likely mediated by additional alpha$_1$-receptor blocking properties or by a previously unknown central mechanism. Prolongation of the QT interval has been observed under higher dosages of ketanserin (cave: increased risk of torsades-de-point tachycardia).

5-hydroxytryptophan$_{1A}$ (5-HT$_{1A}$) agonists

The stimulation of central, medullary serotonin (auto)receptors (5-HT$_{1A}$) leads to decreased sympathetic activation and subsequently to peripheral vasodilation. This mechanism of action contributes − in addition to a blockade of peripheral alpha$_1$ adrenergic receptors − causally to the antihypertensive effects of the "hybrid" substances urapidil and indorsamin (see also Chapter 24).

Stimulators of prostacyclin synthesis:

The (intravenous) administration of prostacyclin leads to a reduction in blood pressure in patients with arterial hypertension. This effect is due to a direct relaxation of the vascular smooth musculature. Because the administration of prostacyclin is only possible intravenously and is associated with significant side effects at higher dosages, the administration of prostacyclin can not be considered a suitable method for the treatment of arterial hypertension.

A stimulation of prostacyclin synthesis as a participatory cause of the antihypertensive effect has, however, been postulated for orally applicable cicletanine, a furopyridine derivative. Whether and to what degree this mode of action is actually relevant is being debated, especially as diuretic and natriuretic properties stand out at higher dosages (> 100 mg). In addition it has been reported that cicletanine causes a reduction of intracellular calcium ions in the vascular smooth musculature.

The recommended daily dosage is initially 100 mg (maximal 200 mg). If a reduction in the diastolic blood pressure to < 95 mmHg is achieved at this dosage, a trial reduction to 50 mg/day can be attempted. Beta-receptor blockers, ACE inhibitors and calcium antagonists are suitable combination partners for cicletanine.

The most important side effect is the development of hypokalemia.

Decreased renal function (creatinine clearance < 40 ml/min. or serum creatinine > 1.8 mg/100 ml), severely impaired liver function, pregnancy and nursing all represent contraindications for treatment with cicletanine, which has thus far only been licensed in France and Germany.

Endopeptidase inhibitors:

The neutral endopeptidase 24.11 (EC 3.4.24.11; NEP) inactivates nonspecific vasodilatory peptide hormones like ANP (atrial natriuretic peptide), BNP (brain natriuretic peptide) and bradykinin. Inhibition of the endopeptidase prevents or slows the breakdown of this hormone and thus increases its biological effect. In recent years various endopeptidase inhibitors have been synthesized. Some of these are now in clinical development for the indications heart failure and arterial hypertension (e.g., SCH 42495, candoxatril, etc.).

Hybrid substances are also in development, which have both NEP and ACE inhibitory effects (e.g., UK-81,252).

Endothelin receptor antagonists:

Endothelin 1 (ET 1) is formed by the endothelial cells. Its role in the pathogenesis of arterial hypertension is a subject of controversial discussion. A systemic, vasoactive effect appears to be rather unlikely, since the peripheral plasma levels of ET 1 are not raised in uncomplicated hypertension without massive target-organ damage. It is conceivable, however, that ET 1 participates in the local regulation of blood flow.

Various ET receptor antagonists have been synthesized. Clinical investigations on patients with mild to moderate hypertension are only available in the form of acute studies with bosentan, an orally applied ET receptor antagonist. In this study, a reduction of the diastolic blood pressure was only observed after administration of 2000 mg bosentan, a reduction which was comparatively less pronounced than 20 mg enalapril.

To what degree the pharmacological inhibition of endothelin serves as a therapeutic principle for the treatment of arterial hypertension must be made dependent on the results of future studies.

Questionable antihypertensive mechanisms of action:

Endothelin converting enzyme (ECE) inhibitors

The vasoactive substance endothelin is cleaved from its precursor, the so-called big endothelin, by proteolysis. The enzyme responsible for this is a highly specific endopeptidase, also referred to as endothelin converting enzyme (ECE). An inhibition of ECE would thus be a pharmacological possibility for inhibiting the formation of endothelin.

Summary (Chapter 28)

- Urapidil and indorsamin are "hybrid" substances whose antihypertensive effect is due, on the one hand, to a blocking of the peripheral $alpha_1$ receptors and, on the other, to a stimulation of central serotonin ($5\text{-}HT_{1A}$) receptors.

- Cicletanine is an antihypertensive drug marketed in France and Germany, with a mode of action that has not yet been fully explained. Among other explanations, a stimulation of prostacyclin synthesis and diuretic and natriuretic properties are being discussed.

- Whether endopeptidase inhibitors, endothelin receptor antagonists or ECE inhibitors will be developed for the treatment of arterial hypertension can not be determined at this time.

Literature (Chapter 28)

Bianci G, Swales JD. Do we need more anti-hypertensive drugs: lessons from the new biology. Lancet 1995; 345: 1555−1557.

Clozel M, Breu V, Burri K, Cassal JM, Fischli GAG, Hirth G, Löffler BM, Müller M, Neidhart W, Ramuz H. Pathophysiological role of endothelin revealed by the first orally active endothelin receptor antagonist. Nature 1993; 365: 759−761.

Favrat B, Burnier M, Nussberger J, Lecomte JM, Brouard R, Waeber B, Brunner HR. Neutral endopeptidase versus angiotensin converting enzyme inhibition in essential hypertension. J Hypertens 1995; 13: 797−804.

Gregoire JR, Sheps SG. Newer antihypertensive drugs. Curr Opin Cardiol 1995; 10: 445−449.

Gros C, Noel N, Souque A, Schwartz JC, Danvy D, et al. Mixed inhibitors of angiotensin-converting enzyme (EC 3.4.15.1) and enkephalinase (EC 3.4.24.11): rational design, properties, and potential cardiovascular applications of glycopril and alatriopril. Proc Nat Acad Sci USA 1991; 88: 4210−4214.

Kitamura K, Kangawa K, Matsuo H, Eto T. Adrenomedullin. Implications for hypertension research. Drugs 1995; 49: 485−495.

Ogihara T, Raguki H, Masuo K, Yu H, Nagano M, Mikami H. Antihypertensive effects of the neutral endopeptidase inhibitor SCH 42495 in essential hypertension. Am J Hypertens 1994; 7: 943−947.

Schmitt R, Belz GG, Fell D, Lebmeier R, Prager G, Stahnke PL, Sittner WD, Karwoth A, Jones CR. Effects of the novel endothelin receptor antagonist bosentan in hypertensive patients. Ricerca Scientifica ed Educazione Permanente 1995; Suppl. 103: 170.

Van Zwieten PA, Chalmers JP. Different types of centrally acting antihypertensives and their targets in the central nervous system. Cardiovasc Drugs Ther 1994; 8: 787−799.

Yanagisawa M. The endothelin system. A new target for therapeutic intervention. Circulation 1994; 89: 1320−1322.

29 Contraindications and indication restrictions/ drug interactions with antihypertensives

The contraindications and important indication restrictions for the antihypertensive substance classes mentioned in sections 23 to 27 are compiled in the following chart (Table 29.1).

The most important drug interactions with antihypertensive drugs are presented in Table 29.2.

Table 29.1: Contraindications and therapeutic restrictions of antihypertensive drugs

Substance (class)	Contraindication	Therapeutic restriction
DIURETICS (Chapter 23)		
Thiazide diuretics	Acute attack of gout, volume depletion, renal insufficiency (creatinine clearance <20 ml/min)	Diabetes mellitus, gout, hypercalcemia, hypokalemia
Loop diuretics	Acute attacks of gout, volume depletion	Acute renal failure, hepatic coma, gout, hypokalemia
Aldosterone-antagonists, potassium-sparing diuretics	renal insufficiency hyperkalemia	Combination with ACE inhibitors
SYMPATHOLYTICS (Chapter 24)		
Primarily centrally acting sympatholytics:		
Alpha-methyldopa	Acute liver disease	Liver disease
Imidazoline-receptor agonists + guanfacine	Sick sinus syndrome AV block II°/III° AV block I° + bifascicular bundle branch block	Bradycardia, combination with beta-blocker or calcium antagonist of the "verapamil" and "diltiazem-type"
Sympatholytics with central and peripheral action sites:		
Reserpine	Depression, Parkinson's disease, epilepsy	Ventricular ulcer
Urapidil	Pregnancy, nursing period	
Primarily peripherally acting sympatholytics:		
Selective alpha$_1$-adrenergic receptor blockers	Pregnancy, nursing period, heart failure due to aortic or mitral stenosis, children <12 years old	Orthostatic hypotension
Beta-adrenergic receptor blockers (unselective and beta$_1$-selective)	Bronchial asthma, sick sinus syndrome, AV block II°/III° monotherapy in cases of pheochromocytoma, decompensated heart failure*	Chronic obstructive lung diseases (COLD), peripheral arterial occlusive disease (PAOD), Raynaud's syndrome, diabetes mellitus, combination with calcium antagonists of the verapamil and diltiazem type, and centrally acting sympatholytics

Table 29.1 (continued):   Contraindications and therapeutic restrictions of antihypertensive drugs

Substance (class)	Contraindication	Therapeutic restriction
VASODILATORS (Chapter 25)		
Dihydralazine	Severe coronary heart disease, aortic aneurysm, valvular stenoses, hypertrophic cardiomyopathy, nursing period	Lupus erythematosus
Minoxidil	Severe coronary heart disease, exsiccosis, nursing period	Mild to moderate hypertension
CALCIUM ANTAGONISTS (Chapter 26)		
Arylalkylamines ("verapamil type")	Sick sinus syndrome, AV block II°/III°, AV block I° + bifascicular bundle branch block, cardiogenic shock, decompensated heart failure	Chronic constipation, combination with beta-blockers or centrally acting sympatholytics
Dihydropyridines ("nifedipine type")	Pregnancy, cardiogenic shock	Severe venous insufficiency, coronary heart disease**
Benzothiazepines ("diltiazem type")	Sick sinus syndrome, AV block II°/III°, AV block I° + bifascicular bundle branch block cardiogenic shock, decompensated heart failure	Combination with beta-blocker or sympatholytis with central sites of action
INHIBITORS OF THE RENIN-ANGIOTENSIN SYSTEM (Chapter 27)		
Angiotensin-I-converting enzyme (ACE) inhibitors	Pregnancy, nursing period, bilateral renal artery stenoses (RAS) or unilateral RAS with solitary functioning kidney, angioneurotic edema	Collagenosis, volume depletion, combination with potassium-sparing diuretics
Angiotensin-II receptor antagonists	Pregnancy, nursing period, bilateral renal artery stenoses (RAS) or unilateral RAS with solitary functioning kidney	Volume depletion

* Reductions in mortality and morbidity have been demonstrated with some beta-receptor blockers as add-on therapy to preexisting drug regimen in patients with severe heart failure (NYHA III–IV) due to dilated cardiomyopathy
** For short-acting dihydropyridines

Table 29.2:   Selected drug interactions with antihypertensive therapy

Class	Antihypertensive efficacy		Effect on other drugs
	Decreased	Increased	
DIURETICS			
	Cholestyramine Colestipol NSAIDs	Combinations of thiazides with furosemide	Lithium: increase of serum levels and renal toxicity Corticosteroids: hypokalemia
SYMPATHOLYTICS			
Centrally and peripherally acting sympatholytics:			
All	Tricyclic antidepressants		
Guanadrel, Guanethidine	Amphetamines Phenothiazines Cocaine		
Alpha-methyldopa			Lithium: increase of serum levels
Primarily peripherally acting sympatholytics:			
Alpha-adrenergic receptor blockers	Higher incidence of postural hypotension with concomitant antihypertensive drugs (especially diuretics)		
Beta-adrenergic receptor blockers	NSAIDs Rifampin Smoking Barbiturates	Cimetidine Quinidine Phenylpropanolamine Pseudoephedrine Ephedrine Epinephrine	Diltiazem- and verapamil-type calcium antagonists: additive depressant effects on SA- and AV-node Reserpine, clonidine: increased risk of bradycardia and syncope Theophylline, lidocaine, chlorpromazine: increase of serum levels Insulin: Prolongation of hypoglycemia (nonselective beta-blockers)

Table 29.2 (continued):   Selected drug interactions with antihypertensive therapy

Class	Antihypertensive efficacy		Effect on other drugs
	Decreased	Increased	
CALCIUM ANTAGONISTS			
Arylalkylamines ("verapamil-type"):			
	Rifampin Carbamazepine Phenobarbital Phenytoin	Cimetidine	Digoxin, carbamazepine: increased serum levels and toxicity Prazosin, quinidine, theophylline, cyclosporine: increased serum levels
Dihydropyridines ("nifedipine-type"):			
		Cimetidine	Cyclosporine Digoxin, carbamazepine: increased serum levels and toxicity
INHIBITORS OF THE RENIN-ANGIOTENSIN-SYSTEM			
ACE-inhibitors:			
	NSAIDs Antacids	Diuretics Salt depletion	NSAIDs, potassium sparing agents, potassium supplements: hyperkalemia Opiates: potentation of analgesic effect and respiratory depressant effect
Angiotensin II receptor antagonists:			
	NSAIDs Antacids	Diuretics Salt depletion	NSAIDs, potassium sparing agents, potassium supplements: hyperkalemia

Abbreviations:

NSAIDs: Non-steroidal anti-inflammatory drugs
SA-node: Sinoatrial node
AV-node: Atrioventricular node

30 Antihypertensive combination therapies

If antihypertensive drug monotherapy (performed according to the therapeutic guidelines mentioned in Section 21) does not lead to sufficient blood pressure reduction, all of the substances recommended as first line therapy can, in principle, be combined with one another. However, not all combinations are equally as effective, well-tolerated or practical from a pharmacodynamic or hemodynamic point of view.

30.1 The free combination of antihypertensive substances

30.1.1 Diuretics and beta-receptor blockers

The administration of a diuretic and a beta-receptor blocker is a widespread combination therapy in the treatment of arterial hypertension. The essential advantages of this combination are the additional antihypertensive effectiveness when compared to the components alone (this has been shown in countless studies), the many years of clinical experience and the relatively low cost. In addition, it has been shown that a combined administration of these substance classes leads to reduction in mortality and cardiovascular morbidity (stroke, myocardial infarction) in elderly patients with hypertension (Swedish Trial in Old Patients with Hypertension, the "STOP Hypertension Study").

The combination diuretic/beta-receptor blocker is not optimal from a pharmacological point of view, because diuretics do not typically trigger any clinically relevant tachycardia, which could be positively influenced by a beta-receptor blocker. In addition, beta-receptor blocker do not generally trigger any fluid retention, which, in turn, would make the combined application of a diuretic appear beneficial.

30.1.2 Diuretics and ACE inhibitors

The combination of thiazide diuretics and ACE inhibitors has a very high antihypertensive effectiveness, which may be primarily due to the diuretic-induced activation of the renin angiotensin system (RAS). In patient populations with low-grade RAS activity ("low-renin hypertension", e.g., in African-American or elderly hypertensive patients) and an unsufficient blood pressure reduction under a monotherapy with ACE inhibitors, the therapeutic responsiveness is significantly increased by a pretreatment or combination treatment with a diuretic. The combination is additionally positive due to the fact that the (dose-related) loss of potassium under a diuretic can be compensated by the potassium-sparing properties of an ACE inhibitor (reduced formation of aldosterone).

The risk of an excessive blood-pressure reduction — especially at the start of therapy (first-dose hypotension) — should be considered.

The combination of a potassium-sparing diuretic and an ACE inhibitor is not optimal, since hyperkalemia can occur.

30.1.3 Diuretics and calcium antagonists

Since both diuretics and calcium antagonists have diuretic and natriuretic properties, their combined administration in the treatment of arterial hypertension is not considered optimal. Even though an additional antihypertensive effect can be expected compared to monotherapy with either individual component, this added efficacy is rather mild, as has been shown in different studies.

30.1.4 Beta-receptor blockers and ACE inhibitors

Beta-receptor blockers inhibit the release of renin from the juxtaglomerular apparatus (see also Figure 27.1). The resulting, more or less pronounced suppression of the RAS is not a positive pre-condition for the blood-pressure reducing effectiveness of an ACE inhibitor from a pharmacological point of view, because ACE inhibitors have a more pronounced effect with an activated RAS (see above). In addition, the negative chronotropic effect of the beta-receptor blockers is not a property, which would support its combined administration with an ACE inhibitor, since vasodilatation under ACE inhibitor administration does not trigger reflex tachycardia.

Although the respective mechanisms of action do not represent a positive support for a rationally justified, combined use of these substances, numerous studies do exist, which at least sufficiently document their therapeutic safety. The antihypertensive effect is only slightly stronger than under monotherapy with either of the substances alone.

The combination of beta-receptor blockers and ACE inhibitors may possibly be beneficial in the treatment of patients with coronary artery disease and after myocardial infarction ("secondary prevention").

30.1.5 Beta-receptor blockers and calcium antagonists

The combined administration of a beta-receptor blocker and a calcium antagonist of the dihydropyridine type is advantageous from a pharmacological point of view, because the renin-inhibiting and negative chronotropic properties of beta-receptor blockers counteract both the (low-level) stimulation of the RAS and the vasodilatory-related reflex tachycardia of the calcium antagonists.

An additive, antihypertensive efficacy has been substantiated in numerous studies for the combination of beta-receptor blockers and calcium antagonists of the dihydropyridine type.

Representatives of other classes of calcium antagonists (benzothiazepines or 'diltiazem-type'-calcium antagonists, phenylalkylamines or 'verapamil-type'-calcium antagonists) are less recommended as partners for combination therapy with beta-receptor blockers. Despite their effective blood-pressure reduction, clinically relevant bradycardia and asystole can occur (see also, Chapter 25).

30.1.6 Calcium antagonists and ACE inhibitors

The diuretic and natriuretic properties of the calcium antagonists increase the antihypertensive efficacy of the ACE inhibitors, so that the combination of both substance classes makes pharmacological sense. An additional advantage is that, due to the safety profile of the monosubstances, no negative influence on other cardiovascular risk factors is expected.

30.1.7 Other combinations

Further combination possibilities are beta and selective alpha$_1$-receptor blockers, as well as diuretics and alpha$_1$-receptor blockers. If the combined administration (especially not recommended in mild to moderate hypertension) of a calcium antagonist and an alpha$_1$-receptor blocker is being considered, a long-lasting alpha$_1$-receptor blocker (e.g., doxazosin) should be chosen to lower the risk of an excessive reduction in blood pressure. In every case, the patient's blood pressure should be monitored over several hours in the physician's practice upon the first administration of this combination.

30.2 Fixed combinations

The administration of fixed combination preparations represents an alternative to the gradual adjustment of hypertension. A primary normalization of blood pressure is achieved more often with these preparations than with monotherapy, because they contain substance combinations, which (ideally) show an additive antihypertensive effect. The prescription of a fixed combination thus makes it possible to limit the antihypertensive therapy to the daily intake of a single tablet or capsule in many cases, thus possibly improving patient compliance.

The disadvantage of this form of application is, among others, the risk of "overtreatment".

30.2.1 Low-dose, fixed combinations as initial therapy

Fixed combinations of beta-receptor blockers and diuretics (betaxolol/chlorthalidone and bisoprolol/hydrochlorothiazide) in very low dosages of the individual components have been approved for the first time as initial antihypertensive therapy by the U.S. health authorities (Food and Drug Administration, Washington, D.C.). It has been shown in multi-factorial studies that the antihypertensive efficacy of these fixed combinations is equal to or even greater than that of higher dosages of the component parts when administered individually. In addition, the side effect profile for both substance classes, which is known to be dosage dependent, is positively influenced by the (combined) administration of very low dosages.

Summary (Chapter 30)

- A combination of two (or more) first-line antihypertensive drugs is recommended, if blood pressure is not sufficiently controlled under antihypertensive monotherapy.

- All of the first-line antihypertensive agents (i. e. diuretics, beta-adrenergic receptor blockers, calcium antagonists, ACE inhibitors, alpha$_1$-adrenergic receptor blockers) can be combined with each other, as can other substance classes not classified as first-line antihypertensives.

- Not all possible combinations are equally effective in and suited for the individual patient. Special care must therefore be taken to choose combinations which, for various reasons, appear to be most rational.

- Starting antihypertensive treatment with fixed low-dose combinations is an attractive alternative to the stepped-care approach as initial therapy for hypertension; so far, only combinations of a beta blocker and a diuretic are approved as first-line antihypertensive treatment in the USA.

Literature (Chapter 30)

Brown MJ, Dickerson JEC. Alpha-blockade and calcium antagonism: an effective and well-tolerated combination for the treatment of resistant hypertension. J Hypertens 1995; 13: 701–707.

Fenichel RR, Lipicky RJ. Combination products as first-line pharmacotherapy. Arch Intern Med 1994; 154: 1461–1468.

Kaplan NM. Implications for cost-effectiveness. Combination therapy for systemic hypertension. Am J Cardiol 1995; 76: 595–597.

Kendall MJ. Approaches to meeting the criteria for fixed dose antihypertensive combinations.

Focus on metropolol. Drugs 1995; 50: 454–464.

Menard J, Bellet M. Calcium antagonists-ACE inhibitors combination therapy: objectives and methodology of clinical development. J Cardiovasc Pharmacol 1993; 21 (suppl 2): S49–S54.

Waeber B, Brunner HR. Main objectives and new aspects of combination treatment of hypertension. J Hypertens 1995; 13 (suppl 2): S15–S19.

31 Drug treatment of arterial hypertension with complicating conditions

Arterial hypertension is not infrequently associated with coexisting conditions, whereby the potential impact on these conditions caused by antihypertensive active agents must be taken into consideration when deciding on a therapy. This leads to the generally valid statement that the goal of blood pressure normalization can not be bought with a detrimental effect on the complicating condition. Whereas one can not always attain a synergistic effect of medication on hypertension and the complicating condition, it is possible in nearly all cases, with the variety of antihypertensive agents available today, to attain therapeutic neutrality towards the complicating condition.

Particular consideration must be given to already manifest end-organ damage to the heart, brain and kidney. Furthermore, when selecting an antihypertensive agent, one must consider cardiovascular risk factors (hyperlipidemia, hyperinsulinemia/insulin resistance or manifest diabetes mellitus) which, similar to hypertension itself, can cause premature end-organ damage. Particularly in hypertensive, postmenopausal women with loss of bone mass caused by an estrogen deficiency (postmenopausal osteoporosis) one must ensure that a long-term antihypertensive therapy neither accelerates the bone loss, nor has a negative influence on the osteoprotective effect of any simultaneously prescribed hormone replacement therapy.

Summary

- The goal of drug treatment of arterial hypertension is not the correction of the arterial blood pressure per se, but the reduction of mortality and morbidity.

- Drug treatment of arterial hypertension must therefore not negatively influence concomitant diseases or cardiovascular risk factors.

31.1 Antihypertensive therapy and heart disease

31.1.1 Therapy and hypertensive heart disease

There is a positive correlation between the duration and severity of arterial hypertension and the development of left ventricular hypertrophy. Furthermore it can still be attested that left ventricular hypertrophy (LVH), when progressing over an ample period of hypertension without drug therapy, almost always leads to dilatation of the ventricle and to clinically manifest congestive heart failure. With regard to this, the Framingham Study also provided evidence that hypertensive heart disease is by far the most common cause of congestive heart failure.

31.1.1.1 Therapy for asymptomatic hypertensive heart disease

The pathological development of untreated hypertensive heart disease, which typically begins with diastolic dysfunction of the left ventricle and progresses via the intermediate stage of left ventricular hypertrophy to congestive heart failure, myocardial ischemia, cardiac dysrhythmia and sudden cardiac death, has already been covered (Section 5.3.2). When selecting an antihypertensive agent in a patient with proven LVH (electrocardiography, echocardiography, radiological and/or nuclear medical imaging procedures) it must be taken into consideration that the therapeutic goal is not only correcting increased blood pressure but also regressing the LVH. Due to the risk of developing heart insufficiency (see above), the regression of LVH is globally considered a therapeutic necessity in cases of coexisting arterial hypertension, though there has not yet been any proof that this actually achieves a decrease in mortality and morbidity. Whereby all currently available first line medications (diuretics, beta and selective alpha$_1$ blockers, calcium antagonists,

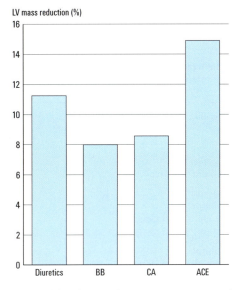

Figure 31.1: Effects of first-line antihypertensive agents on the reduction of left ventricular (LV) mass in patients with hypertension and left ventricular hypertrophy. Data based on a metaanalysis of 109 treatment studies comprising 2357 patients. Confidence intervals of LVM reduction: Diuretics 5.6 to 17 %, BB 4.8 to 11.2 %, CA 5.1 to 11.8 % and ACE 9.9 to 20.8 %. Abbreviations: BB = beta adrenergic blockers; CA = calcium antagonists; ACE = ACE inhibitors

(Data adapted from Dahlöf B et al., Am J Hypertens 1992; 5: 95−110).

ACE inhibitors) lead to a reduction of left ventricular hypertrophy, there are differences in efficacy (Figure 31.1). The differing influence on hypertensive heart disease despite comparable reductions in blood pressure could indicate that the regression of left ventricular hypertrophy is at least partially independent of pressure.

The most effective are possibly substances that lower the blood pressure by reducing the activity of the sympathetic nervous system (sympatholytic drugs) or by inhibiting the formation (ACE inhibitors) or the binding of angiotensin II (Ang II) to its receptor (Ang II receptor antagonists). This experience indicates that the experimentally documented trophic qualities of Ang II and catecholamines (see also Chapter 27) are of considerable significance in the genesis of hypertensive LVH. In the meantime, contrary to earlier assumptions, it has been shown that long-term therapy with diuretics also leads to regression of left ventricular hypertrophy (Veterans Cooperative Study, SHEP Study, TOMHS Study; see also Figure 31.1).

Analogous to the old stepped-care approach used in the treatment of hypertension, a similar stepped-care approach has been recommended for the treatment of asymptomatic hypertensive heart disease which has therapeutic goals based on the principles of possibly reversing the LVH on the one hand and simultaneously correcting blood pressure on the other hand (Table 31.1).

Since, in principle, all first-line antihypertensive medications can be used for the treatment of hypertension with concomitantly existing LVH (see above), the doctor in charge has sufficient leeway, despite the schematic recommendations, to meet the particular needs of the individual patient.

Table 31.1: "Stepped-care" approach for the treatment of (compensated) hypertensive heart disease*

Therapeutic procedure	Substance(s)
Step 1:	Calcium antagonist** or ACE inhibitor
Step 2:	Calcium antagonist** plus ACE inhibitor
Step 3:	Calcium antagonist** plus ACE inhibitor plus clonidine/alpha methyldopa
Step 4:	Calcium antagonist** plus ACE inhibitor plus clonidine/alpha methyldopa plus diuretic and/or Beta adrenergic receptor blocker and/or Vasodilator

 * Modified according to Strauer and Motz (1988 and 1993)
** Only long-acting calcium antagonists are recommended

31.1.1.2 Therapy of hypertensive heart disease with angina pectoris symptoms

The goal of drug therapy applied against hypertensive heart disease with coexisting angina pectoris is on the one hand the prevention of discomfort and, on the other hand, a regression of the hypertrophied myocardium. In addition to the therapeutic stepped-care approach recommended for the treatment of asymptomatic hypertensive heart disease (Table 31.1, Section 31.1.1.1), patients with symptomatic angina pectoris should also be treated with medication effective as antianginal agents (beta adrenergic receptor blockers, nitrates, NO donors) (Table 31.2). In cases of angiographically documented coronary macroangiopathy it is recommended, if appropriate for the indication, to undertake a revascularization either operatively (coronary bypass grafting) or through the use of a PTCA (percutaneous transluminal coronary angioplasty) (Table 31.2).

Table 31.2: Therapy for hypertensive heart disease

Stage of hypertensive heart disease	Therapy
Asymptomatic hypertensive heart disease	"Stepped-care" approach (see Table 31.1)
Hypertensive heart disease with symptomatic angina pectoris	
— Coronary macroangiopathy	Revascularisation or medicinal therapy with beta-receptor blockers, calcium antagonists* and nitrates and/or NO-donors
— Coronary microangiopathy	"Stepped-care" approach (see Table 31.1) and — Beta-receptor blockers — ACE inhibitors — Nitrates and/or NO-donors
Hypertensive heart failure	ACE inhibitor Diuretics Digitalis

* Long-acting calcium antagonists
NO = nitric oxide

31.1.1.3 Therapy for symptomatic heart failure as a terminal stage of hypertensive heart disease

Since a correction of the ventricular morphology can no longer be expected in this stage of hypertensive heart disease, and any further reduction in wall thickness of the dilated heart is therapeutically undesirable, treatment should strive for a recompensation of the manifest heart failure. As a rule, treatment is initiated with ACE inhibitors or heart glycosides (Table 31.2) and then ensues according to the usual guidelines for the treatment of heart insufficiency in the clinical stages III-IV (according to the classification of the NYHA) (sodium restriction, ACE inhibitors, glycosides, diuretics).

Summary (Section 31.1.1)

- The goal of therapeutic efforts in treating asymptomatic hypertensive heart disease is the correction of blood pressure and the regression of left ventricular hypertrophy.

- All antihypertensive first line drugs recommended for the initial treatment of hypertension (diuretics, beta and selective alpha$_1$-receptor blockers, calcium antagonists, ACE inhibitors) effectively reduce blood pressure and result in regression of left ventricular hypertrophy.

- The effective reduction of left ventricular hypertrophy through the long-term administration of sympatholytic drugs and ACE inhibitors is possibly due not only to their efficacy in lowering blood pressure, but additionally due to an inhibition of trophogenic hormones (catecholamines, Ang II).

- The additional administration of nitrates or other antianginal agents is necessary in cases of coexisting angina pectoris. If high-grade macroangiopathic stenoses of the coronary arteries are the cause for this condition, revascularization is always to be recommended, in so far as this is permitted by morphology and the localization of the stenoses.

- The treatment of decompensated hypertensive heart failure is aimed at cardiac recompensation, and follows the general guidelines for the treatment of congestive heart failure. In this stage of the disease, a regression of the myocardial wall thickness of the dilated ventricle is not necessary and not desirable.

31.1.2 Antihypertensive therapy and coronary artery disease

Whereas an increase in systolic arterial blood pressure requires an increase in the left ventricle oxygen demand, an increase in diastolic blood pressure impairs the coronary blood flow during diastole and therewith the supply of the myocardium. The presence of coronary artery disease with arterial hypertension therefore requires an optimal correction of both the systolic and diastolic blood pressure. Beta blockers and calcium antagonists have proven themselves as effective antihypertensive agents in patients with hypertension and concomitant coronary artery disease. Among the dihydropyridine calcium antagonists, long-acting substances or combinations with a slow release of the active agent should be given precedence to avoid a rapid drop in blood pressure and the triggering of reflex tachycardia. Short-acting dihydropyridines are already contraindicated with unstable angina pectoris or status post recent myocardial infarction (Chapter 26). − ACE inhibitors lower mortality and morbidity with coronary artery disease, if administered during long-term therapy after an acute myocardial infarction ("secondary prevention"; see also Section 27.2.2).

Diuretics can induce hypokalemia, which can present a particular risk for patients with coronary artery disease due to the increased tendency for ventricular ectopy. Antihypertensive agents that can trigger a reflex tachycardia, and therewith an increased myocardial oxygen demand, should only be used in combination. First and foremost among these are the vasodilators, which — should they be used despite the above-mentioned reservations — must be combined with beta blockers. Centrally effective sympatholytic drugs can also be used against reflex tachycardia if there is a contraindication to beta blockers.

Summary (Section 31.1.2)

- The presence of coronary artery disease requires optimal correction of the systolic and diastolic blood pressure.

- Beta blockers and long-acting calcium antagonists (or those with sustained release) have proven themselves effective as antihypertensive first line medication for patients with hypertension and coexisting coronary artery disease. Short-acting, first generation calcium antagonists should not be prescribed for coronary artery disease.

- ACE inhibitors reduce mortality and morbidity among patients with coronary artery disease after an acute myocardial infarction.

- A regular control of the potassium level is advisable during the administration of diuretics, since hypokalemia will advance the tendency for ventricular arrhythmia particularly among patients with coronary artery disease.

- A combination of a beta blocker or a centrally acting sympatholytic drug is advisable with the administration of vasodilators in order to avoid reflex tachycardia.

31.1.3 Antihypertensive therapy and cardiac dysrhythmias

Ventricular ectopic activity is not uncommon among patients with arterial hypertension, particularly in the presence of myocardial alterations in the sense of hypertensive heart disease and/or coexisting micro- or macroangiopathic coronary artery disease. Hypokalemia, which can result from an antihypertensive therapy with diuretics, increases the tendency for ventricular ectopia and must therefore be corrected (potassium supplementation, changing substance class, combination with a potassium-sparing substance).

The therapeutic attempt with a (relatively) selective beta$_1$ blocker is justified after subjective reports of ventricular extrasystole (up to stage IVa according to the

LOWN classification), since these substance classes are effective as both antihypertensive and antiarrhythmic agents.

A specific antiarrhythmic therapy of ventricular ectopia is indicated for life-threatening tachyarrhythmia. Drug treatment of non-life-threatening cardiac dysrhythmia has been handled extremely restrictively since the publication of the CAST study results because of the potential pro-arrhythmic effect of all antiarrhythmic agents and the continued lack of proof on lowering mortality and morbidity. However, if the introduction of a specific antiarrhythmic therapy is necessary, the effect that some antiarrhythmic drugs have on lowering the blood pressure should be taken into account; if necessary, the existing antihypertensive medication should be reduced.

Supraventricular arrhythmia also occurs among hypertensive patients more often than among normotensive patients. Beta blockers and calcium antagonists of the verapamil or diltiazem type are the preferred medication in such cases.

Summary (Section 31.1.3)

- Ventricular ectopic activity occurs more often in hypertensive patients than among the normal population.

- Subjective reports of disturbing, non-life-threatening ventricular extrasystole (up to LOWN IVa) should be countered by the administration of a beta blocker, since this substance class is effective both as an antihypertensive and an antiarrhythmic agent.

- Beta blockers and calcium antagonists of the verapamil or diltiazem type are to be used in supraventricular arrhythmia and hypertension.

31.2 Antihypertensive therapy and cerebrovascular diseases

31.2.1 Antihypertensive therapy in acute stroke

Hypertensive blood pressure values immediately after the onset of a stroke are usually the result of a (stress related) excessive release of catecholamines and therefore often only of a temporary nature. Quite often the values will spontaneously correct themselves within a few hours. A drug therapy during the acute phase of stroke should only ensue with blood pressure values over 200 mmHg systolic and/or 110−120 mmHg diastolic. The lowering of blood pressure must progress very cautiously and slowly, since cerebral autoregulation is canceled in an acute stroke. Sudden drug-induced drops in blood pressure can intensify ischemia and increase the infarct area. The therapeutic goal for hypertension is the reduction of the mean arterial blood pressure by a maximum of 25% of the base-line value within the first 24 hours; values under 160/100 mmHg should definitely be avoided. The administration of sodium nitroprusside can ensue for excessive increases of blood pressure with diastolic values over 130 mmHg, and should be administered intravenously by means of an infusion pump under intensive-care conditions. Since sodium nitroprusside can possibly increase intracranial pressure, many experts now recommend the administration of labetalol.

In any case, labetalol has become the drug of choice for lower blood pressure values that nonetheless require treatment, since it apparently does not increase intracranial pressure, possibly improves the autoregulation of the cerebral blood flow and does not induce any unforeseen decreases in blood pressure. The administration of labetalol can also be regulated quite well, particularly through parenteral application with an infusion pump (0.5 to 2 mg/kg/min). Alternatively, labetalol can be injected intravenously in intervals of about 15 to 20 minutes.

ACE inhibitors can lead to distinct decreases in blood pressure among volume depleted patients or patients with undiagnosed renal artery stenosis, thereby aggravating intracerebral blood flow. If this is nevertheless the substance class that is chosen, treatment should start with only half of the normally recommended first dose.

No drug therapy is necessary for only moderately increased blood pressure (systolic $< 180-200$ mmHg and/or diastolic $< 105-110$ mmHg), since a spontaneous drop is often observed within the first few hours after stroke (see above).

31.2.2 Antihypertensive therapy as primary prevention of cerebrovascular accidents

Up to now it has only been shown for beta blockers and diuretics that long-term antihypertensive drug treatment can reduce the incidence of stroke in both patients with diastolic (primary prevention: STOP 1 study; EWPHW study; MRC II study; etc.) and with isolated systolic (SHEP study) hypertension.

Though it is assumed that the long-term administration of ACE inhibitors or selective alpha$_1$ -adrenergic receptor blockers increases the tolerance of cerebral autoregulation in relation to (nocturnal) drops in blood pressure, there are no study results to document any preventive effect these substance classes can have on the incidence of lethal and non-lethal cerebrovascular events. Appropriate data at least for ACE inhibitors (and calcium antagonists) can be expected after the completion of the HOT- and the ALLHAT-Study (for other presently ongoing studies see also Table 26.2).

31.2.3 Antihypertensive therapy as prevention of recurrent stroke (secondary prevention)

If hypertensive blood pressure values persist after acute stroke, antihypertensive medication should be administered continuously. In order to avoid a worsening of cerebrovascular blood flow, the blood pressure should be lowered gradually without intervals of clinically relevant hypotension. Caution should be taken especially with the condition of older patients after stroke due to their inherently worse cerebral autoregulative tolerance with relation to hypotension if, during drug therapy, blood pressure falls to values below 160/90 mmHg.

Since there are not yet any known study results available documenting a therapeutic advantage for one of the substance classes recognized as first line medication with regard to the secondary prevention of stroke, the criteria for the choice of an antihypertensive agent does not principally differ from the (individual) criteria that must categorically be taken into consideration in the choice of antihypertensive medication. − Prevention studies with appropriate end points (cerebrovascular mortality and morbidity) will have to determine if the advantages derived from experimental studies indicating benefits for ACE inhibitors and alpha$_1$-adrenergic blockers with regard to intracerebral autoregulation (Section 31.2.2) have any clinical relevance. The same is true for the administration of calcium antagonists, preferred by some authors.

Summary (Section 31.2)

- Increased blood pressure values after onset of an acute stroke are usually the result of a reactive release of catecholamines and are temporary in nature.

- A drug-induced reduction of blood pressure is often not necessary and may even be detrimental to cerebral blood flow.

- Blood pressure should only be reduced through medication slowly and under continuous supervision with blood pressure values over 200 mmHg systolic or 110 mmHg diastolic; sudden drops in blood pressure in the acute phase of a stroke are more of a risk to the patient than moderately elevated blood pressure values.

- Excessively elevated blood pressure should be reduced slowly (via an infusion pump) under intensive care supervision with labetalol or sodium nitroprusside.

- An approximate target value within the first 24 hours is the maximum reduction of blood pressure requiring treatment by about 25% of the initial value (mean arterial blood pressure) or to a minimum of 160/100 mmHg.

- As of yet there is only evidence that beta blockers and diuretics are suitable for primary prevention of cerebrovascular disease among patients with hypertension. The preventive effectiveness of ACE inhibitors and calcium antagonists is one of the end points of studies that are currently still underway.

- If blood pressure values remain continuously elevated after the acute phase of stroke, an antihypertensive therapy with one of the first line medications should be initiated with caution. Particularly in the treatment of older patients, however, the reduction of blood pressure to values under 160/90 mmHg after a stroke should be avoided.

31.3 Antihypertensive therapy and peripheral arterial occlusive disease

A reduction in blood pressure in the case of advanced, peripheral arterial occlusive disease (PAOD) (> stage II according to Fontaine's classification) is always accompanied by the danger that the blood flow in the stenotic or in the poststenotic sections of affected arteries will be further aggravated. Antihypertensive medication that can lead to a constriction of the periphery (beta blockers) should therefore be used with caution. − Diuretics can lead to hemoconcentration; the resulting increase in blood viscosity and the drop in blood pressure may further adversely influence the peripheral blood flow, which is diminished in any case.

Vasodilatory substances such as ACE inhibitors, long-acting calcium antagonists and long-acting, selective alpha$_1$-adrenergic receptor blockers should be given preference in cases that include the coexistence of an PAOD. In advanced cases of stenosis, however, there is the risk that the distension of the healthy, peripheral vessels can lead to a worsening of blood flow in the area of the stenosis through the so-called 'steal effect'.

Following these comments it must be said that the drug treatment of hypertension with PAOD may be problematic and must be adapted specifically to the individual case. Tight controls and an in-depth questioning of the patient with regard to subjective discomforts (walking distance without pain, claudication intervals, cold extremities, etc.) are essential in monitoring a PAOD anyway, but also urgently advisable after the initiation of antihypertensive drug therapy.

Summary (Section 31.3)

- Any reduction in blood pressure can further worsen the arterial blood supply in cases of peripheral arterial occlusive disease (PAOD).

- Long-acting, vasodilating antihypertensive agents (ACE inhibitors, calcium antagonists and possibly alpha-$_1$ receptor blockers) are best tolerated with a coexisting PAOD.

31.4 Antihypertensive therapy and renal insufficiency

The lowering of blood pressure to values of 130/85 mmHg among patients with hypertension delays the progression of already existent kidney damage and must therefore be consistently implemented.

Drug therapy for hypertension with renal insufficiency differs only slightly from the general treatment of high blood pressure. However, one must take into account the increasing accumulation of renally eliminated substances during the reduction of the glomerular filtration rate, as well as the decreasing effectiveness of thiazide diuretics.

A regular control of serum creatinine, BUN and potassium, essential among patients with renal insufficiency anyway, must ensue during the initial phase of an antihypertensive therapy with particularly tight controls.

31.4.1 Antihypertensive monotherapy

The treatment of arterial hypertension with coexisting renal insufficiency should also first be initiated with a monotherapy. In principal, all substance classes that are generally used in the treatment of arterial hypertension are suitable for this.

31.4.1.1 Diuretics

The treatment of arterial hypertension with coexisting renal insufficiency with diuretics is pathophysiologically sensible due to the reduced capacity of the kidneys to excrete sodium. The administration of thiazide diuretics is only effective up to a glomerular filtration rate (GFR) of 30 ml/min (corresponding to a serum creatinine concentration of 2 mg/dl); any further reduction in kidney function, however, nullifies the antihypertensive effects of these diuretics so that loop diuretics (furosemide, pretanide, etc.), which are effective up to a GFR of 5 ml/min, should be prescribed additionally or alone.

Potassium-sparing diuretics should be used with restraint with renal insufficiency; due to the risk of hyperkalemia they are contraindicated at any GFR below 30 ml/min.

31.4.1.2 Beta-adrenergic receptor blockers

Hydrophilic beta-receptor blockers (Table 31.3) are renally eliminated so that, to avoid an accumulation of the substances, an appropriate adjustment of the dosage (50−25% of the initial dose) should be made during any decrease in kidney function.

31.4.1.3 Calcium antagonists

Although calcium antagonists primarily induce a dilatation of the afferent arteriole, thereby theoretically increasing the intraglomerular pressure, clinical studies have failed to document any further aggravation of preexisting renal insufficiency. The observation that at least some existing cases of proteinuria were favorably influenced indicates that this was either the result of a reduction in systemic blood pressure, or of other intrarenal active mechanisms of calcium antagonists which have, as of yet, not been fully clarified. − The slight natriuretic effects are advantageous because the renal capacity to exrete sodium decreases with increasing renal insufficiency (see above as well).

Table 31.3:   Adaptation of dosage of hydrophilic beta receptor blockers in renal insufficiency

Substance	Creatinine-clearance (ml/min)	Serum-creatinine (mg %)	Dosage range (mg/day)
Atenolol	>30 10–30 <10	<2.5 2.5–5 >5.0 Removed by hemodialysis	25–100 12.5–50 (50%) 6.25–25 (25%)
Nadolol	>30 10–30 <10	<2.5 2.5–5 >5.0 Removed by hemodialysis	20–240 10–120 (50%) 5–60 (25%)
Sotalol	>30 10–30 <10	<2.5 2.5–5.0 >5.0 Removed by hemodialysis	160–480 80–240 (50%) 40–120 (25%)

In conclusion it should be assumed that calcium antagonists are suited for the treatment of hypertension in patients with renal insufficiency. Dose adjustment is not necessary.

31.4.1.4 ACE inhibitors

ACE inhibitors dilate the efferent renal arteriole and lead thus to a reduction in the increased intraglomerular pressure caused by hypertension. This intrarenal effect on the one hand and the reduction in systemic blood pressure on the other hand explain, at least in part, the reduction in proteinuria observed under treatment with ACE inhibitors. Whether or not ACE inhibitors are better than other antihypertensive agents at protecting the kidney from further damage continues to be controversial, since there is still a need for appropriate long-term studies with a sufficiently large number of patients.

An increase in the serum creatinine concentration at the start of treatment with ACE inhibitors is usually only temporary in nature and therefore requires no change in substance classes. Any increase in the creatinine level, however, must be closely monitored, since there are rare instances of ACE inhibitors triggering acute renal failure in cases of preexisting renal insufficiency; the cause for this is often the existence of an undiagnosed bilateral renal artery stenosis or a renal artery stenosis in patients with a solitary functioning kidney.

ACE inhibitors are eliminated either renally or by both renal and hepato-biliary excretion (Table 27.1). Since one must be prepared for a toxic effect at high serum concentrations particularly of renally eliminated ACE inhibitors, the dosage for such cases must be adjusted to the severity of renal insufficiency (with a creatinine clearance < 40 ml/min 50% of the lowest recommended dose, < 10 ml/min

25−33%). In cases with moderate renal insufficiency, no dose adjustment is necessary for ACE inhibitors that are eliminated via both renal and hepatobiliary routes (e. g. fosinopril and others; see also Table 27.1); should the creatinine clearance drop to below 10 ml/min, however, these substances should also be used with caution.

As a rule, the initiation of an antihypertensive therapy especially for patients with more severe renal insufficiency, should be done under hospitalized conditions, since there is usually an activated renin-angiotensin-system due to the underlying disease, and one must reckon with strong drops in blood pressure following the first dose of ACE inhibitors. In any case, diuretics should be discontinued about 2−3 days before the initial dose in order to avoid any further potential hypotensive effect. In order to reduce the risk of first-dose hypotension among patients with impaired kidney function, it is advisable to initiate therapy with 50 percent of the lowest recommended dosage for patients with healthy kidneys.

If the therapy can not be initiated under hospitalized conditions, the patient must be monitored as an outpatient for at least 3−4 hours after the initial dose.

For ACE inhibitors that are eliminated through hemodialysis, the administration of the medication should ensue on dialysis days after the completion of the dialysis treatment.

31.4.1.5 Sodium nitroprusside

Sodium nitroprusside is only used in the course of treatment for hypertension during a hypertensive crisis or, temporarily, for malignant hypertension. When metabolized it first forms thiocyanide and then thiocyanate, the latter of which is eliminated renally and, as an overdose, can lead to metabolic acidosis, convulsions, coma and delirium. In cases of coexisting renal insufficiency the treatment must be limited to 2−3 days (initial dose: 25 g/min; maximum dose: 500 g/min.); control of the plasma thiocyanide levels is advisable.

31.4.1.6 Further substances effective as antihypertensive agents

The remaining sympatholytic drugs (reserpine, imidazoline receptor agonists, guanfacine, alpha-methyldopa and the selective alpha$_1$-receptor blockers) and vasodilators such as (di-)hydralazine or, in cases of severe hypertension, minoxidil are also suitable for reducing blood pressure among patients with renal insufficiency. These substances do not require dose adjustment.

31.4.2 Antihypertensive combination therapy

The necessity of aggressively reducing blood pressure in patients with hypertension and coexisting renal insufficiency has already been covered repeatedly.

The logical conclusion for treatment is that drug therapy must be expanded to a dual or multiple drug therapy if monotherapy fails to attain a correction of blood pressure (< 140/90 mmHg, better: 130/85 mmHg). A combination therapy should always include a diuretic, due to the sodium retention associated with renal insufficiency. If minoxidil (cave: fluid retention) is necessary for the treatment of severe hypertension, the additional administration of a beta blocker is also necessary to compensate for reflex tachycardia caused by vasodilation.

Summary (Section 31.3)

- The treatment of arterial hypertension with concomitantly existing renal insufficiency must ensue "aggressively" and aim for a reduction in blood pressure to 130/85 mmHg; it is, however, not significantly different from the generally recommended antihypertensive therapy.

- The dosage of renally eliminated substances (some beta blockers, the majority of ACE inhibitors) must be adjusted to the severity of renal dysfunction.

- Benzothiazides are only effective as antihypertensive agents for a GFR > 30 ml/min. Therefore, in cases where the kidney function continues to decrease, supplemental or additional loop diuretics must be administered.

- Due to the risk of developing hyperkalemia, potassium-sparing diuretics are contraindicated for a GFR < 30 ml/min.

- Antihypertensive therapy should be initiated with low doses (50% of the initial dose for patients with normal kidney function) to avoid first dose hypotension due to the increased likelihood of a stimulated renin angiotensin system in renal dysfunction; any previous therapy with diuretics should therefore, if possible, be interrupted.

- Initial creatinine increases after the administration of ACE inhibitors with impaired kidney function are usually temporary in nature; however, particularly tight controls of the laboratory chemical parameters are necessary in these cases.

- If antihypertensive monotherapy fails to correct blood pressure, the drug treatment should be expanded to a dual or multiple combination; this combination should contain a diuretic.

31.5 Antihypertensive therapy and metabolic diseases

For the majority of patients, arterial hypertension is not the sole cardiovascular risk factor, but only part of a total risk profile that additionally consists of metabolic disorders involving carbohydrates, lipids and/or purines, and has been described by some authors as a so-called "metabolic syndrome." − Therefore, when selecting medication, in order to be able to reduce the total cardiovascular risk, one must also take into consideration the effect the antihypertensive agent would have on the already mentioned metabolic parameters. At any rate, the "purchase" of a successful reduction in blood pressure at the cost of an unfavorable influence on a different risk factor must be avoided.

31.5.1 Antihypertensive therapy and diabetes mellitus

Diabetes mellitus (type I and type II) is quite often associated with arterial hypertension and also represents an independent cardiovascular risk factor. Since coexisting hypertension significantly accelerates the development of diabetic nephropathy and retinopathy, a correction of blood pressure in diabetics (if possible to < 130/85 mmHg) is of the utmost importance.

Patients with diabetes mellitus type II (about 90% of all diabetics), who are usually overweight, should first attempt to lose weight, since this can favorably influence both the underlying insulin resistance and the hypertension. Dietary measures should particularly concentrate on a reduction in fat intake, and the favorable adjustment of the metabolism should be supported by increasing physical activity.

Table 31.4:   Antihypertensive treatment in diabetic patients with hypertension*

	Type I and type II diabetes, younger patients	Type II diabetes, elderly patients
Therapeutic goal	"Aggressive" BP-reduction (<140/90 mmHg)	Slow BP reduction (<160/90 mmHg)
Non-drug therapy	Salt (NaCl) restriction Increase of physical activity	Weight loss Salt (NaCl) restriction Increase of physical activity Reduction of alcohol consumption
Drug therapy Monotherapy	ACE-inhibitors Beta$_1$-blockers Calcium antagonists	ACE-inhibitors Calcium antagonists Thiazide diuetics (+ potassium sparing agents) Beta$_1$-blockers
Combination therapy	All combinations permitted	All combinations permitted

* Adapted from Klaus D, Med Klin 1994; 89: 330–338 (in accordance with the Recommendations of the German Society of Hypertension and the German Society of Diabetes (Second edition, 1993)
BP = blood pressure

A restriction of sodium consumption (6 g/day) and of possible alcohol consumption (< 30 g/day) is also advisable.

Whereas a slow drop in the blood pressure of patients with hypertension and diabetes mellitus type II is acceptable — starting with general non-drug treatment measures (life-style modifications) — a rapid correction of the blood pressure in patients with diabetes mellitus type I, who are usually young and slim, is important, and almost without exception only possible through drug therapy (Table 31.4).

Since the progressive development of diabetes-induced end-organ damage can be deferred with a good therapeutic correction of the diabetic metabolic situation, preference should be given to antihypertensive agents that do not impair glucose tolerance.

31.5.1.1 Diuretics

Glucose tolerance can be impaired through the use of thiazide diuretics in higher or conventional doses as a result of hypokalemia and suppressed insulin secretion. If, for individual reasons, one decides on a treatment with thiazide for hypertensive diabetics, it should be administered in low doses. — Loop diuretics are often helpful in insulin-dependent diabetes with already manifest nephropathy in order to effectively counter the ever-present sodium retention.

Whereas diuretics have a solid value as combination partners in an antihypertensive therapy for hypertensive diabetics, their acceptance for use as a monotherapy for this target group is generally met with reservation or rejection by most professional associations because of the described effects on the carbohydrate metabolism.

31.5.1.2 Beta adrenergic receptor blockers

Beta blockers also appear to impair glucose tolerance; discussions on causes for this cover a reduction in insulin sensitivity, an inhibiting influence on the release of insulin and a stimulation of glucagon secretion.

Among diabetics who receive oral hypoglycemic agents or insulin for their condition, nonselective beta blockers, in particular, can trigger hypoglycemia, since the blockade of $beta_2$ receptors in the liver and skeletal muscles inhibits the mobilization and release of glucose. With regard to this, particular consideration should be given to the fact that beta blockers mask the typical characteristics of hypoglycemia (tachycardia, palpitations), with which most diabetics are familiar. The administration of $beta_1$-selective receptor blockers appears to reduce the risk of hypoglycemia, so that it is not necessary to categorically avoid prescribing beta blockers for diabetes mellitus.

Distinct orthostatic problems can occur if sympatholytic drugs are used to reduce blood pressure among hypertensive diabetics with severe peripheral neuropathy.

31.5.1.3 ACE inhibitors, calcium antagonists

At the current point in time, it is still not possible to definitely judge any particular value that ACE inhibitors and calcium antagonists might hold in the treatment of hypertensive diabetics, since there is still a lack of appropriate prospective long-term studies with large numbers of patients.

With regard to ACE inhibitors, several studies have shown that a correction of high blood pressure not only leads to a reduction in micro-albuminuria and to a delay in the progression of diabetic nephropathy in type I diabetics, but also to a reduction in insulin resistance in type II diabetics, which also results in an improvement in glucose utilization.

A reduction in albuminuria among hypertensive diabetics has also been documented for calcium antagonists, though not uniformly. Calcium antagonists do not negatively influence glucose tolerance.

There is however not yet any proof that ACE inhibitors or calcium antagonists specifically reduce morbidity and mortality among hypertensive diabetics through their effect in reducing the blood pressure. A comparison oriented towards these end points with other antihypertensive substance classes therefore fails to justify any overall preference in the selection of a drug therapy. If, however, one is able to observe a certain partiality for ACE inhibitors and calcium antagonists particularly for patients with diabetes mellitus type I over the past few years, this is rationalized less by (the as of yet unproved) advantages of these substance classes (in the sense of a reduction of mortality and morbidity), but rather in the disadvantages of diuretics and nonselective beta-receptor blockers (unfavorable influence in glucose tolerance).

31.5.1.4 Other substance classes effective as antihypertensive agents

With regard to diabetes mellitus, there are no specific restrictions in indication for the use of all other substances effective as antihypertensive agents.

31.5.1.5 Recommendations by professional societies (USA, Germany)

Recommendations made by the Joint National Committee on Detection, Evaluation and Treatment of High Blood Pressure (USA), made in their most recent report (JNC V, 1993), cite the necessity of lowering blood pressure in patients with diabetes mellitus to 130/85 mmHg or lower. None of the available antihypertensive substance classes (beta blockers, diuretics, calcium antagonists, ACE inhibitors, alpha$_1$-selective adrenergic blockers) are listed as contraindicated or given preference.

The 1989 guidelines drawn up by the German Hypertension Society in cooperation with the German Diabetes Society largely corresponded with the US recommendations of 1993, which at that time appraised all available first-line antihypertensive medications as being principally of equal value for the treatment of hypertensive diabetic patients. In the current, revised version, ACE inhibitors, low-doses of selective beta$_1$-adrenergic receptor blockers and calcium antagonists are recommended as preferred substance classes for the treatment of younger patients with diabetes mellitus types I and II. The administration of a diuretic is only recommended as a combination partner to follow the insufficient reduction in blood pressure during monotherapy. − The recommendations for the treatment of older hypertensive individuals with type II diabetes (> 60 years) do not, however, exclude diuretics as monotherapy, so that all first-line medications can continue to be appraised as largely of equal value in the treatment of this population group (see Table 31.4).

31.5.2 Antihypertensive therapy and dyslipidemia

Increases in the total cholesterol in serum (> 200 mg/dl) are accompanied by an increased cardiovascular risk. Whereas an atherogenic effect is attributed to cholesterol of the low-density lipoprotein fraction (LDL), impressions up to now have been that high-density lipoproteins (HDL$_3$) exhibit a cardioprotective effect. − Therefore, the lipid status of every patient should be determined before initiating a drug therapy. While choosing antihypertensive medication for hypertensive patients with an additionally existing hypercholesterolemia, preference should be given to substance classes which (i) do not increase the LDL fraction and (ii) do not cause a reduction in the potentially cardioprotective HDL fraction. Calcium antagonists and ACE inhibitors fulfill these requirements, selective alpha$_1$-receptor blockers and centrally-acting sympatholytic drugs even appear to exercise a positive influence on the lipoprotein profile (increase in HDL cholesterol).

In contrast, monotherapy with benzothiazide and loop diuretics produces an increase in the total cholesterol level as well as of LDL and VLDL; the HDL cholesterol level remains unchanged. However, more recent studies indicate that this is dose-dependent, so that a slight increase in the atherogenic lipoprotein fractions could be expected under the low doses common today. In most controlled studies with 2.5 mg indapamide, a diuretic similar to benzothiazide in mode and site of action, but different with regard to chemical structure, no unfavorable effects on the lipid metabolism were observed, despite the achievement of a reduction in blood pressure.

A worsening of the lipoprotein profile has also been observed in selective and nonselective beta blockers: although the LDL fraction remained unchanged under the administration of beta blockers, there was a drop in the level of HDL. Furthermore, an increase in triglycerides was observed. At the current level of knowledge, it can not be determined for sure whether or not this effect on the blood lipids during long-term therapy with beta blockers is actually clinically relevant. − Additionally, there was no effect on the plasma lipids observed in a therapy with beta receptor blockers with ISA (intrinsic sympathomimetic activity; Table 24.2).

The popular demand for so-called metabolically neutral antihypertensive drugs should therefore not inevitably lead to the exclusive use of newer first line medications, since one has yet to produce solid evidence of a clinical relevance of changes in plasma lipids (effect on mortality and morbidity in comparison to meta-bolically neutral antihypertensive agents) in the course of long-term therapy with beta blockers or diuretics. The results of the STOP-2 study might possibly provide more clarity in this matter.

However, any further worsening of the lipid metabolism should be avoided in hypertension with severe lipidemia, so that even today the concept of metabolical neutrality should be taken into account in the selection of an antihypertensive agent.

31.5.3 Hyperuricemia

Although a preexisting hyperuricemia can be aggravated by antihypertensive ther-apy with benzothiazide diuretics or related sulfonamides and with loop diuretics, these substances are not contraindicated for slight elevations of the serum uric acid. – Hypertensive patients with renal insufficiency under treatment with diuret-ics, however, should have regular inspections of the serum uric acid level. It is only advisable to check the uric acid level of hypertensive patients with healthy kidneys if there are symptoms typical of gout.

Summary (Section 31.5)

- Antihypertensive therapy with diabetes mellitus is not fundamentally dif-ferent from other general guidelines; however, diuretics should be used with particular caution, since they can negatively effect glucose tolerance. Treat-ment with nonselective beta blockers should be completely avoided.

- A correction of the arterial blood pressure to < 135/85 mmHg is important (particularly in younger) hypertensive diabetics, since this can delay the manifestation of diabetic end-organ damage to the kidneys, eyes and vascu-lar system.

- The most important causal therapy for patients with diabetes mellitus type-II is weight loss, since there is a positive correlation between the level of body weight and hypertension on the one hand and insulin resistance on the other hand.

- Antihypertensive therapy, usually drug therapy, should be immediately initi-ated for patients with diabetes mellitus type I who are diagnosed with hyper-tension. Monotherapy with diuretics is not advisable, since it negatively in-fluences glucose tolerance.

- Preference should be given to metabolically neutral medication or antihyper-tensive agents that favorably influence the distribution of lipoproteins (calcium antagonists, ACE inhibitors, selective alpha$_1$-receptor blockers) for the treatment of hypertensive patients with clinically relevant hyperlipidemia.

31.6 Antihypertensive therapy and osteoporosis

Normal bone metabolism is marked by a balance between bone loss and bone formation. The development of osteoporosis is the result of a long-term disorder in this metabolism that can rest categorically on two different pathomechanisms:

1. An increased activity of all cells involved in bone turnover:
The loss of bone mass that follows the loss of ovarian function is associated with an increase in the rates of bone resorption and bone formation, with the former exceeding the latter (high-turnover bone loss). High-turnover bone loss, being typical for the early phase of the postmenopause, primarily affects the spongiosa, to a lesser degree the cortical substance. Due to the rapid bone loss, it is often already clinically manifest between the ages of 50 and 60.

2. A progressive decline in the supply of osteoblasts in proportion to the demand for them contrasts with the activity of the osteoclasts:
A progressive decline in the supply of osteoblasts is accompanied by slow bone loss (low turnover bone loss) in the spongiosa and cortical substance and is characteristic of age-induced osteoporosis, which effects men and women equally. Clinical manifestation of this form of osteoporosis usually occurs after the age of 70.

In the USA, 1.5 million people suffer bone fractures annually as a result of osteoporotic changes in the skeleton. In the course of their lives, women and men loose up to 50% or respectively 30% of their spongiosa and 30% or respectively 20% of their cortical bone mass. Since the loss of bone mass among women occurs particularly quickly in the early phase of postmenopause and leads to clinical manifestation already before the age of 60, the promotion of preventive measures for this patient population is particularly urgent. Estrogen in low doses, calcitonin and biphosphonates are examples for long-term drug interventions that can prevent bone loss. Whereas it is at least known of estrogen replacement therapy that low doses tend to reduce systolic blood pressure and favorably influence lipid metabolism, little is known about the effect of antihypertensive agents on bone metabolism. Since the prevention of osteoporosis has been defined as an urgent goal, it would be desirable to use antihypertensive agents to treat female patients in the early phase of postmenopause, often suffering rapid bone loss, that possess an osteoprotective or at least "osteoneutral" effect. Furthermore it must be ensured that simultaneous therapies do not weaken the osteoprotective effect of estrogen or other substances. – Unfortunately, there have hardly been any controlled studies conducted to examine the effects that antihypertensive agents have on this important concomitant disorder. No professional societies, national or international, have yet taken on this problem.

Thiazide diuretics:

Clinical studies examining the influence of substances effective as antihypertensive agents on the development or results of osteoporosis have, as of yet, only been completed for thiazide diuretics. In a prospective study (La Croix, 1990), it was shown that there was a lower incidence of hip fractures among older patients (> 65 years) of both sexes that received thiazide diuretics, for various reasons, than among patients who received no thiazides. Smaller studies investigating the effect of a two-year thiazide therapy on bone density in postmenopausal women also tend to show a favorable influence by thiazide diuretics. The beneficial effect of chlorthalidone on bone mass in postmenopausal women with isolated systolic hypertension was already mentioned elsewhere (see also Figure 23.1).

Calcium antagonists:

In a very small study with primary hypertensive patients, the bone density remained unchanged after a 12-month therapy with a calcium antagonist, whereas the density increased slightly under the administration of a thiazide diuretic. Some reservations do exist about the long-term administration of a calcium antagonist for manifest osteoporosis, however, due to an observed increase in the parathyroid hormone (PTH) level in this study.

ACE inhibitors:

The effect of ACE inhibitors on the bone turnover has, as of yet, only been examined in one study using an animal model of human postmenopausal osteoporosis (ovariectomized rat). In this study the osteoprotective effect of estrogen therapy was not weakened by the simultaneous administration of an ACE inhibitor; no unfavorable effect on the bone turnover was observed when the ACE inhibitor was given alone (without concomitant estrogen replacement).

In conclusion, the only data available concerning the treatment of hypertension in patients with a coexisting manifest osteoporosis pertains to thiazide diuretics, which would justify a certain therapeutic preference for this substance class, particularly for the treatment of older patients. Experimental data that indicates a neutral or antiresorptive effect on bone production for ACE inhibitors will have to be confirmed by clinical studies in human beings.

Summary (Section 31.6)

- Ideally, the treatment of postmenopausal women with a higher risk of osteoporosis and of patients with already manifest osteoporosis and coexisting hypertension should ensue with antihypertensive agents that are themselves osteoprotective or osteoneutral.

- Antihypertensive therapy and the drug treatment of osteoporosis must be compatible and, ideally, complement one another.

- A weakening of antihypertensive effects by a concomitant osteoporosis therapy is as undesirable as a negative influence on the osteoprotective effect by the concomitantly administered antihypertensive agent.

- There can be no recommendation for any of the antihypertensive substance classes recognized as first line medications based on the criteria listed above; however, a certain preference for thiazide diuretics in the treatment of hypertension and coexisting, manifest osteoporosis does appear to be justified.

- The clinical relevance of the neutral or antiresorptive effects of an ACE inhibitor on bone production as shown in experimental studies can not currently be assessed.

31.7 Conclusive observations on the selecting criteria for drug treatment of arterial hypertension with complicating conditions

The preferred use and undesirable side effects of current antihypertensive agents are summarized in Table 31.5.

Table 31.5: Antihypertensive drug treatment in the presence of coexisting diseases

Substance (class)	Preferred application in cases of	Cautions or contraindications
DIURETICS (Chapter 23)		
Thiazide diuretics*, Loop diuretics	– CHF – Renal insufficiency* – Osteoporosis	– PAOD – Severe lipid metabolism disorders – Symptomatic hyperuricemia/gout – Diabetes mellitus
Potassium sparing diuretics	– CHF	– Renal insufficiency
Aldosterone-antagonists	– Primary and secondary aldosteronism	– Renal insufficiency
SYMPATHOLYTICS (Chapter 24)		
Imidazoline-receptor agonists	– Tachycardia – LVH	– Bradycardia, in particular in elderly patients – Sick sinus syndrome
Alpha-methyldopa	– Pregnancy – LVH	
Beta-adrenergic receptor blockers	– CAD – LVH	– COLD/asthma – Decompensated cardiac insufficiency – AV-blocks II°b/III° – PAOD – Diabetes mellitus
Selective alpha$_1$-receptor blockers	– CHF – Severe lipid metabolism disorders	– Orthostatic dysregulation

Table 31.5: (continued)

Substance (class)	Preferred application in cases of	Cautions or contraindications
VASODILATORS (Chapter 25)		− Decompensated cardiac insufficiency − Severe CAD − Idiopathic edema − Ventricular tachyarrthythmia
CALCIUM ANTAGONISTS (Chapter 26)		
Dihydropyridines ("nifedipine-type")	− CAD** − COLD/asthma − Generalized atherosclerosis*** − Severe lipid metabolism disorders − PAOD	− PAOD (> stage IIb, Fontaine's classification) − Decompensated cardiac insufficiency
Phenylalkylamines ("verapamil-type")	− CAD − Supraventricular tachycardia − Generalized atherosclerosis** − Severe lipid metabolism disorders	− AV blocks (IIb°/III°)
Benzothiazepines ("diltiazem-type")	As with verapamil	As with verapamil
INHIBITORS OF THE RENIN ANGIOTENSIN SYSTEM (Chapter 27)		
ACE inhibitors	− CHF − LVH	− Bilateral renal artery steno-ses and unilateral artery stenosis with a solitary functioning kidney
Ang II-receptor antagonists	As with ACE inhibitors?	As with ACE inhibitors

*   Thiazide diuretics: loss of antihypertensive efficacy when GFR is ≤30 ml/min.

**   Recommendation valid only for long-acting calcium antagonists or sustained release formulations.

*** Antiatherogenic effects of calcium antagonists have to date only been convincingly demonstrated in animal experiments (rabbit etc.).

Abbreviations:
AV = atrioventricular; CAD = coronary artery disease; CHF = congestive heart failiure; COLD = chronic obstructive lung disease; LVH = left ventricular hypertrophy; PAOD = peripheral arterial occlusive disease

Literature (Chapter 31)

Bianci S, Bigazzi R, Baldari G, Campese VM. Microalbuminuria in patients with essential hypertension: effects of several antihypertensive drugs. Am J Med 1992; 93: 525−528.

Dahlöf B, Pennert K, Hansson L. Rversal of left ventricular hypertrophy in hypertensive patients. A metaanalysis of 109 treatment studies. Am J Hypertens 1992; 5: 95−110.

Deutsche Liga zur Bekämpfung des hohen Blutdruckes e.V. Deutsche Hypertonie Gesellschaft. Empfehlungen für die Behandlung des Hochdrucks bei Diabetes, 2. Aufl., 1993.

Garner L. Natrium nitroprusside treatment in patients with acute strokes. Arch Intern Med 1986; 146: 1454.

Giles TD, Sander GE, Roffidal LE, Quiroz AC, Mazzu AL. Comparative effects of nitrendipine and hydrochlorothiazide on calciotropic hormoncs and bone density in hypertensive patients. Am J Hypertens 1992; 5: 875−879.

Harlos J, Götz R, Heidland A. Antihypertensiva und Proteinurie. Nieren Hochdruckkrkht 1993; 22: 573−582.

Hatton R, Stimpel M, Chambers TJ. Angiotensin II is generated from angiotensin I by bone cells and stimulates osteoclastic bone resorption in vitro. Endocrinology 1996, in press.

Klaus D. Gehirnerkrankungen bei Hochdruck. Med Klin 1993; 88: 701−709.

Klaus D. Hochdruck bei Diabetes mellitus. Ursachen, Verlauf und Behandlung. Med Klin 1994; 89: 330−338.

Kloner RA. Nifedipine in ischemic heart disease. Circulation 1995; 92: 1074−1078.

Lacroix AZ, Wienpahl J, White LR, Wallace RB, Scherr PA, George LK, Cornoni-Huntley J, Ostfeld AM. Thiazide diuretic agents and the incidence of hip fracture. N Engl J Med 1990; 322: 286−290.

Lewis EJ, Hunsicker LC, Bain RP, Rohde RD. The effect of angiotensin-converting-enzyme inhibition on diabetic nephropathy. N Engl J Med 1993; 329: 1456−1462.

Liebson PR, Grandits GA, Dianzumba S, Prineas RJ, Grimm RH, Neaton JD, Stamler J for the Treatment of Hypertension Study Research Group. Comparision of five antihypertensive monotherapies and placebo for change in left ventricular mass in patients receiving nutritional-hygienic therapy in the Treatment of Mild Hypertension Study (TOMHS). Circulation 1995; 91: 698−706.

Lindsay R, Marshall B, Haboubi A, Herrington BS, Tohme J. Increased axial bone mass in women with hypertension: role of thiazide therapy. J Bone Miner Res 1987; 2 (suppl 1): S29.

Madhavan S, Stockwell D, Cohen H, Alderman MH. Renal function during antihypertensive treatment. Lancet 1995; 345: 749−751.

Manolagas SC, Jilka RL. Mechanism of disease: Bone marrow, cytokines, and bone remodeling. Emerging insights into the pathophysiology of osteoporosis. N Engl J Med 1995; 332: 305−311.

Marmot MG, Poulter NR. Primary prevention of stroke. Lancet 1992; 339: 344−347.

Mori S, Sadoshima S,Fujii K, Ibayashi S, Iino K, Fujishima M. Decrease in cerebral blood flow with blood pressure reductions in patients with chronic stroke. Stroke 1993; 24: 1376−1381.

Opie LH, Messerli FH. Nifedipine and mortality. Grave defects in the dossier. Circulation 1995; 92: 1068−1073.

Pettinger WA, Lee HC, Reisch J, Mitchell HC. Long-term improvement in renal function after short-term strict blood pressure control in hypertensive nephrosclerosis. Hypertension 1989; 13: 766−772.

Parving HH, Andersen AR, Smidt UM, Svendsen PA. Early aggressive antihypertensive treatment reduces rate of decline in kidney function in diabetic nephropathy. Lancet 1983; 1: 1175−1179.

Psaty BM, Heckbert SR, Koepsell TD, Siscovick DS, Raghunathan TE, Weiss NS, Rosendaal FR, Lemaitre RN, Smith NL, Wahl PW, Wagner EH, Furberg CD. The risk of myocardial infarction associated with antihypertensive drug therapies. JAMA 1995; 274: 620−625.

Smith U (ed). Hypertension and glucose tolerance − effects of antihypertensive therapy. J Intern Med 1991; 229 (suppl 2): 1−128.

Poulsen OB, Jarden JO, Vorstrup S, Godtfredsen J. Effect of captopril on the cerebral circulation in chronic heart failure. Eur J Clin Invest 1986; 16: 124−132.

Phillips SJ. Hypertension and the brain. Arch Intern Med 1992; 152: 938−945.

Stein PP, Black HR. Drug treatment of hypertension in patients with diabetes mellitus. Diabetes Care 1992; 15: 1875−1891.

Stimpel M, Jee WSS, Ma Y, Yamamoto N, Chen Y. Impact of antihypertensive therapy on postmenopausal osteoporosis: effects of the angiotensin converting enzyme inhibitor moexipril, 17β-estradiol and their combination on the ovariectomy-induced cancellous bone loss in young rats. J Hypertens 1995; 13: 1852−1856.

Strauer BE. Diagnostische und therapeutische Probleme bei hypertensiver Herzkrankheit. Z Kardiol 1993; 82 (Suppl. 4): 17−24.

Talbert RL. Drug dosing in renal insufficiency. J Clin Pharmacol 1994; 34: 99−110.

Teo KK. Risk and management of hypertension-related left ventricular hypertrophy. Drugs 1995; 50: 959−970.

Thadani U, Whitsett TL (Editorial). Beta-adrenergic blockers and intermittent claudication. Time for reappraisal. Arch Intern Med 1991; 151: 1705−1707.

Weidmann P, De Courten M, Ferrari P. Effect of diuretics on the plasma lipid profile. Europ Heart J 1992; 13 (Suppl. G): 61−67.

Working Group on Managment of Patients with Hypertension and High Blood Cholesterol. National Education Programs Working Group Report on the management of patients with hypertension and high blood cholesterol. Ann Intern Med 1991; 114: 224−237.

Yusuf S. Calcium anatgonists in coronary artery disease and hypertension. Time for reevaluation ? Circulation 1995; 92: 1079−1082.

Zanchetti A. Hyperlipidemia in the hypertensive patient. Am J Med 1994; 96 (suppl 6A): 3S−8S.

Zanchi A, Brunner HR. Is antihypertensive therapy expected to be different in postmenopausal women ? In: Safar M, Stimpel M, Zanchetti A (eds): Hypertension in Postmenopausal Women. Springer Verlag, Berlin-Heidelberg-New York 1994, 65−71.

32 Antihypertensive therapy in special situations

32.1 Therapy for hypertensive crises

Tremendous increases in blood pressure require a reduction. This reduction may, depending on the cause, be conducted either by the immediate and controlled administration of parenteral antihypertensives, (hypertensive "emergency"), or a gradual reduction over a period of 24−48 hours with oral substances (hypertensive "urgency").

Blood pressure exacerbations that are accompanied by symptoms of hypertensive encephalopathy (severe headaches, vomiting, impaired vision, confusion, loss of consciousness), or cardiac decompensation (pulmonary edema, angina, ventricular tachy- or bradyarrythmia) and/or acute renal failure (oliguria) represent hypertensive emergencies.

Absolute blood pressure values (> 120 mmHg diastolic) can be used as guidelines, but do not serve as criteria. During pregnancy, for example, diastolic blood pressure values greater than 100−110 mmHg can be associated with clinical signs of eclampsia (Section 33.3.3), while diastolic values of 120−130 mmHg and more are tolerated without any symptoms by some patients with a long-standing hypertension.

The first and foremost rule for the treatment of blood pressure exacerbations, with or without signs of end-organ damage, is a cautious and controlled reduction in blood pressure. Especially (though not exclusively) in elderly patients, too aggressive a therapy can cause the perfusion pressure to fall below the minimum required for the normal function of the end organs. The resulting inadequate perfusion can result in further damage to the brain, the myocardium, and/or the kidneys and thus be as harmful to the patient as the increased blood pressure. A reasonable target is to lower the mean arterial blood pressure by approximately 25 % (or to reduce the diastolic blood pressure to 105−110 mmHg) in the course of the first two hours of "emergency" treatment, or within the first 24 hours of "urgent" treatment. Due to the heterogeneity of the illnesses associated with hypertension, a differentiated therapy is often not possible. The following demands are therefore made of antihypertensive medications used in the treatment of hypertensive crises:

- Efficacy in primary and secondary hypertension,
- rapid onset of action,
- careful and calculable reduction in blood pressure,
- increase of blood flow in the endangered organs (brain, heart and kidneys) through the most selective vascular dilatation possible, and
- the lowest possible risk of drug-induced hypotension.

32.1.1 Treatment of hypertensive crises with no sign of end-organ damage

In treating a hypertensive crisis where end-organ damage is neither manifest nor imminent, seclusion and elimination of external irritants (noise, light, excitement) are therapeutic measures that should be attempted before administering antihypertensive medication. If no reduction in blood pressure is observed within $20-30$ minutes, orally administered antihypertensives with a quick onset of action are recommended (Table 32.1).

Nifedipine, a dihydropyridine calcium antagonist, has proven the treatment of choice. Nifedipine is administered orally in $5-10$ mg doses. The capsule must be chewed and its contents swallowed. It takes effect in $5-10$ minutes and reaches

Table 32.1: Drugs for the treatment of hypertensive urgencies and emergencies

Drugs	Route of administration	Dosage (mg)	Onset (min)	Comments, precautions
Urgency:				
Nifedipine	Sublingual Buccal Oral	$5-20$	$5-10$ $5-10$ $15-20$	Headache, tachycardia, hypotension, flushing, dizziness, angina pectoris
Nitrendipine phiola	Sublingual	$5-10$	$5-10$	See nifedipine
Clonidine	Oral	$0.075-0.3$	$30-60$	Sedation, dry mouth; not in patients with AV block II°/III°, bradycardia, sick sinus syndrome
Nitroglycerin spray, capsula	Sublingual	$0.8-2.4$	$5-10$	Headache, nausea, vomiting
Captopril	Oral	$6.25-50$	$30-60$	Severe hypotension in high renin states
Emergency:				
Sodium nitroprusside	IV infusion	$0.5-10$ µg/kg/min	Immediate	Nausea, vomiting, hypotension; risk of cyanide thiocyanate intoxication (levels must be monitored)
Labetalol	IV bolus every $5-10$ min IV infusion	$20-80$ $0.5-2$ mg/min	$5-10$ $5-10$	Hypotension, nausea, scalp tingling, bronchospasm

Table 32.1:   (continued)

Drugs	Route of administration	Dosage (mg)	Onset (min)	Comments, precautions
Nitroglycerin	IV infusion	5−100 µg/min	1−2	Headache, nausea; tolerance development
Clonidine	IV	0.075 to 0.30	10	See above
Urapidil	IV bolus	25−50	2−5	Headache, dry mouth, nausea, hypotension
Nicardipine	IV infusion	5 mg/h	5−15	Hypotension, headache, flushing, angina pectoris
Prefered use in the treatment of eclampsia:				
Dihydralazine	IV bolus	6.25 to 25	10−20	Hypotension, nausea, headache, fetal distress, tachycardia, angina pectoris
Hydralazine	IV bolus	5−10	10−20	See dihydralazine
For treatment of catecholamine excess:				
Phentolamine	IV bolus	2.5−10 mg	Immediate	Hypotension, tachycardia, headache, paradoxical pressure response

maximum effectiveness in 30−40 minutes. If no reduction in blood pressure is observed within 10 minutes of intake, a second, equivalent dose can be administered. The greatest danger in administering nifedipine in a hypertensive crisis is that the blood pressure may drop too rapidly. This can precipitate ischemia in the already poorly perfused tissue areas supplied by severely stenotic arteries (myocardial ischemia in the case of coronary artery disease, cerebrovascular accident /TIA in the case of carotid stenosis(es), renal failure or worsening of renal function in the case of renal artery stenosis).

Orally administered nitrendipine (5 mg) is just as well suited for the treatment of hypertensive crisis, but has not been approved in all countries. Nitroglycerin (as a sublingual capsule or as a spray) can have advantages for patients with known or suspected coronary artery disease, since it causes an immediate dilatation of the coronary vessels. Onset of action occurs within about 5−10 minutes. Repeated doses are possible if the reduction in blood pressure is inadequate. − Captopril (6.25−50 mg) works just as quickly. It may, however, result in excessive reduction of the blood pressure in patients with hypovolemia or undetected renal artery stenoses.

A further recommended option in the treatment of hypertensive crisis is the oral administration of the combined beta-/alpha-blocker labetalol.

If none of the orally administered antihypertensives named produces a satisfactory reduction in blood pressure, an attempt with an intravenously administered substance is justified. Clonidine (0,075−0,15 mg; onset of action in ca. 10 min.), urapidil (initially 12.5 mg; onset of action in 5−10 min.), and enalaprilat (1.25 mg) are examples of such substances.

If the patient experiences no volume depletion, the additional administration of a diuretic (e.g. furosemide 20−40 mg i.v.; see Section 31.1.2) is recommended.

It should be kept in mind that excessive decreases in pressure endanger the patient. Cerebral, myocardial and renal ischemia with subsequent end-organ damage can be caused by a sudden, drug-induced hypotension, particularly in elderly patients or those with long-standing, poorly controlled hypertension (see also Section 31.1). Even after blood pressure has been successfully reduced by use of one of the drugs mentioned, the patient's condition should be monitored for another 4−6 hours in order to counteract a possible over-reduction or a renewed increase in the blood pressure.

Generally it is not necessary to immediately hospitalize the patient if the blood pressure can be reduced with one of the drugs mentioned, and if no symptoms or signs of imminent or manifest end-organ damage are observed. If the successfully employed antihypertensive comes in a form that permits long-term therapy, or there is another such drug from its substance class, the patient can be released from the hospital and treated with this drug. If a specific therapy is in progress prior to a hypertensive crisis, it should be expanded to include a further antihypertensive with a different mode of action (Chapter 21 and/or 30).

The patient's blood pressure should be checked again within the following 24−48 hours.

It is recommended that a differential-diagnostic clarification be performed sometime thereafter. This should be performed preferably under in-patient conditions (Chapters 13−18).

32.1.2 Therapy for hypertensive emergencies

The immediate introduction of antihypertensive therapy in cases of excessive increases of blood pressure is necessary where clinical signs of imminent or already manifest end-organ damage have been observed:

− severe headaches, nausea/vomiting, impaired vision, confusion, impairment to or loss of consciousness, neurological signs (hypertensive encephalopathy),
− pulmonary edema, angina, cardiac arrhythmia (left ventricular decompensation, acute myocardial ischemia)
− oliguria/anuria (acute renal failure)

As mentioned in Section 32.1, it is desirable to maintain intensive care monitoring in such cases. This makes it possible, on the one hand, to control the decrease in blood pressure within one to two hours without sudden hypotension, and on the other hand, to support the functions of the endangered or damaged end organs or to treat the end organs. Mean arterial blood pressure should not be reduced below 20−25% of the initial value or diastolic blood pressure below 105−110 mmHg. Treatment is normally performed intravenously (by means of an adjustable infusion pump) (Table 32.1). Continuous monitoring of intraarterially measured blood pressure is obligatory. The necessity of a particularly careful approach to apoplectic insult and excessive increases in blood pressure was covered thoroughly in Section 31.2.

Sodium nitroprusside is easily controllable and is therefore the substance still most widely used in the acute treatment of a hypertensive emergency. Its antihypertensive action occurs within minutes and continues for only 2−3 minutes after the discontinuation of the infusion. The dosage, which normally starts at 0.2−0.5 µg/kg/min, can be slowly increased every 5−7 minutes. When the target blood pressure is achieved (see above), the therapeutic dosage should be maintained for at least another 24 hours, and corrected where necessary. Where cerebral symptoms persist despite the successful reduction in blood pressure, it should be kept in mind that sodium nitroprusside can increase intracranial pressure through dilatation of the cerebral vasculature. On the other hand, sodium nitroprusside is metabolized to thiocyanate, so that doses of more than 2 µg/kg/min, particularly in cases of deteriorating renal function, accumulate, and may cause cerebral symptoms (fatigue, vomiting, confusion, hallucination, toxic psychoses, etc.) resembling those of hypertensive encephalopathy. A significant deterioration in clinical condition with the development of a metabolic acidosis and cardiac arrhythmia are differential-diagnostic indicators of a possible thiocyanate toxicity. The infusion should then be interrupted. Sodium thiosulfate generally leads to rapid improvement. If sodium nitroprusside must be administered for more than 24 hours, daily measurement of the plasma level is desirable. In cases of high dose administration or kidney dysfunction, daily measurement of the plasma level is obligatory. Since nitroprusside results in both arterial and venous dilatation, not only cardiac afterload but preload as well are reduced. Where coronary artery disease already exists, a reduction in stroke volume and cardiac output can, despite a simultaneous increase in heart rate, result in a worsening of the disease and cause acute ischemia.

Since nitroglycerin improves coronary circulation, it is increasingly used for emergency blood pressure reduction in patients with known coronary artery disease. To achieve the desired blood pressure reduction, the dose should be increased at five-minute intervals through the use of an adjustable infusion pump. The development of tolerance after 24−48 hours of therapy should be considered in treatment.

Labetalol, a combined beta-/alpha-blocker (Section 24.3) is finding increasing acceptance as a treatment for hypertensive exacerbations in cases of apoplectic insult (Section 31.2). Since in its oral form it is also suitable as a long-term treatment, labetalol has the advantage that there is no substance change in switching from parenteral to oral treatment. There is therefore no danger of a renewed deterioration in the blood pressure. Due to its beta-receptor blocking properties, labetalol is nevertheless contraindicated in known cases of bronchial asthma and in pheochromocytoma (without previous selective alpha-blockade). Caution is also recommended in borderline cases of compensated or decompensated heart failure and high grade atrioventricular (AV) blocks.

Nicardipine, a dihydropyridine calcium antagonist, is another option for the intravenous treatment of a hypertensive emergency. Nicardipine is initially administered in a dose of $5-15$ mg/hour, and can be increased by $1-2.5$ mg/hour at 15 minute intervals.

Because it improves circulation in the uterus, (di-)hydralazine is indicated for eclampsia (1 mg/min). To avoid reflex tachycardia, (di-)hydralazine is best administered in combination with a low dose, beta$_1$-selective blocker (atenolol, metoprolol, acebutalol). Fluid retention makes the additional administration of a diuretic necessary. Increased intracranial pressure is a further disadvantage to dihydralazine.

Since hypertensive emergencies often go hand-in-hand with sodium and water retention, which can be further exacerbated by vasodilatory substances, treatment should be combined with an accompanying diuretic ($20-125$ mg furosemide). The additional introduction of a diuretic is naturally not indicated for patients who,

Table 32.2:   Treatment recommendations for specific hypertensive emergencies

Hypertensive emergency	Recommended treatment	Drugs to avoid
Hypertensive encephalopathy	Labetalol, sodium nitroprusside, nimodipine, nicardipine;	Clonidine, beta-blockers, alpha methyldopa, reserpine;
Stroke	No treatment, labetalol, sodium nitroprusside;	Alpha methyldopa, reserpine, clonidine, (di)hydralazine;
Intracerebral hemorrhage	No treatment, labetalol, sodium nitroprusside;	Alpha methyldopa, reserpine, clonidine, (di)hydralazine;
Myocardial ischemia or infarction	Nitroglycerin, sodium nitroprusside, labetalol;	(Di)hydralazine, "nifedipine-typ"-calciumantagonists, minoxidil;
Left ventricular failure/ acute pulmonary edema	Sodium nitroprusside and loop diuretics, nitroglycerin and loop diuretics, enalaprilate;	(Di)hydralazine, labetalol and other beta-blockers;
Aortic dissection	Sodium nitroprusside or trimethaphan and beta-blockers;	(Di)hydralazine, minoxidil;
Eclampsia	(Di)hydralazine, diazoxide, labetalol, calcium antagonists;	Trimethaphan, diuretics, sodium nitroprusside;
Catecholamine excess/ pheochromocytoma	Phentolamine, calcium antagonists, sodium nitroprusside;	Beta-blockers as initial therapy;
Malignant hypertension	Sodium nitroprusside, labetalol, urapidil, calcium antagonists;	

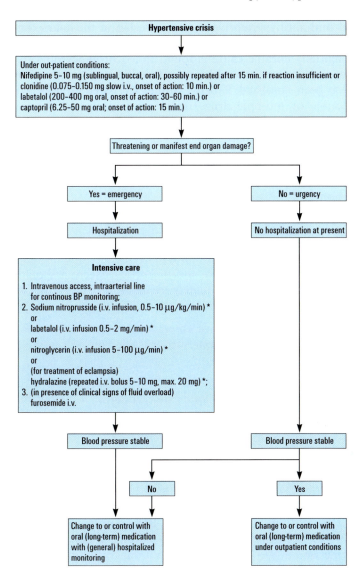

Figure 32.1: Management of hypertensive crisis

due to pressure induced diuresis or massive vomiting, have lost considerable fluid and are therefore volume depleted.

Often it is impossible to determine the cause of a hypertensive emergency during the acute situation. Should it nonetheless be known, based on previous history or unequivocal clinical symptoms, then a medicinally differentiated therapeutic approach is recommended (Table 32.2).

Intravenous and oral antihypertensive therapy overlap in the course of switching from one to the other. Blood pressure is continuously monitored throughout the process. If a potentially curable cause is found (pheochromocytoma, renal artery stenosis, etc.), causal therapy should be introduced as soon as possible after the blood pressure has been stabilized. Patients with exacerbated primary hypertension often require double or multiple drug treatments in order to normalize blood pressure. These should be phased in slowly over a period of several weeks and should vary according to the cause.

(See also flow chart Figure 32.1).

Summary (Section 32.1)

- A hypertensive crisis may or may not involve clinical signs of imminent and/ or previously manifest end-organ damage.

- A hypertensive crisis with concomitant of encephalopathy, decompensating left heart failure, acute renal failure and/or aortic dissection should be categorized as an emergency; and adequately treated under intensive-care conditions.

- The drug treatment of hypertensive emergencies is normally accomplished intravenously by means of sodium nitroprusside, nitroglycerin, labetalol, among others.

- A reduction in diastolic blood pressure below a value of 105−110 mmHg, or in mean arterial pressure to a value more than 25% below that of the initial pressure within the first two hours must be avoided. Blood pressure measurement should preferably be carried out intraarterially and closely monitored.

- After a hypertensive emergency, a slow normalization of blood pressure, taking into account the underlying illnesses, is desirable (2−6 weeks).

- A hypertensive crisis without clinical symptoms of imminent or manifest end-organ damage (hypertensive urgency) demands immediate therapeutic intervention, but need not be classified as an emergency. It may therefore be treated first on an outpatient basis by administrating oral (nifedipine or sublingual nitroglycerin, clonidine, captopril, labetalol) or intravenous (urapidil, labetalol, clonidine) antihypertensive medication.

- The medicinal reduction of blood pressure should take place gradually over a period of 24−48 hours (target blood pressure as in hypertensive emergency).

- An aggressive reduction in blood pressure should be absolutely avoided, since iatrogenic hypotension can lead to an acute underperfusion of the end organs, and thereby endanger the patient at least as much as a hypertensive episode.

32.2 Antihypertensive therapy for malignant hypertension

According to the WHO guidelines, malignant hypertension is defined as severe hypertension with bilateral retinal exudates and hemorrhaging (WHO, 1978). Although in most cases diastolic blood pressure exceeds $120-130$ mmHg, the absolute height of the blood pressure is not a decisive factor.

As a consequence of chronic high blood pressure, cerebral autoregulation moves to a new and higher tolerance level. On the one hand it acts as a defense against high systemic pressure, but on the other hand there is a significant impairment of the ability to compensate for sudden decreases in blood pressure. Since abrupt decreases in blood pressure in cases of malignant hypertension can lead to disastrous consequences, the utmost caution is dictated in the introduction or augmentation of antihypertensive therapy. A gradual reduction in diastolic blood pressure to 110 mmHg in the course of the first 48 hours is adequate and should not be exceeded, so that orally administered intermediate or long-acting antihypertensives can be introduced. Frequent controls are essential. The patient should be seen daily or every other day, to the extent possible in the initial weeks of treatment, unless it has already been decided to clarify the cause under hospitalized conditions.

Summary (Section 32.2)

- In cases of malignant hypertension, blood pressure must be reduced slowly and gradually.

- Sudden hypotension is poorly compensated for in cases of malignant hypertension, and can lead to severe cerebral ischemia.

- Antihypertensive therapy can be accomplished with intermediate or long-acting, orally administered first-line medications.

- Where the cause of the malignant hypertension is unclear, hospitalization should be considered.

32.3 Therapy resistant hypertension

It has been observed that, despite combinations of three antihypertensive drugs, blood pressure reduction is either insufficient or wholly lacking in $2-5\%$ of all cases treated medicinally. The designation "therapy resistant hypertension" is only applicable, however, if certain conditions are excluded:

- The patient takes medication partially, erroneously, or not at all.
- The approved dosage of one or all prescribed medications has been exhausted.
- Medications interact negatively (Table 29.2).

- The patient is taking drugs or other substances which (potentially) increase blood pressure (Chapter 17).
- A secondary hypertension exists.
- Chronic alcohol consumption exists.

Moreover obesity significantly reduces the efficacy of antihypertensive therapy, so that a medication augmentation or increase in dosage will not only have the desired result, but may even lead to an increase in side-effects. For such patients, therefore, strict weight-loss is the primary, and possibly the only promising therapeutic measure. The unsatisfactory response to an antihypertensive medication, as a consequence of one or more of the factors mentioned above, is therefore designated "pseudo-resistance."

The Report of the Joint National Committee on Detection, Evaluation and Treatment of High Blood Pressure (JNC V, 1993) designates hypertension as resistant "if the blood pressure in a patient who is adherent to treatment can not be reduced to less than 160/100 mmHg by an adequate and appropriate triple-drug regimen prescribed in nearly maximal doses when the pretreatment blood pressure was greater than 180/115 mmHg. If the pretreatment blood pressure was less than < 180/115 mmHg before treatment, resistance should be defined as failure to achieve normotension (< 140/90 mmHg)".

For older patients with isolated systolic hypertension the JNC V defines therapy resistance in a patient who is adherent to treatment "as failure of an adequate triple-drug regimen to reduce systolic blood pressure to less than 170 mmHg if the pretreatment value was greater than 200 mmHg or to less than 160 mmHg and by at least 10 mmHg if pretreatment systolic blood pressure was 160 to 200 mmHg."

A number of potent antihypertensive drug-combinations exist for the treatment of therapy resistant hypertension (Table 32.3). Only those drugs whose various

Table 32.3: Antihypertensive drug combinations for the treatment of therapy resistant hypertension*

Basic combination			Recommended add-on medication
1.		Diuretic	
	plus	beta-receptor blocker	
	plus	calcium antagonist	ACE inhibitor**
2.		Diuretic	
	plus	beta-receptor blocker	
	plus	ACE inhibitor	Calcium antagonist
3.		Diuretic	
	plus	beta-receptor blocker	
	plus	(di-)hydralazine	Alpha$_1$-receptor blocker
4.		Diuretic	
	plus	beta-receptor blocker	Minoxidil

  * For definition see text
 ** Reduced dosage in patients with renal insufficiency (creatinine clearance <30 ml/min)

pharmacological mechanisms of action complement one another should be combined (see also Chapter 30). The currently most effective antihypertensive drug in the treatment of resistant hypertension is minoxidil (Section 25.2.2). Since minoxidil on the one hand causes reflex tachycardia, and on the other hand induces fluid retention, it is necessary to combine it with a beta blocker and with a diuretic.

If a renewed increase in previously, controlled blood pressure is observed despite adherence to treatment, the target organ may have developed a resistance to one or more of the antihypertensives being used. Switching from the base medication to an adequate alternative substance frequently leads to a renewed normalization of blood pressure (see also Table 19.3).

Summary (Section 32.3)

- True resistance to an antihypertensive combination therapy is extremely rare.

- The diagnosis of therapy resistance always demands the exclusion of the variety of causes of "pseudoresistance" (secondary hypertension, non-adherence to treatment, inadequate application of medication, false or inadequate medication, obesity, alcohol consumption etc.).

- Effective antihypertensive multiple drug combinations that as a rule lead to blood pressure normalization are available for the treatment of difficult-to-control (therapy-resistant) hypertension. Minoxidil, among others, has proven itself, but must nevertheless always be combined with a beta blocker (reflex tachycardia) and a diuretic (fluid retention).

32.4 Antihypertensive therapy before, during and after surgery

Patients with arterial hypertension demonstrate greater intraoperative blood pressure fluctuation than normotensive patients. The overall surgical risk is nevertheless only higher for hypertensive patients, if previous cardiac damage exists (coronary artery disease, recurrent, silent myocardial ischemia, left ventricular hypertrophy).

Long-term elevated blood pressure should be normalized before surgery. Patients with known, drug-controlled arterial hypertension should take their antihypertensive medication as usual on the day of surgery. It has been shown that beta blockers, whether used in continuing an existing therapy or introduced prior to surgery, reduce the overall operative risk. A sudden withdrawal of antihypertensive drug therapy is not recommended, since intraoperatively large hemodynamic fluctuations − in particular after a high-dose, long-term therapy with beta blockers or clonidine − and rebound hypertension can occur. Diuretics, which should not be taken on the day of surgery, are an exception since they reduce intravascular volume. Possible potassium loss, often a consequence of long-term treatment with diuretics, must be compensated, since they can cause severe ventricular arrhythmias, especially in patients with coexisting cardiac diseases.

When a patient is first diagnosed with mild to moderate hypertension (USA: stages 1 and 2) several days prior to a planned operation, a 1−2 day preoperative, antihypertensive treatment with a selective beta$_1$-receptor blocker is recommended (for contraindications see Table 29.1). A postponement of the operation is generally unnecessary.

If a targeted therapeutic stabilization of an as yet untreated hypertension is not possible due to time constraints (emergency!), then an antihypertensive with a rapid onset of action should be introduced prior to surgery. These are primarily preventive measures, since in- and extubation, as well as recovery from general anesthesia represent extreme stress factors which not infrequently lead to acute blood pressure exacerbations in cases of untreated hypertension. Nifedipine can be used preoperatively as an oral, sublingual antihypertensive. The preventive effect of calcium antagonists (and ACE inhibitors) against stress-induced, sympathoadrenally related hypertensive reactions during the operation is considered to be minimal. Many anesthesiologists therefore prefer the beta blocker esmolol, which takes effect immediately after administration, and remains effective at a maximum 20−30 minutes after discontinuance.

The intraoperative adjustment of blood pressure is governed by preoperative blood pressure values, by coexisting diseases (myocardial damage, peripheral occlusive vascular disease, carotid stenosis, etc.) and by surgery-specific conditions. The anesthesiologist must assure that, on the one hand, stress-inducing procedures (intubation, etc.; see above) do not cause any hypertensive blood pressure imbalances and, on the other hand, that antihypertensive medication and (primarily hypotensive-acting) anesthetics do not interact with each other to create sudden decreases in blood pressure.

Endotrachial aspiration and extubation at the end of the operation can also cause spontaneous blood pressure exacerbation. As noted above, such sympathoadrenally related blood pressure reactions can for the most part be prevented by the administration of a beta blocker (esmolol).

If blood pressure is significantly elevated postoperatively, antihypertensive therapy can initially be administered intravenously. Labetalol, esmolol, sodium nitroprusside and nicardipine are recommended. Oral antihypertensive drugs should be substituted as quickly as possible.

Summary (Section 32.4)

- Patients with arterial hypertension are at greater risk of hemodynamic fluctuation during an operation than are normotensive patients. A higher overall surgical risk applies, however, only to hypertensive patients with concomitant heart diseases.

- Hypertension should, to the extent possible, be controlled prior to surgery.
- Previously prescribed antihypertensive medication should be continued and administered as usual on the morning of the operation.
- The prophylactic administration of selective, short-acting beta blockers is recommended for patients with hypertension since in- and extubation, endotracheal aspiration and surgical manipulation lead to sympathoadrenally mediated increases in blood pressure which can bring about a hypertensive crisis in cases of preexisting arterial hypertension.
- Significantly higher postoperative blood pressure values can initially be treated intravenously. Oral medication should, however, be substituted as quickly as possible.

Literature (Chapter 32)

Bussmann WD, Kenedi P, von Mengden HJ, Nast HP, Rachor N. Comparision of nitroglycerin with nifedipine in patients with hypertensive crisis or severe hypertension. Clin Investig 1992; 70: 1085−1088.

Calhoun DA, Oparil S. Treatment of hypertensive crisis. N Engl J Med 1990; 323: 1177−1183.

Cucchiara RF, Benefiel DJ, Matteo RS, DeWood M, Albin MS. Elevation of esmolol in controlling increases in heart rate and blood pressure during endotracheal intubation in patients undergoing carotid endarterectomy. Anaesthesiology 1986; 65: 528−531.

Deutsche Liga zur Bekämpfung des hohen Blutdruckes e.V. Deutsche Hypertonie Gesellschaft. Empfehlungen zur Hochdruckbehandlung in der Praxis und zur Behandlung hypertensiver Notfälle. 11. Aufl., 1994.

Fagan TC. Acute reduction of blood pressure in asymptomatic patients with severe hypertension. An idea whose time has come − and gone. Arch Intern Med 1989; 149: 2169−2170.

Ferguson RK, Vlasses PH. Hypertensive emergencies and urgencies. JAMA 1986; 255: 1607−1613.

Ferguson RK, Vlasses PH. How urgent is „urgent" hypertension ? Arch Intern Med 1989; 149: 257−258.

Fujii K, Ueno BL, Baumbach GL, Heistad DD. Effect of antihypertensive treatment on focal cerebral infarction. Hypertension 1992; 19: 713−716.

Hirschl MM. Guidelines for the drug treatment of hypertensive crisis. Drugs 1995; 50: 991−1000.

Jaker M, Atkin S, Soto M, Schmid G, Brosch F. Oral nifedipine vs oral clonidine in the treatment of urgent hypertension. Arch Intern Med 1989; 149: 260−265.

Ledingham JGG, Rajagopalan B. Cerebral complications in the treatment of accelerated hypertension. Q J Med 1979; 48: 25−41.

Prisant LM, Carr AA, Hawkins DW. Treating hypertensive emergencies. Controlled reduction of blood pressure and protection of target organs. Postgrad Med 1993; 93: 92−110.

Ram CVS. Hypertensive crisis. In: Kaplan NM, Ram CVS (eds). Individualized therapy of hypertension. Marcel Dekker, New York, 1995, 223−255.

Weiss SJ, Longnecker DE. Perioperative hypertension: an overview. Coron Art Dis 1993; 4: 401−406.

Zeller KR, Kuhnert LV, Metthews C. Rapid reduction of severe asymptomatic hypertension. a prospective, controlled study. Arch Intern Med 1989; 149: 2186−2189.

33 Antihypertensive therapy for select populations

In the various populations diagnosed with arterial hypertension, certain individual characteristics have to be taken into consideration when choosing a medication and establishing its dosage, its introduction and/or performance of the antihypertensive therapy.

33.1 Antihypertensive therapy in the childhood

33.1.1 The treatment of secondary forms of hypertension

Here as with adult patients, the treatment of potentially curable secondary forms of hypertension aims at the removal (pheochromocytoma, adrenal adenoma) or correction (renal artery stenosis, stenosis of the aortic isthmus) of the primary causes. In cases of renal parenchymal hypertension, an optimal, medicinal therapeutic approach should be adopted ($<$ 95th percentile) in order to counter additional deterioration of kidney function resulting from damage caused by the increased blood pressure.

33.1.2 The treatment of primary hypertension

The goal of antihypertensive therapy in children and adolescents is the reduction of blood pressure below the applicable 95th percentile (Figure 11.1). As in the treatment of adult hypertensive patients, immediate drug therapy is recommended in cases of

- severe hypertension ($>$ 99th percentile), as well as in cases of
- mild to moderate hypertension (95th−99th percentile), where hypertension-induced end-organ damage is present.

The therapeutic recommendations for mild to moderate primary hypertension (95th−99th percentiles), in the absence of end-organ damage, above all comprise non-medicinal actions (weight reduction, sodium restriction, physical exercise, etc., see Chapter 20) and long-term observation.

Only when blood pressure values register persistently higher than 10 mmHg above the 95th percentile (moderate hypertension), despite non-pharmacological measures, does antihypertensive drug treatment become advisable. The same substance classes recognized as first-line medications for adults are valid here as well (beta blockers, diuretics, calcium antagonists, ACE inhibitors, alpha$_1$-receptor blockers).

Due to their longer track records, beta blockers and diuretics are given preference in some countries.

Dosages are based on body weight, and therefore to be individually adjusted (Table 33.1). The patient should be slowly weaned from antihypertensive medication

Table 33.1:   Dosage of antihypertensive drug therapy in children with sustained hypertension*

Substance	Dosage (mg/kg per day)	Dosage interval (hours)
DIURETICS		
– Hydrochlorothiazide	1–2	12–24
– Chlorthalidone	0.5–2	24
– Furosemide**	1–5	8–12
SYMPATHOLYTICS		
Sympatholytics with primarily central sites of action		
– Clonidine	0.005–0.03	8–12
– Alpha-methyldopa	5–40	6
Sympatholytics with primarily peripheral sites of action		
– Alpha$_1$-receptor blockers: Prazosin	0.02–0.5	8
– Beta-receptor blockers:		
Propanolol	1–6	8–12
Metoprolol	1–4	12
Atenolol	1–2	24
VASODILATORS		
– (Di-)Hydralazine	1–5	8–12
– Minoxidil	0.05–1	12
CALCIUM ANTAGONISTS		
Phenylalkylamines		
– Verapamil	2–10	8–12
Dihydropyridines		
– Nifedipine	0.25–2	8–24***
– Nitrendipine	0.5–1	12–24
INHIBITORS OF THE RENIN ANGIOTENSIN SYSTEM		
ACE inhibitors		
– Captopril:		
Children and adolescents	0.5–3.0	12
Newborns and infants	0.01–1.0	
– Enalapril	0.15–0.6	12–24

* The medications listed in this table are not universally approved in all countries
** Only in cases of impaired renal function
*** According to pharmaceutical formulation (sustained release; gastrointestinal therapeutic systems, GITS; etc.)

Table 33.2:   Dosage of antihypertensive drugs for the treatment of hypertensive emergencies
in children*

Substance	Dosage (mg/kg)	Onset of action
Oral/sublingual:		
Nifedipine s. l. or p. o.	0.25−0.5	Few minutes
Captopril p. o.		
Newborns and infants	0.01−0.25	Minutes
Children and adolescents	0.1−0.2	Minutes
Intravenous:		
Sodium nitroprusside	0.5−8 µg/kg/min	Immediately
Labetalol	1−3	Minutes
(Di-)Hydralazine	0.1−0.5	Minutes
Urapidil	1−4	Minutes
Clonidine	0.003−0.006	Minutes
Phentolamine**	0.1−0.2	Immediately

  * The medications listed in this table are not universally approved in all countries
** In cases of catecholamine excess (pheochromocytoma)

over a period of 1−2 years through gradual reductions in dose. This period should
be accompanied by frequent examinations of the blood pressure.

The treatment of severe hypertension (more than 30 mmHg above the 95th percentile) and of hypertensive crises displays no fundamental peculiarities during childhood and adolescence (Table 33.2).

Summary (Section 33.1)

- The treatment of arterial hypertension in childhood is not fundamentally
  different from treatment for the same illness in adulthood.
- Dosages of antihypertensive medications in childhood are based on body
  weight, and therefore to be individually adjusted.

33.2 The antihypertensive treatment
of elderly hypertensive patients

Elderly patients (> 65 years old) with arterial hypertension particularly profit from
a reduction in blood pressure. Several large, prospective studies have determined
that reductions not only in combined systolic-diastolic hypertension (STOP-hypertension, MRC study, EWPHE study), but as well in isolated systolic hypertension
(SHEP study) lead to a reduction in the significantly higher mortality and morbidity in elderly patients. The reduced incidence of stroke among elderly hypertensive

patients following a successful reduction in long-term elevated blood pressure, has been known for some time (Figures 33.1 and 33.2).

Long-term elevated blood pressure values > 140 mmHg systolic and/or > 90 mmHg diastolic are also considered hypertensive in older patients. Possibly false-high blood pressure measurements occasionally caused by advanced sclerosis of major arteries (brachial, radial, etc.) must, however, first be excluded.

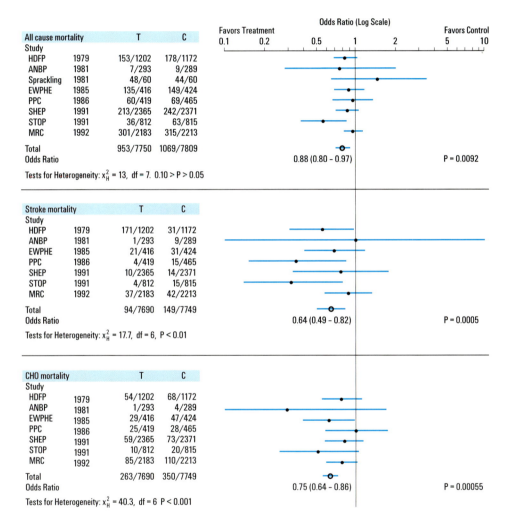

Figure 33.1: Results of meta-analysis of mortality end points from large trials performed in elderly patients with hypertension. Left: Absolute numbers. Right: Odds ratios and 95 % confidence intervals. ANBP = Australian National Blood Pressure Study; EWPHE = European Working Party on High Blood Pressure in the Elderly; HDFP = Hypertension Detection and Follow-up Program; MRC = Medical Research Council; PPC = Practice in Primary Care; SHEP = Systolic Hypertension in the Elderly Program; STOP = Swedish Trial in Old Patients with Hypertension; VA = Veterans Administration Cooperative Study on Antihypertensive Agents. (From Insua JT et al., Ann Intern Med 1994; 121: 355−362)

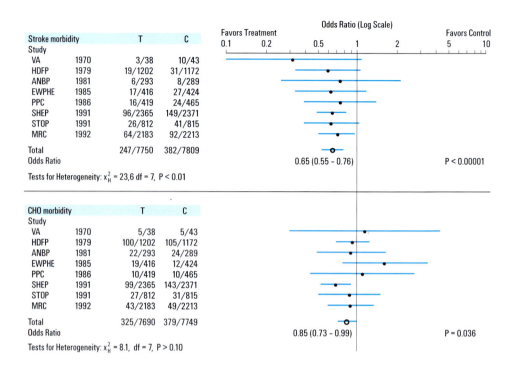

Figure 33.2: Results of meta-analysis of morbidity end points from large clinical trials performed in elderly patients with hypertension. Left: Absolute numbers. Right: Odds ratios and 95 % confidence intervals. ANBP = Australian National Blood Pressure Study; EWPHE = European Working Party on High Blood Pressure in the Elderly; HDFP = Hypertension Detection and Follow-up Program; MRC = Medical Research Council; PPC = Practice in Primary Care; SHEP = Systolic Hypertension in the Elderly; STOP = Swedish Trial in Old Patients with Hypertension; VA = Veterans Administration Cooperative Study on Antihypertensive Agents. (From Insua JT et al., Ann Intern Med 1994; 121: 355–362)

The goal of treatment in elderly hypertensive patients is also the reduction of diastolic blood pressure to < 90–85 mmHg, and systolic blood pressure below roughly 140–160 mmHg. Since it has been shown in recent years that systolic hypertension is in itself a cardiovascular risk factor, there is no longer any doubt that isolated systolic hypertension requires treatment.

The blood pressure values discussed serve merely as guidelines. Whether a further reduction of diastolic pressure is beneficial or damaging is a question that the HOT study may answer.

33.2.1 Mild to moderate combined and isolated systolic hypertension (stages 1 and 2)

The treatment of mild to moderate combined systolic/diastolic or isolated systolic hypertension (USA: Stages 1 and 2) in elderly patients follows the general guidelines for antihypertensive therapy. Therefore non-drug treatment (Chapter 22) is the therapy of choice (as it is for younger patients). If this does not result in normalization of blood pressure within 6 months, the introduction of drug therapy is recommended. In the elderly, this should be handled carefully (50% of the standard initial dosage) and slowly (over a period of weeks or months), since larger reductions in blood pressure are poorly compensated for due to frequently slowed cardiovascular reflexes. Frequent blood pressure examinations, which should not only be performed while seated or supine, but while standing as well, are especially informative in the early phases of drug treatment. If subjective and/or objective side-effects should occur, a change in medication should be taken into consideration earlier than would be the case for younger patients.

When introducing antihypertensive drug therapy it should also be noted, that elderly patients more frequently suffer arteriosclerotic stenoses of their organ-supplying arteries than do younger patients. Drug-induced systemic decreases in pressure can therefore lead to reduced perfusion in organs supplied by the stenotic vessel. The patient then has to be specifically queried about recurrences of chest pain (coronary stenosis?), pain caused by climbing stairs (peripheral occlusive arterial disease?), or dizziness and/or impaired vision (carotid stenosis?).

For the reduction of systolic blood pressure, the Joint National Committee on Detection, Evaluation, and Treatment of High Blood Pressure (JNC V) especially recommends a gradual approach, meaning that where initial values exceed 180 mmHg, a subsequent reduction to < 160 mmHg should be sought; and likewise where initial values lie between 160 and 179 mmHg, a reduction of 20 mmHg. If the blood pressure reached is well-tolerated, a further reduction can be attempted to values lie between 140 and 160 mmHg, preferably by means of general antihypertensive measures.

33.2.2 Severe hypertension (stages 3 and 4)

Medicinal treatment for severe arterial hypertension in the elderly does not, in general, require any special form of treatment. Multiple-drug therapy is generally required to achieve the desired blood pressure. Despite, or perhaps because of the severity of the condition, drug therapy must be introduced very carefully, since it can be assumed that cerebral autoregulatory tolerance for decreases in blood pressure is significantly diminished. A gradual reduction in blood pressure spread out over months is therefore desirable. Therapeutic steps, meaning increases in dosage or additions of second and third medications to the existing array, should be spread over intervals of 2−5 weeks and be oriented on the time span within which the maximum efficacy of the medications can be expected to be attained.

33.2.3 Choice of antihypertensive drugs for elderly patients with hypertension

The choice of medication for elderly patients is, as for younger patients, based primarily on individual circumstances. Concomitant illnesses and the day-to-day needs of the patient should be taken into account. Diuretics, beta-receptor blockers, calcium antagonists and ACE inhibitors are therefore viewed as fundamentally interchangeable in the treatment of elderly hypertensives. Selective alpha$_1$-receptor blockers as well as combinations of beta- and alpha$_1$-receptor blockers are equally well suited, but the pros and cons of treating with these substances should be carefully weighed due to the danger of orthostatic hypotension.

33.2.4 Therapeutic problems in cases of borderline hypertension

The necessity for medicinally treating elderly patients with borderline hypertension (90−94 mmHg diastolic and/or 140−159 mmHg systolic) can not be uniformly evaluated. On the one hand, the usefulness of reducing blood pressure to below 90 mmHg has been unequivocally demonstrated; on the other hand, the risk of "over-treatment", particularly in elderly patients, is higher. The general consensus is, however, that a further reduction in blood pressure by non-drug treatment/life-style modifications must be conscientiously pursued. If drug therapy is selected to reduce diastolic blood pressure below 90 mmHg in elderly patients − they being more frequently affected by severe arteriosclerosis than younger ones − extreme caution is recommended, since a simultaneous reduction in systolic blood pressure to below 140 mmHg can trigger ischemia in end organs poorly supplied by stenotic arteries.

Summary (Section 33.2)

- The goal of therapy in elderly patients with combined systolic-diastolic or isolated systolic hypertension is the reduction of blood pressure to below 90 mmHg diastolic and to below 140 mmHg systolic.
- If blood pressure normalisation is not achieved within six months by antihypertensive non-drug treatment, medicinal monotherapy must be attempted.
- Drug induced hypotension is frequently observed in elderly patients; therefore the usual initial dosage should be halved.
- The choice of first-line antihypertensive medication should be based on individual criteria. Diuretics, beta-receptor blockers, calcium antagonists, ACE inhibitors and selective alpha$_1$-receptor blockers are all equally well suited for the treatment of elderly patients.
- The treatment of severe hypertension (USA: Stages 3 and 4) in patients over 65 years old is based on the usual therapeutic recommendations; nevertheless blood pressure must be especially carefully and slowly reduced.

33.3 Antihypertensive therapy for women

Approximately half of all hypertensive patients are women. Whereas primary hypertension is seldom encountered in premenopausal women in comparison with men of the same age, its incidence following menopause increases steadily until, above the age of 60, the number of women with hypertension exceeds the number of men. Black women in North America display a particularly high incidence of arterial hypertension which, when contrasted with that of white women, is more pronounced, is more frequently accompanied by other cardiovascular risk factors, and more often already involves end-organ damage.

Since exogenous estrogen substitution after menopause lowers cardiovascular risk, it is supposed that endogenous estrogen production prior to menopause protects a woman's body against the development of cardiovascular diseases. Lower androgen production as well as menstrually-induced reduction in blood volume are further factors which protect younger women as much against the development of hypertension and other cardiovascular diseases.

33.3.1 Treatment of hypertension prior to menopause

The most common cause of hypertension among women prior to menopause is probably the ingestion of oral contraceptives (Section 17.1.1). This, as well as any other causes of secondary hypertension, must therefore first be excluded.

Primary hypertension affects women prior to menopause far more seldom (see above), and with more favorable hemodynamic characteristics (lower total peripheral resistance, less pronounced increase in blood pressure during isometric exercise), than it affects men of the same age. Furthermore, the myocardial adaptive processes, such as left ventricular hypertrophy, associated with increased cardiovascular risk in premenopausal women with mild to moderate hypertension are less pronounced than those of men of the same age. Since these gender-specific differences disappear with menopause, it is conjectured that estrogen possesses both vaso- and cardioprotective properties. Whether or not this premenopausal protection justifies a less aggressive treatment for hypertension has yet to be evaluated. A conscientious reduction of blood pressure to below 140/90 mmHg is therefore desirable even in this patient population. If nonpharmacologic measures/life-style modifications aimed at the reduction of blood pressure fail consistently over a long period of observation, then, following the standard guidelines for the treatment of hypertension, medicinal antihypertensive therapy should be instituted.

33.3.2 Antihypertensive treatment of postmenopausal women

Although postmenopausal women develop all the known cardiovascular risk factors on equal terms with men, the prevalence of coronary artery disease is higher for men of any age than it is for women. This observation, however, does not justify a less conscientious treatment of cardiovascular risk factors, including hypertension, in women than in men.

33.3.2.1 Gender-independent criteria for the selection of medication

The choice of antihypertensive therapy for postmenopausal women is determined in part by factors which also influence the same choice for men. Among those factors are

- disorders of lipometabolism, in particular increases in LDL or decreases in HDL cholesterol,
- truncal obesity, mostly encountered along with
- disorders of carbohydrate metabolism, such as increasing insulin resistance with subsequent hyperinsulinemia,

as well as concomitant diseases:

- manifest diabetes mellitus,
- renal insufficiency, and
- myocardial hypertrophy.

33.3.2.2 Gender-specific criteria for the selection of medication

Certain gender-specific characteristics must furthermore be taken into consideration when choosing medication:

- Osteoporosis induced by a lack of estrogen,
- interaction with simultaneously administered hormone replacement therapy and/or with other osteoprotective substances (biphosphonates, etc.).

While the effects of the available antihypertensive drugs on cardiovascular risk factors and on the diseases that primarily accompany hypertension are well known with respect to the overall hypertensive population (see sections 31.1−31.5), the long-term effects of antihypertensive medication on bone loss, in particular that brought about through lack of estrogen, have to date only been evaluated for thiazide diuretics. As stated in section 31.6, a decreased incidence of bone loss was observed in most studies where thiazide diuretics were administered over the long-term. In a longitudinal study (duration: ca. 7.5−10 years) of 993 postmenopausal women averaging 63 years of age, the group treated with a combination of thiazide diuretics and estrogen evidenced a significantly higher bone density than the groups treated with thiazide or estrogen alone. The lowest bone density measurements were obtained in the untreated control group. The detection of Ang II-receptors on osteoblasts as well as on the endothelial cells of bone marrow capillaries raises the suspicion that the renin angiotensin system (RAS) may be locally involved in the regulation of bone metabolism. The extent to which long-term treatment with ACE inhibitors or other inhibitors of the RAS might influence the bone turnover is unclear (see also Section 31.6).

33.3.2.3 Therapeutic consequences

Since the majority of postmenopausal women with arterial hypertension are overweight, appropriate life-style modifications known to lower high blood pressure (weight loss, low-fat diet, abstinence from alcohol and nicotine, reduction in salt intake, physical exercise, etc.; see also Chapter 20) form the vanguard of therapeutic measures. If these yield no satisfactory result, medicinal treatment should be instituted, preferably drawing on the available first-line antihypertensive drugs, whose selection should take into account the particulars of the individual patient. Gender-specific criteria come into play in cases of treatment-demanding, postmenopausal osteoporosis, whose simultaneous appearance calls for the administration of thiazide diuretics (possibly in combination with ACE inhibitors).

> Summary (Sections 33.3.1 and 33.3.2)
>
> - The treatment of primary hypertension in women prior to menopause follows the usual guidelines for antihypertensive therapy.
>
> - The medicinal treatment of postmenopausal women requires that attention be given to their overall cardiovascular risk, which — possibly as a consequence of the lack of estrogen — does not differ from that of men.
>
> - Where hypertension and postmenopausal osteoporosis requiring treatment coexist, their respective long-term medicinal therapies should complement one another.
>
> - While it is anticipated that estrogen hormone replacement therapy will beneficially influence cardiovascular risk factors, the effect of antihypertensive therapy on postmenopausal bone loss has been investigated very little to date.
>
> - Among the currently available antihypertensive drugs, only thiazide diuretics display a definite osteoprotective effect.

33.3.3 Antihypertensive therapy during pregnancy

The goal of antihypertensive therapy in pregnancy is the prevention of eclampsia. The most important preventive action is the frequent measurement of blood pressure during pregnancy.

33.3.3.1 Non-drug treatment of hypertension during pregnancy

The following strategies for non-drug treatment are recommended for high blood pressure during pregnancy:

- Decreased physical activity; in cases of severe hypertension, bed rest (goal: reduction of arterial blood pressure, improvement of placental blood flow).

- No restriction of salt intake, since this may lead to a further reduction in the already decreased intravascular volume with deterioration of placental blood flow and, in the specific condition, to a further blood pressure increase (renin-stimulation?). Women with a known salt-sensitive form of hypertension who should have been adhering to a salt-restricted diet prior to pregnancy, are exempted from this recommendation.

— No reduction in weight.

— Absolute abstention from alcohol and nicotine.

Thus, the general therapeutic recommendations for pregnant women vary fundamentally from those for individuals not in pregnancy (Chapter 22).

33.3.3.2 Preeclampsia (pregnancy-specific hypertension)

Despite its unknown pathogenesis, pregnancy-specific hypertension should be categorized as a secondary form of hypertension, since it is possible to treat it causally by delivery. In many instances this approach is not possible due to the immaturity of the fetus, so that either general measures alone (see section 33.3.3.1) or additional medicinal therapy have to be introduced. The benefit of antihypertensive drug therapy in cases of pregnancy-specific hypertension has not been proven; therefore most experts recommend it only when maternal blood pressure reaches diastolic values of > 100 mmHg.

The medication of choice in the treatment of hypertension during pregnancy is, as it has been, alpha methyldopa (Section 24.1.1). An initial twice-daily dose of 250 mg is recommended, and may be increased, where necessary, to as much as 2 g. In a study performed in the 70's on women with mild hypertension (140/90 mmHg to 155/100 mmHg), fewer premature births and lower perinatal mortality were observed in those taking alpha methyldopa than in those taking a placebo. Although in certain cases this study provided a maximum daily dose of 4 g of methyldopa, the follow-up of more than seven years revealed no evidence of diminished neurological function or intellectual development.

Beta-receptor blockers should be classified as therapy of second choice during pregnancy, whereby only beta$_1$-selective substances are recommended. Treatment with beta-receptor blockers should be carried out with the lowest possible dosages (atenolol up to a maximum of 100 mg/d, metoprolol up to a maximum of 200 mg/d, acebutol up to a maximum of 400 mg/d), and should be resorted to in the course of the first trimester only when absolutely indicated, since its administration in this phase of pregnancy may cause fetal growth retardation. Bradycardia induced by beta-receptor blockers can lower hypoxia tolerance and endanger the fetus, particularly during delivery.

Various smaller comparative studies have shown labetalol to be more effective than alpha methyldopa in lowering elevated blood pressure during pregnancy. Although this combined beta-/alpha$_1$-receptor blocker can be administered orally as well as intravenously, and although it displayed no serious fetal side-effects in the studies mentioned, its use can not be recommended without reservations, since in certain cases a causal relationship between its intake and maternal liver damage could not be ruled out.

Verapamil is also recommended for the treatment of hypertension during pregnancy.

If satisfactory blood pressure reduction can not be achieved through monotherapy with one of the antihypertensives mentioned, (di-)hydralazine can additionally be administered (25 mg/d to 300 mg/d). Monotherapy with (di-)hydralazine is less well suited, since its efficacy becomes impaired with time as a result of progressive sodium retention and reflex tachycardia.

None of the other antihypertensive drugs commonly used in the treatment of primary and secondary hypertension should be used during pregnancy. This holds especially true for ACE inhibitors (contraindicated), dihydropyridine-type and diltiazem-type calcium antagonists, and reserpine.

Diuretics further reduce the already diminished plasma volume anyway, and so can lead to a deterioration in placental circulation. Diuretics should therefore only be administered in those women, who had been already treated successfully with these substances prior to pregnancy, and in those, who are known to have a salt-sensitive form of hypertension.

33.3.3.3 Treatment of (imminent) eclampsia

The triad of hypertension, proteinuria and edema is characteristic of preeclampsia. The additional presence of neurological symptoms (headaches, blurred vision, changes in consciousness) is characteristic of imminent eclampsia and is interpreted as a precursor to manifest eclampsia; eclampsia is defined as the occurrence of general convulsions and severe, sometimes comatose, changes in consciousness in a preeclamptic patient, which can not be attributed to other causes.

Imminent and manifest eclampsia with severe hypertension (diastolic > 120 mmHg) therefore represent a hypertensive emergency which demands immediate antihypertensive therapy − wherever possible, in intensive care.

Hypertensive crises in cases of imminent (preeclampsia) or manifest eclampsia are treated with (di-)hydralazine.(Di-)hydralazine must be administered intravenously and should, after an initial dose of 6.25 mg, be dispensed via perfusor. As an alternative, diazoxide (repeated intravenous bolus, 30 mg) or urapidil (12.5 mg intravenously; urapidil is not approved in all countries !) are recommended. The goal is a slow reduction in diastolic pressure. Excessively rapid and/or deep reductions in blood pressure should be avoided, since these may lead to a deterioration in uterine blood flow. Sedative (diazepam) and anticonvulsive therapy with magnesium sulfate should follow. Where (di-)hydralazine fails to adequately reduce blood pressure, or where reflexive tachycardia occurs, beta$_1$-selective receptor blockers in low doses can be added.

The additional introduction of loop diuretics is reserved for acute left ventricular decompensation. Other medications useful in the treatment of hypertensive crises with widely varying origins cannot, because of the danger to the fetus, be administered (sodium nitroprusside).

33.3.3.4 Chronic, preexisting hypertension
      (pregnancy-independent hypertension)

In patients with preexisting mild to moderate arterial hypertension (USA: Stages 1 and 2) and normal to slightly diminished kidney function (serum creatinine

< 1.5–2.0 mg/dL), pregnancy presents no specific danger either to the mother or the child. Hypertension and more severe renal insufficiency mean increased risk of renal failure, the development of preeclampsia, and in the end, perinatal morbidity and mortality. Pregnancy is ill advised where severe hypertension (USA: Stages 3 and 4) is present.

The goal of therapy is the normalization of blood pressure (< 140/90 mmHg). If blood pressure can not be lowered to diastolic levels < 100 mmHg by nonpharmacologic treatment, then the need for medicinal therapy is unequivocal. Conversely, therapeutic approaches vary where diastolic values lie between 90–99 mmHg despite non-drug treatment. Whereas, for example, the German Hypertension Society finds it necessary in such cases to resort to medication in order to normalize blood pressure, other professional associations (e.g. Working Group on High Blood Pressure in Pregnancy; National Heart, Lung and Blood Institute – NHBLI, USA) are far more hesitant since, on the one hand, its value to mother and child has not been determined, and, on the other hand, antihypertensive therapy might lead to a reduction in placental blood flow, and thus to endangerment of the fetus. On this basis, I find Cunningham and Lindheimer (N Engl J Med, 1992) to be convincing with their recommendation to institute medicinal therapy where blood pressure lies between 90–99 mmHg only when further risk factors exist (renal insufficiency, end-organ damage, etc.).

Antihypertensive agents recommended for the treatment of pregnancy-independent/primary hypertension are naturally the same as those named in section 33.3.3.2.

33.3.3.5 Acute blood pressure elevation during delivery

Acute blood pressure elevations up to 105 mmHg immediately before or during delivery can be tolerated, without resort to antihypertensive medication. Greater increases in blood pressure should, however, be treated with short-acting antihypertensive drugs, since where arterial blood pressure exceeds 170/110 mmHg (and/or mean pressures exceed 130 mmHg), cerebrovascular autoregulatory compensation mechanisms are diminished and the danger of cerebral ischemia or of cerebral hemorrhage increases exponentially. The goal is a reduction of blood pressure to values between 90–104 mmHg diastolic. Drugs with a rapid onset of action such as (di-)hydralazine, diazoxide, sublingual nifedipine, labetalol or clonidine are recommended in such cases.

33.3.3.6 Antihypertensive therapy after delivery

Persistently high blood pressure values for more than a week after delivery indicate the presence of primary hypertension, the treatment of which depends on its severity. In moderate to severe hypertension (USA: Stages 3 and 4), medicinal treatment should begin prior to the patient's release. If hypertension was not known to exist prior to pregnancy, and if the therapy selected succeeded in reducing blood pressure, an attempt at suspending medication is warranted after several weeks.

33.3.3.7 Antihypertensive therapy while nursing

If the mother intends to breast-feed her child, the possible passage of the chosen medication into the mother's milk should be taken into consideration. In mild to moderate hypertension (stages 1 and 2), it is best to refrain from drug therapy while nursing; in more severe cases of hypertension (stages 3 and 4), treatment with alpha methyldopa is recommended. In such cases, once past the nursing period, a switch to one of the first-line antihypertensive drugs is recommended, even where blood pressure has already been successfully normalized.

Summary (Section 33.3.3)

- The primary therapeutic goal in cases of hypertension during pregnancy is the prevention of eclampsia.

- The most important general measure in pregnant women with hypertension is a reduction in physical activity. In more severe hypertension temporary bed rest is established as a means to improve placental blood flow. Reductions in sodium intake and weight are not recommended.

- Drug therapy is indicated above a diastolic value of 100 mmHg whenever pregnancy-induced hypertension (preeclampsia) is known to exist. The same holds true for the treatment of primary hypertension where it is known to have existed prior to pregnancy.

- The decision to treat diastolic blood pressure values below 100 mmHg with medication must be reached on a case-by-case basis. Such treatment is nevertheless advisable wherever kidney function is diminished or where end-organ damage exists.

- The medication of choice for long-term antihypertensive therapy during pregnancy is alpha methyldopa. With certain restrictions, selective beta$_1$-receptor blockers, labetalol or verapamil can also be recommended.

- Imminent or manifest eclampsia should be viewed as hypertensive emergencies which should be treated medicinally using, primarily, (di-)hydralazine. Urapadil is recommended as an alternative in some countries (e.g. Germany). Medicinal sedation and the introduction of anticonvulsive therapy should be carried out simultaneously.

33.4   Ethnic influences on the selection of antihypertensive therapy

33.4.1 Antihypertensive therapy for black hypertensives

In contrast to white Americans, black US citizens (African-Americans) demonstrate a higher incidence of mild (+30%), moderate (+200%) and severe (+280%)

hypertension. It has yet to be clarified whether or not this higher incidence of hypertension in the black population is the consequence of genetic and/or environmental influences. A higher incidence of salt sensitivity among African-American hypertensives in contrast to white hypertensives is seen by some authors as a consequence of a natural selection effected during the time of slavery and passed on to subsequent generations of black Americans. The basis for this hypothesis is the assumption that, in the course of their abduction and transport to America, primarily those Africans survived the months-long crossing (the so-called "middle passage") who best compensated for the salt loss induced by the sun, diarrhea and strenuous slave labor through elevated renal sodium retention. This acquired ability predisposes affected individuals whose social environment encourages higher salt intake to develop hypertension. Further characteristics noted more frequently − in the USA, at least − among black rather than white hypertensives include insulin resistance, obesity (particularly in women) and a lesser secretion of renin both before and after stimulation.

If the nonpharmacologic measures laid out in Chapter 20, valid for black as well as white hypertensives, fail, then drug treatment is called for. To date only thiazide diuretics have yielded a reduction in African-American morbidity and mortality (Hypertension Detection and Follow-up Program, HDFP). Despite the efficacy of diuretics in the treatment of African-American hypertensive patients, their known unfavorable impact on glucose tolerance should be taken into account, the more so, since insulin resistance and hyperinsulinemia are more often seen in this, rather than in the white population. − Calcium antagonists are reputedly as effective as diuretics and are therefore often the preferred first-line medication for African-American hypertensives with coexisting obesity and disorders of the lipid and carbohydrate metabolism.

Various studies have indicated that beta-receptor blockers and ACE inhibitors are less effective among black hypertensives. This is probably only true for those patients whose renin secretion is actually lower. The combined administration of these substance classes with a low dose of a thiazide diuretic leads in any event to a therapeutic response rate not at all different from that of white hypertensives.

No ethnically-based differences in effectiveness have yet been demonstrated for alpha-receptor blockers.

33.4.2 Antihypertensive therapy for other ethnic groups

Pathogenic peculiarities that could influence the choice of antihypertensive non-drug or drug therapy have not been reported to date for hypertension in members of other ethnic groups (Asian, Hispanics). Therapy therefore follows the general guidelines for the treatment of hypertension.

Summary (Section 33.4)

• Drug treatment of arterial hypertension in black (African-American) patients and in members of other ethnic groups normally follows the generally accepted guidelines.

• Beta-receptor blockers and ACE inhibitors are less effective as monotherapies among black hypertensive patients than white hypertensive patients. A low renin secretion is a possible cause.

• A reduction of cardiovascular morbidity and mortality among African-American patients with hypertension has, as yet, only been shown for thiazide diuretics. All other antihypertensive substance classes are presently still lacking this proof.

33.5 Antihypertensive therapy for obese patients

Almost 50% of overweight patients have elevated arterial blood pressure, while, at the same time, up to 50% of hypertensives are overweight. In contrast to normal-weight patients with primary hypertension, obese patients display certain peculiarities that need to be taken into account when treating hypertension. The list of peculiarities includes increased insulin resistance and secretion, increased sympathetic activity, increased tubular sodium reabsorption with subsequent expansion of intravascular volume, disturbed homeostasis of endothelially-released vasoactive substances (especially nitric oxide), moderately increased peripheral arterial resistance, and an increased incidence of lipid metabolism abnormalities. Left ventricular hypertrophy develops more quickly, and the transition to an ill-boding ventricular dilatation is abetted by the simultaneous occurrence of increased blood pressure (increased cardiac afterload) and expanded intravascular volume (increased cardiac preload) (see also Figure 9.2).

Weight loss, inasmuch as possible in connection with an increase in physical activity, reduces or normalizes not only the hormonal and metabolic parameters named, but blood pressure as well. For that reason, weight loss is the most important therapy of hypertension in obese patients. Unfortunately, due to unsatisfactory compliance on the part of most patients, significant weight loss can not be achieved and antihypertensive drug treatment has to be introduced.

Since obesity-related hypertension is typically characterized by an expanded intravascular volume and an only slightly elevated peripheral vascular resistance, direct vasodilators (Chapter 27) are not recommended for its treatment, since they may lead to further fluid retention.

From the hemodynamic perspective, diuretics are well suited for the treatment of hypertension, since they reduce the intravascular volume of obese patients. Unfortunately, diuretics not only worsen the impaired glucose tolerance of obese patients, but also further increase the mostly elevated atherogenic lipoprotein fractions (especially LDL cholesterol) as well. Therefore, higher dosages of diuretics are, if at all, recommended only as an adjunct therapy, and not as a monotherapy, for overweight patients with high blood pressure.

Despite their inhibiting influence on the sympathetic nervous system, the preceding remarks concerning diuretics also apply to beta blockers without ISA, since they also worsen the impaired glucose tolerance and, by decreasing HDL cholesterol, further increase the atherogenic risk in obese patients. Whether beta$_3$-receptors are additionally blocked particularly by nonselective beta-receptor blockers is unknown; a reduced expression of beta$_3$-receptors or their blockade is suspected to be causally involved in the development of obesity.

The primary goal for treating obese, hypertensive patients is a reduction of the overall increased cardiovascular risk. For that reason, only those antihypertensive first-line medications are recommended that impair neither carbohydrate nor lipid metabolism. Selective alpha$_1$-receptor blockers reduce atherogenic LDL cholesterol, on the one hand, and improve glucose tolerance on the other. Calcium antagonists have neither a significant influence on the plasma lipids, nor on the carbohydrate metabolism. The slight natriuretic effect, which the above-mentioned sodium retention counteracts, is nonetheless beneficial. ACE inhibitors are also recommended, since, like calcium antagonists, they are classed as "metabolically neutral" antihypertensive drugs.

Summary (Section 33.5)

- Almost 50% of obese adults are hypertensive; and, conversely, almost 50% of hypertensive patients are overweight.

- Moreso than normal weight hypertensives, obese hypertensives display increased sympathetic activity, insulin resistance, expanded intravascular volume and abnormalities of the lipid metabolism. The myocardial adaptations seen in obesity-associated hypertension result from both an increased arterial blood pressure (increased afterload) and an expanded intravascular volume (increased preload).

- Weight reduction and an increase in physical activity are the most important therapeutic measures and normalise not only hypertension, but the altered hormonal and metabolic parameters as well.

- Calcium antagonists, ACE inhibitors and alpha$_1$-blockers are the preferred first-line medications in the treatment of hypertension in obese patients, since these substance classes have no detrimental influence on other coexisting cardiovascular risk factors.

Literature (Chapter 33)

Beard K, Bulpitt C, Mascie-Taylor H, O'Malley K, Sever P, Webb S. Management of elderly patients with sustained hypertension. Br Med J 1992; 304: 412−416.

Campese VM, Parise M, Karubian F, Bigazzi R. Abnormal renal hemodynamics in black salt-sensitive patients with hypertension. Hypertension 1991; 18: 805−816.

Cholley BP, Shroff SG, Sandelski J, Korcarz C, Balasia BA, Jain S, Berger DS, Murphy MB, Marcus RH, Lang RM. Differential effects of chronic oral antihypertensive therapies on systemic arterial circulation and ventricular energetics in African-American patients. Circulation 1995; 91: 1052−1062.

Cunningham FG, Lindheimer MD. Hypertension in pregnancy. N Engl J Med 1992; 326: 927−932.

Dahlöf B, Lindholm LH, Hansson L, Schersten B, Ekbom T, Wester PO. Morbidity and mortality in the Swedish Trial in Older Patients with Hypertension (STOP-Hypertension). Lancet 1991; 338: 1281−1285.

Deutsche Liga zur Bekämpfung des hohen Blutdruckes e.V. Hochdruck in der Schwangerschaft und während der Stillperiode. 2. Aufl., 1991.

Fischer T, Schmieder RE, Aepfelbacher FC, Messerli FH. Antihypertensive therapy in hypertensive postmenopausal women. In: Messerli FH (ed): Hypertension in potmenopausal women. Marcel Dekker New York, 1995: 241−266.

Frishman WH, Chesner M. Beta-adrenergic blockers in pregnancy. Am Heart J 1988; 115: 147−152.

Frohlich ED. Obesity hypertension. Converting enzyme inhibitors and calcium antagonists. Hypertension 1992; 19 (suppl I): I-119-I-123.

Gallery EDM. Hypertension in pregnancy. Practical management recommendations. Drugs 1995; 49: 555−562.

Garavaglia GE, Messerli FH, Schmieder RE, Nunez BD, Oren S. Sex differences in cardiac adaptation to essential hypertension. Europ Heart J 1989; 10: 1110−1114.

Glynn RJ, Field TS, Rosner B, Hebert PR, Taylor JO, Hennekens CH. Evidence for a positive linear relation between blood pressure and mortality in elderly people. Lancet 1995; 345: 825−829.

Harris RZ, Benet LZ, Schwartz JB. Gender effects in pharmacokinetics and pharmacodynamics. Drugs 1995; 50: 222−239.

Hsueh WA, Buchanan TA. Obesity and hypertension. Endocrinol Metab Clin N Amer 1994; 23: 405−427.

Insua JT, Sacks HS, Lau T-S, Lau J, Reitman D, Pagano D, Chalmers TC. Drug treatment of hypertension in the elderly: a meta-analysis. Ann Intern Med 1994; 121: 355−362.

Kando JC, Yonkers KA, Cole JO. Gender as a risk factor for adverse events to medications. Drugs 1995; 50: 1−6.

Kaplan NM. The treatment of hypertension in women. Arch Intern Med 1995; 155: 563−567.

Laville M, Lengani A, Serme D, Fauvel JP, Ouandaogo BJ, Zech P. Epidemiological profile of hypertensive disease and renal risk factors in Black Africa. J Hypertens 1994; 12: 839−843.

Lever AF, Ramsay LE. Treatment of hypertension in the elderly. J Hypertens 1995; 13: 571−579.

Lowe SA, Rubin PC. The pharmacological management of hypertension in pregnancy. J Hypertens 1992; 10: 201−207.

Messerli FH, Garavaglia GE, Schmieder RE, Sundgaard-Riise K, Nunez BD, Amodeo C. Disparate cardiovascular findings in men and women with essential hypertension. Ann Intern Med 1987; 107: 158−161.

MRC Working Party. Medical Research Council trial of treatment of hypertension in older adults: principal results. Br Med J 1992; 304: 405−412.

National High Blood Pressure Education Program (NHBPEP). Working group report on high blood pressure in pregnancy. US Department of Health and Human Services, National Institutes of Health, National Heart, Lung, and Blood Institute. NIH Publication No. 90−3029, 1990.

Ounsted M, Cockburn J, Moar VA, Redman CWG. Maternal hypertension with superimposed pre-eclampsie: effect on child development at 7 1/2 years. Br J Obstet Gynecol 1983; 90: 644−649.

Pines A, Fisman EZ, Levo Y, Drory Y, Ben-Ari E, Motro M, Ayalon D. Menopause-induced changes in left ventricular wall thickness. Am J Cardiol 1993; 72: 240−241.

Proudler AJ, Hasib Ahmed AI, Crook D, Fogelman I, Rymer JM, Stev-enson JC. Hormone replacement therapy and serum angiotensin-converting enzyme activity in postmenopausal women. Lancet 1995; 346: 89−90.

Report by the Management Committee of the National Heart Foundation of Australia.

Treatment of mild hypertension in the elderly. Med J Aust 1981; 2: 398−402.

Roberts JM, Redman CWG. Pre-eclampsia: more than pregnancy-induced hypertension. Lancet 1993; 341: 1447−1454.

Rutledge DR. Race and hypertension. Drugs 1994; 47: 914−932.

Safar M, Stimpel M, Zanchetti A (eds.). Hypertension in postmenopausal women. Springer Verlag, Berlin-New York-Tokyo, 1994.

Saunders E, Weir MR, Kong BW, Hollifield J, Gray J, Vertes V, Sowers JR, Zemel MB, Curry C, Schoenberger J, Wright JT, Kirkendall W, Conradi EC, Jenkins P, McLean B, Massie B, Berenson G, Flamenbaum W. A comparision of the efficacy and safety of a beta-blocker, a calcium channel blocker, and a converting enzyme inhibitor in hypertensive blacks. Arch Intern Med 1990; 150: 1707−1713.

Schmieder RE, Gatzka C, Schächinger H, Schobel H, Rüddel H. Obesity as a determinant for response to antihypertensive treatment. Br Med J 1993; 307: 537−540.

Seedat YS. Varying responses to hypotensive agents in different racial groups: black versus white differences. J Hypertens 1989; 7: 515−518.

SHEP Cooperative Research Group. Prevention of stroke by antihypertensive drug treatment in older persons with isolated systolic hypertension. Final results of the Systolic Hypertension in the Elderly Program (SHEP). JAMA 1991; 265: 3255−3264.

Sibai BM, Mabie WC, Shamsa F, Villar MA, Anderson GD. A comparison of no medication versus methyldopa or labetalol in chronic hypertension during pregnancy. Am J Obstet Gynecol 1990; 162: 960−977.

Sibai BM. Diagnosis and management of chronic hypertension in pregnancy. Obstet Gynecol 1991; 78: 451−461.

Sinaiko AR. Pharmacologic management of childhood hypertension. Ped Clin N Am 1993; 40: 195−212.

Staessen J, Bulpitt C, Clement D, De Leeuw P, Fagard R, Fletcher A, Forette F, Leonetti G, Nissinen A, O'Malley K, Tuomiletho J, Webster J, Williams BO. Relation between mortality and treated blood pressure in elderly patients with hypertension: report of the European Working Party on High Blood Pressure in the Elderly. Br Med J 1989; 298: 1552−1556.

Stimpel M, Jee WSS, Ma Y, Yamamoto N, Chen Y. Impact of antihypertensive therapy on postmenopausal osteoporosis: effects of the angiotensin converting enzyme inhibitor moexipril, 17β-estradiol, and their combination on the ovariectomy-induced cancelleous bone loss in young rats. J Hypertens 1995; 13: 1852−1856.

Studer JA, Peipho RW. Antihypertensive therapy in the geriatric patient: II. Review of the alpha-1-adrenergic blocking agents. J Clin Pharmacol 1993; 33: 2−13.

Wasnich RD, Davis JW, Ross PD, Vogel JM. Effect of thiazide on rates of mineral loss: a longitudinal study. Br Med J 1990; 301: 344−347.

Wasnich RD, Davies JW, He YF, Petrovich H, Ross PD. A randomized, double-masked, placebo-controlled trial of chlorthalidone and bone loss in elderly women. Osteoporosis Int 1995; 5: 247−251.

34 Specific therapy for secondary forms of hypertension

34.1 Therapy for renoparenchymal hypertension

For all forms of renoparenchymal hypertension, blood pressure should be reduced to values lower than 140/90 mmHg (better: 130/85 mmHg) to avoid damage to other end organs on the one hand and, on the other hand, to delay the progression of renal failure. − There has been significant documentation of a delay in renal failure through normalization of blood pressure specifically in the treatment of diabetic nephropathy (see as well Section 31.5.1).

34.1.1 Non-drug treatment

Therapy for renoparenchymal hypertension differs only slightly from the treatment of primary hypertension. Whereas "salt sensitivity" is found in only part of the patients with primary hypertension, renoparenchymal hypertension always accompanies a progressive loss of the renal ability to excrete sodium. A restriction of common salt in the diet to less than 6 g per day is therefore categorically desirable for all patients affected by renoparenchymal hypertension. Due to the particular significance of sodium reduction in this form of hypertension, the compliance of the patient should be monitored through the determination of sodium excretion in the urine. Furthermore, a diet low in protein (0.6−0.8 g/kg/day) and phosphate is recommended.

A normalization of body weight, restriction of alcohol consumption, reduction of any additional cardiovascular risk factors and moderate physical activity are also important general measures to support or facilitate the correction of blood pressure in patients with renoparenchymal hypertension.

34.1.2 Drug therapy

The drug therapy for renoparenchymal hypertension essentially follows the general guidelines for the treatment of high blood pressure. All currently available first line medication can therefore first be applied as monotherapy and then be supplemented with further antihypertensive agents only if the reduction of blood pressure is insufficient. The dosage of substances that undergo renal elimination (some beta blockers, ACE inhibitors) must, of course, be reduced with decreasing GFR (Section 31.4).

Diuretics take a particular place in the treatment of renoparenchymal hypertension since they counteract the progressive loss of renal capacity to excrete sodium. Thiazide diuretics are effective up to a serum creatinine level of 2.0 mg/dl; if the renal function continues to decline, thiazides should be replaced or supplemented with loop diuretics. Potassium sparing diuretics should also not be given with mild renal dysfunction; for creatinine values over 1.8 mg/dl they are contraindicated anyway.

ACE inhibitors reduce albuminuria and proteinuria in diabetic nephropathy and non-diabetic renal disease. Long term studies have also documented a delayed progression in renal insufficiency for diabetic nephropathy with the administration of ACE inhibitors. Many experts today grant this substance class particular significance in the treatment of renoparenchymal hypertension, since a reduction in protein excretion has also been observed after the administration of ACE inhibitors in patients with normotensive blood pressure. A final conclusion will only be possible, however, once long-term studies with a large numbers of patients are available, especially since it has long been known that conventional antihypertensive agents used to reduce blood pressure can also delay the development of end-stage renal failure.

A reduction in blood pressure in renal hypertension is often initially associated with a slight increase in the serum creatinine, which in most cases may be the result of a temporarily restricted perfusion of the kidney as a limited autoregulative reaction; it is not necessary to discontinue antihypertensive treatment. However, particularly at the beginning of therapy with ACE inhibitors, close monitoring of renal retention values is necessary in order to assure the timely recognition of any possible drug-induced impairment of the intrarenal circulation in undiagnosed, bilaterally stenosed renal arteries or in unilateral renal artery stenosis with a functional single kidney. Regular control of the serum potassium should also be made, since a dangerous hyperkalemia can develop during increasing azotemia and the simultaneous administration of ACE inhibitors.

34.1.3 Dialysis treatment

Hypertensive blood pressure values are found in about 80% of patients with end-stage renal failure, most of which can be easily normalized in the course of a dialysis procedure through a reduction in volume. In 10–20% of cases of end-stage renal failure, a normalization of blood pressure can not be achieved, or only achieved at the price of side effects due to dehydration, so that antihypertensive drug therapy must also be pursued in this stage of renal failure.

Details on different dialysis procedures should be taken from literature specializing in nephrology.

34.1.4 Nephrectomy

Whereas it has not yet been possible to apply a curative therapy to bilateral renal disease, unilateral renal disease can be classified as potentially curable. Therefore, in cases of unilateral renal disease and a healthy contralateral kidney, a nephrec-tomy of the affected kidney should be taken into consideration.

Summary (Section 34.1)

- Restriction of sodium (< 6 g/day) and the adherence to a low protein diet are important general therapeutic measures for renoparenchymal hypertension.

- Antihypertensive drug therapy essentially follows the general treatment guidelines for arterial hypertension.

- Various medications require the adjustment of dosage to the increasing loss of renal function.

- First choice agents in the treatment of renoparenchymal hypertension are thiazide diuretics, which, however, are only effective up to a serum creatinine level of < 2 mg/dl and must be replaced or supplemented with loop diuretics if the renal function continues to decline.

- In end-stage renal failure, a normalization of blood pressure values is usually attained, without complications, through consistent volume control within the frame of dialysis treatment.

- Renal hypertension based on unilateral renal disease should be seen as poten-tially curable.

34.2 Therapy for renovascular hypertension

Renovascular hypertension is the most frequent, potentially curable form of hyper-tension. Specific treatment of this form, when diagnosed early, can prevent end-organ damage caused by hypertension and save the poststenotic, hypoperfused kidney from progressive loss of function. Renovascular hypertension is considered cured when, after the correction of renal artery stenosis, the diastolic arterial blood pressure measures 90 mmHg or less without the additional administration of anti-hypertensive agents. The definition of an "improved hypertension" after interven-tion measures is used unsystematically and complicates the comparison of indivi-dual studies.

The following opportunities present themselves for the treatment of renovascular hypertension:

- Percutaneous transluminal angioplasty(PTA)/vasodilatation,
- surgical revascularization, and
- long-term antihypertensive drug treatment.

Since intervention measures (PTA, surgery) can, in principle, produce a cure, they should be taken into consideration for every patient. The expected rate of success, however, should be carefully measured against the risk of intervention; in individual cases — especially with elderly, multimorbid patients — drug therapy is therefore, in some circumstances, more useful.

34.2.1 Percutaneous transluminal angioplasty (PTA)

When compared with a surgical revascularization, PTA has the following advantages:

- No need for general anesthesia,
- low rate of complications,
- shorter stay in hospital, and
- lower costs.

34.2.1.1 Success rate

Success rates for a PTA vary, but may lie at about 50% for fibromuscular renal artery stenosis (Fig. 34.1 a+b) and at a maximum of only 19% for arteriosclerosis. An improvement of hypertension following PTA has been observed in about 90% of the patients with fibromuscular-related renal artery stenoses, but should be interpreted with all previously mentioned reservations. Unilateral, arteriosclerotic occlusions that do not occur in the region of the vascular ostium have a comparatively higher "improvement rate" for hypertension after PTA.

The therapeutic success rate of PTA for bilateral, arteriosclerotic renal artery stenoses distally located is, firstly, extremely low and, secondly, the rate of complications climbs significantly. If there is angiographic evidence of such changes, a PTA is only indicated for cases where the more favorable prognosis of an operation is not attainable due to the general condition of the patient (Figure 34.2 a+b).

PTA has also been reported as having a 50% cure rate for hypertension among patients with Takayasu's arteritis and an afflicted renal artery (or arteries). Takayasu's arteritis is a chronic inflammatory disease of unknown etiology that affects the aorta, its connecting branches and the pulmonary arteries, causing stenotic lesions. Whereas this disease is seldom observed in North America or Europe, it is a relatively common cause of renovascular hypertension in Asian countries (see also Figure 13.1).

Contraindications to PTA include aneurysms of the aorta and additional occlusions of segmental arteries.

Figure 34.1: Arteriographies of a right-sided, fibromuscular renal artery stenosis (medial fibroplasia) in a female patient (37 years of age at the time of diagnosis) with therapy resistant hypertension.
(a) Arteriogram before PTA: Typical "string-of-beads" stenosis of the right renal artery
(b) Arteriogram after successful PTA: Normalization of blood pressure after PTA justifies retrospectively the diagnosis of renovascular hypertension
(Source: Courtesy of van Offern P, General Hospital Merheim, Cologne, Germany)

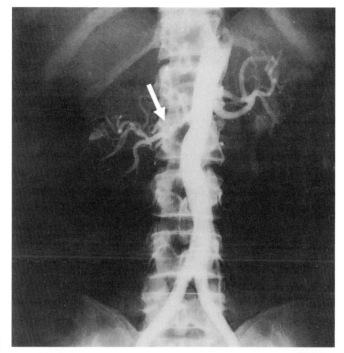

a)

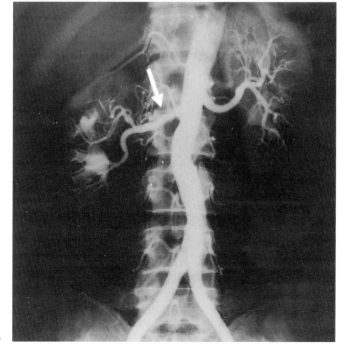

b)

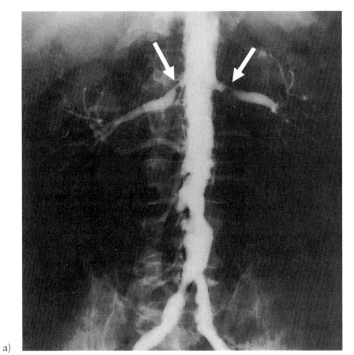

a)

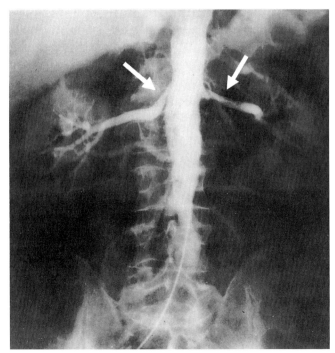

b)

34.2.1.2 PTA complications

The most common complications occurring during PTA are hematomas, occlusion or dissection of the renal artery or lesser arterial segments caused by arterial puncture, renal infarction, or contrast-media induced renal damage. Specialized centers register a resulting complication rate of about 5%. Restenosis is seen in 5% of the fibromuscular cases and 10−30% of cases involving arteriosclerotic vascular changes.

34.2.2 Surgical treatment of renovascular hypertension

The preferred method for the surgical treatment of renovascular hypertension is the placement of an aortorenal bypass, which is generally accomplished through the use of a saphenous vein graft. The more extensive arteriosclerotic changes, however, often demand alternative solutions (splenorenal, hepatorenal or iliorenal bypass).

The cure rate following a surgical correction of renal artery stenosis is 40−45%, the "improvement rate" (= a reduction in the amount of antihypertensive agents required) 40−50%. The long term success, however, may be considerably lower.

In patients with bilateral, renal arterial occlusions and renal failure, a dramatic improvement in renal function can, in individual cases, be achieved through operative revascularization. This is possible if one kidney has collateral vascular access and the size (> 8 cm) indicates that damage can be reversed.

The complete vascular status of patients should be determined prior to operation, particularly among patients with arteriosclerotic changes of the renal artery, in order to rule out stenoses of the coronary arteries and of the arteries supplying the brain.

34.2.3 Percutaneous renal embolization

Percutaneous renal embolization has been introduced among patients with severe renovascular hypertension who have undergone futile, repeated PTA or surgical revascularization as an alternative to nephrectomy, leading to a cure of hypertension among the majority of patients thus treated in a still limited collective.

Figure 34.2: Arteriographies of bilateral renal artery stenoses in a 65-year old patient with severe hypertension
(a) Before PTA: Arteriogram of high-grade, arteriosclerotic stenoses of both renal arteries with typical poststenotic dilatation . − Note also high-grade arteriosclerosis of the abdominal aorta infrarenally as well as of both iliac arteries communes.
(b) After PTA: Significant improvement of the right renal artery stenosis, and nearly-to-normal lumen of the left renal artery. Though hypertension was not cured after PTA, dosage and number of antihypertensive drug therapy could be reduced after PTA retrospectively indicating the hemodynamic relevance of the renal artery stenoses.
(Source: Courtesy of van Offern P, General Hospital Merheim, Cologne, Germany)

34.2.4 Drug treatment of renovascular hypertension

Drug treatment of renovascular hypertension is only indicated in those cases where revascularization measures (PTA, operation) are impossible (inoperability, no statement of consent by the patient, contraindication, etc.).

The selection of antihypertensive agents to initiate therapy follows the usual guidelines for the treatment of hypertension and must, in part, be adapted to the increasing dysfunction of the kidney.

ACE inhibitors have proven themselves particularly effective in the drug treatment of renovascular hypertension, but since ACE inhibitors produce a dilatation of the efferent arteriole and therewith obstruct the autoregulative capabilities of the kidney suffering from hypoperfusion, the use of these potent antihypertensive agents is accompanied by the risk of functionally induced renal insufficiency. ACE inhibitors should therefore only be applied in the presence of bilateral renal artery stenosis or of unilateral renal artery stenosis with a functioning solitary kidney if treatment with other antihypertensive drugs has failed to produce a satisfactory correction of blood pressure and if close monitoring of the renal function is assured.

Summary (Section 34.2)

- Hypertensive patients with angiographic evidence of renal artery stenosis should primarily be treated with a revascularization procedure (PTA or bypass surgery).

- If no contraindications exist, the recommended first choice of intervention is PTA.

- The existence of extensive morphologic alterations in the renal arteries, also affecting segmental arteries, should be treated primarily with surgical revascularization. – Any stenotic processes of the coronary arteries and the arteries supplying the brain should be ruled out or corrected prior to operation.

- Drug treatment for renovascular hypertension should only have a supportive function (inadequate reduction of blood pressure after attempts at revascularization), or ensue if operational risks are untenable or if revascularization measures failed completely or were not possible in the first place. Otherwise, it follows the general guidelines of treatment for hypertension.

- ACE inhibitors should only be applied in the presence of bilateral renal artery stenosis or of unilateral artery stenosis with a functioning solitary kidney if other antihypertensive agents have failed and close monitoring can be assured.

34.3 Treatment of post-transplant hypertension

34.3.1 Drug therapy

Drug therapy for post-transplant hypertension does not differ significantly from the usual treatment for hypertension. The necessary substitution of loop diuretics for thiazide diuretics and the contraindication of potassium sparing diuretics must be observed with progressive renal dysfunction. Furthermore, the dosage of hydrophilic beta blockers should be adjusted to the extent of renal dysfunction.

The administration of ACE inhibitors for cases of renal artery stenosis of the transplanted kidney (functionally = solitary kidney) should only be allowed if close monitoring is assured.

34.3.2 Nephrectomy of the native kidney

The native kidney left in situ is apparently one of the most common causes for the development of post-transplant hypertension. Despite the current possibility of substituting erythropoietin, most treatment centers are extremely restrictive when it comes to the routine prophylactic removal of the native kidney at the time of transplantation, as well as a later nephrectomy following the development of an (often severe) post-transplant hypertension. Currently, it is impossible to provide any generally valid guidelines concerning nephrectomy in host-related post-transplant hypertension.

34.3.3 PTA or surgical revascularization for treatment of transplant renal artery stenosis

A renal artery stenosis of the transplanted kidney is responsible for post-transplant hypertension in 5–10% of the patients. A PTA is the preferred treatment in these cases. Stenoses developing in the anastomotic area can be more successfully treated by surgical revascularization. – Drug treatment with ACE inhibitors may deteriorate renal perfusion leading to a progressive loss of graft function.

Summary (Section 34.3)
- Hypertension resulting from parenchymal processes of the transplanted kidney (chronic rejection, diabetic nephrosclerosis, recurrent glomerulonephritis) should be treated according to the general guidelines for antihypertensive drug therapy. A reduction in volume (diuretics) is usually advantageous, as well as an inhibition of the (mostly) activated renin-angiotensin-system (beta blockers, ACE inhibitors).

- If the cause of hypertension is assumed to be an increase in the release of renin from the native kidney, and if attempts at drug therapy do not result in a normalization of blood pressure, a nephrectomy should be considered.

- A stenosis of the artery that supplies the transplanted organ can be corrected with a PTA; the surgical revascularization of stenoses occurring in the anastomotic area is more successful than a PTA.

- Drug therapy for renovascular related post-transplant hypertension with ACE inhibitors should only ensue if close monitoring of the renal function can be assured.

34.4   Treatment of pheochromocytoma

34.4.1 Hypertensive crisis

The intravenous administration of the nonselective alpha-receptor blocker phentolamine (bolus or infusion) has proven effective in the treatment of hypertensive crises in the presence of a pheochromocytoma. The use of urapidil (Section 24.2.2), also through parenteral administration, has not yet been approved for all countries. − An alternative treatment is the intravenous administration of sodium nitroprusside (for details see also Section 32.1.2).

Due to the extreme risk of intense drops in blood pressure, treatment of a hypertensive crisis should, when possible, ensue under intensive care conditions.

34.4.2 Treatment of benign pheochromocytomas

In the presence of benign pheochromocytomas, the surgical removal of the tumors is always advisable, since, in the majority of cases, a lasting normalization of blood pressure can be attained.

Since there is principally always the risk of massively releasing catecholamines during the operation through manipulations on the tumor, leading to almost uncontrollable increases in blood pressure, it is recommended that pharmacological blockade of the alpha receptors, preferably with phenooxybenzamine, be initiated about one to two weeks before the planned operation.

After the removal of the tumor, the vasoconstrictive influence of the catecholamine subsides, so that the hypotensive effect of the reduced intravascular volume is no longer compensated. In order to prevent extreme drops in blood pressure intra- and postoperatively, it is therefore recommended that plasma expanders or whole blood conserves be used about 12−18 hours before the operation and during the operation to compensate for the reduced blood volume usually observed with pheochromocytomas. In doing so, the loss in volume caused by the operation should be surpassed in quantity.

Hypertensive blood pressure values after the excision of the pheochromocytoma indicate the presence of a further, as of yet undiscovered catecholamine producing tumor; since the complete pharmacological blockade of alpha receptors suppresses this important clinical symptom, most specialized clinics forgo increasing the dosage until the occurrence of orthostatic complaints.

Occasionally, tachyarrhythmia or cardiac dysrhythmia requires the administration of a beta blocker (such as atenolol, metoprolol), which, however, is only permitted if the therapy was already initiated with an alpha receptor blocker. The sole administration of beta blockers in the presence of a pheochromocytoma is contraindicated, since the vasodilatation caused by the beta blockers increases the sensitivity for catecholamine induced vasoconstriction towards alpha receptors and can thus intensify hypertension.

Inoperable patients or patients unwilling to consent to an operation should receive long-term drug treatment with phenoxybenzamine or other alpha receptor blockers (such as prazosin, doxazosin, terazosin, bunazosin).

The use of alpha-methyl-para-tyrosine has not yet been widely accepted. Due to its inhibitory effect on the tyrosinehydroxylase, and therewith on the synthesis of catecholamines, the administration of this substance should at least be considered as a second choice medication for the long-term therapy for inoperable pheochromocytomas.

34.4.3 Treatment of malignant pheochromocytomas

The primary therapeutic goal in the treatment of malignant pheochromocytomas should also be the operative removal of the tumor. Additionally − particularly in cases of only partial removal or of preexisting metastatic progression − a cytostatic therapy should ensue; the best results observed so far have been with combined chemotherapy of cyclophosphamide, vincristine and dacarbazine. − Should this therapy fail, an attempt with ^{131}I-MIBG in a high dosage (100−200 mCi intravenously using a perfusor over two to four hours) is appropriate, whereby the assimilation of this radionuclide by the tumor must first be ascertained through the administration of a test dose before administration of the therapeutic dose. There have also been reports of therapy successes using alpha-methyl-para-tyrosin, but the effect of this substance on malignant pheochromocytomas may be merely symptomatic in nature.

34.4.4 Postoperative monitoring

A normalization of the urinary catecholamine excretion can be expected already only a few days after the complete removal of a pheochromocytoma. In order to

Table 34.1:   Treatment of pheochromocytoma

Condition	Treatment	Dosage for drug treatment
Hypertensive crisis	Phentolamine	2.5−10 mg i. v.
	Sodium nitroprusside	0.02−0.5 mg/h* i. v.
	Urapidil	25−50 mg i. v.
Preparation for surgery	Phenoxybenzamine	20−120 mg/d p. o.**
	Prazosin	4−10 mg/d p. o.
	Doxazosin	1−16 mg/d p. o.
	Terazosin	1−20 mg/d p. o.
Benign pheochromocytoma	Surgical removal	−
− in case of inoperability	Phenoxybenzamine	20−200 mg/d p. o.
	Prazosin	4−10 mg/d p. o.
	Doxazosin	1−16 mg/d p. o.
	Terazosin	1−20 mg/d p. o.
	Nifedipine	30−60 mg/d p. o.
	Nicardipine	60−120 mg/d p. o.
	Alpha-methyl-paratyrosine	1−4 g/d p. o.
Malignant pheochromocytoma	Surgical removal and/or chemotherapy and/or ^{131}I-meta-iodobenzyl-guanidine (MIBG)	− 100−200 mCi for 90 min i. v.
Tachycardia	Beta$_1$-receptor blockers	Individual***

   *   Using an infusomat/infusion pump under intensive-care conditions
  **   Dosage follows clinical symptoms (orthostatic dysregulation) in cases, where alpha$_1$-receptors are
         to be blocked completely (maximum dose ca. 220 mg/d)
***   According to selected agent and clinical symptoms, but always following pharmacological blockade
         of alpha receptors

rule out incomplete resection of the tumor or an unrecognized second tumor, urinary catecholamines should be determined about a week after surgery. Furthermore, every patient who has undergone the removal of a pheochromocytoma should receive careful endocrinological routine examinations in yearly intervals to rule out the development of a relapse or detect it in a timely manner.

(The therapy for pheochromocytoma is summarized in Table 34.1)

Summary (Section 34.4)

• Hypertensive crises in the presence of a pheochromocytoma should be treated with phentolamine or sodium nitroprusside under intensive care conditions.

- Benign pheochromocytomas should be removed by surgery.

- Treatment with an alpha receptor blocker (preferably phenoxybenzamine, but also prazosin, doxazosin, terazosin, among others) should ensue before operation or if inoperable.

- The treatment of tachyarrhythmia or cardiac dysrhythmia with beta blockers must not ensue before the initiation of alpha receptor blocking.

- Malignant pheochromocytomas should, if possible, also be removed through operation or reduced in size and/or treated with chemotherapy or with ^{131}I-MIBG).

- After the surgical removal of a pheochromocytoma, postoperative endocrinological check-ups should take place a week after the operation and in annual intervals, as a matter of routine.

34.5 Therapy for primary aldosteronism

The goal of treatment of primary aldosteronism is the normalization of blood pressure and of electrolyte disturbances. Based on previous experience, therapeutic procedures recommended for primary aldosteronism differ with regard to the various subtypes of this secondary form of hypertension.

34.5.1 Therapy for idiopathic adrenocortical hyperplasia (idiopathic hyperaldosteronism; IHA)

The treatment of idiopathic adrenocortical hyperplasia (idiopathic hyperaldosteronism; IHA) should be initiated with drug therapy (Table 34.2), since operative procedures for this form of hyperaldosteronism do not lead to the long-term goal of blood pressure and electrolyte normalization. Spironolactone has proven itself as the treatment of choice, having the effect of lowering blood pressure and inhibiting the potassium loss through the competitive displacement of aldosterone at its steroid receptors in the distal tubule. Due to a high rate of side effects (gynecomastia, gastrointestinal complaints, impotence, loss of libido, disruption of the menstrual cycle) I recommend that the maximum dose of 400 mg/day, often necessary at the initiation of treatment, be continuously lowered during the progression of treatment. A daily dose of 50−100 mg should not be exceeded for a long-term therapy with spironolactone. If this dosage does not produce a satisfactory control of blood pressure, the combination with thiazide diuretics is possible. The administration of amiloride and triamterene as alternative potassium sparing diuretics is − due to the lack of an antihypertensive effect with these substances − only meaningful in combination with a thiazide diuretic.

Table 34.2:   Treatment of primary aldosteronism

Diagnosis	Treatment	Daily dosage
IHA	Drug therapy	
	– Spironolactone	50–100 mg
	if necessary combined with hydrochlorothiazide	25–100 mg
	– Triamterene plus	50–100 mg
	hydrochlorothiazide	25–100 mg
	– Amiloride plus	5–10 mg
	hydrochlorothiazide	25–100 mg
	– Trilostane	240–480 mg
	– Calcium antagonists of the dihydropyridine class	*
	(Nitrendipine, nifedipine, amlodipine, isradipine etc)	
DSH	Drug therapy	
	– Dexamethasone	0.5–2.0 mg
	– In cases of unsatisfactory blood pressure control, therapy as in IAH	
Adenoma	Adrenalectomy	–
PAH	Adrenalectomy	–
Carcinoma	Adrenalectomy and (or) medicinal therapy	–
	– o,p'DDD (mitotane)	1.5–10 g

* Dosage as recommended for the individual antihypertensive drugs

Abbreviations:
IHA = idiopathic aldosterone producing (bilateral) corticoadrenal hyperplasia (idiopathic hyperaldosteronism)
DSH = Dexamethasone (glucocorticoid-) suppressible hyperaldosteronism
PAH = Primary aldosterone producing corticoadrenal hyperplasia

The treatment of primary aldosteronism with trilostane is still not widely practiced. Trilostane reduces the steroid-biosynthesis through the inhibition of 3-beta-dehydrogenase, so that a drop in the excessively formed aldosterone and a consecutive normalization of blood pressure and potassium can be observed during therapy with this substance. Although there is only limited experience with trilostane in the long-term therapy for IAH, it appears defensible to attempt a therapy with this medication in the presence of intolerable side effects caused by spironolactone (see above). Treatment ensues in small doses, whereby the therapy goal will normally be reached with a maximum dose of 480 mg/day. Since trilostane does not selectively inhibit the synthesis of aldosterone, regular monitoring of other relevant steroids, particularly of cortisol, should be ensured during the corresponding long-term therapy.

Selective aldosterone synthesis inhibitors, such as 18-ethinyl-deoxycorticosterone, are currently still undergoing preclinical testing and are therefore not available for the treatment of human patients.

A second-choice medication for the long-term treatment of IAH are calcium antagonists of the 1,4-dihydropyridine type (amlodipine, isradipine, nifedipine, nitrendipine, etc.). Whereas a satisfactory reduction in blood pressure can usually be attained through the use of these substances, our experience has shown that a normalization of the increased secretion of aldosterone and resulting hyperkalemia can not be expected.

34.5.2 Therapy for dexamethasone/glucocorticoid-suppressible hyperaldosteronism (DSH)

The autonomy of aldosterone production with dexamethasone-suppressible hyper-aldosteronism (DSH) can be influenced through the exogenous administration of glucocorticoids. In most cases, after only a few days, a normalization of blood pressure, of the hormonal parameters and of the electrolytes is usually observed during therapy with dexamethasone (Table 34.2).

34.5.3 Therapy for aldosterone-producing adrenocortical adenomas (APA)

The treatment of aldosterone-producing adrenocortical adenomas (APA) should primarily aim for the surgical removal of the tumor, since, in most cases, an adrenalectomy of the tumorous side can result in a normalization of blood pressure, or at least an alleviation of hypertension and consequently a significant reduction in antihypertensive medication (Table 34.2). Among surgical procedures, transperitoneal access has proven itself effective — at best as a upper abdominal laparotomy — since this access enables an exploration of both adrenal regions and the abdomen. If the tumor has positively been localized unilaterally and abdominal exploration is not necessary, the operation can ensue extraperitoneally from the translumbar or posterior position. A preoperative drug normalization of blood pressure and electrolytes (particularly potassium) is advisable. The most common method for this is the use of spironolactone (100–400 mg/day). If the maximum daily dosage of 400 mg does not produce an adequate drop in blood pressure, the therapy can be supplemented with the additional administration of thiazide diuretics.

A therapy with slowly increasing dosages of trilostane (see above) can be considered as an alternative. According to our experience, the risk of developing an acute adrenocortical insufficiency ('Addisonian crisis') under treatment with trilostane is relatively low.

A therapy attempt with calcium antagonists (see above) is recommended in case of intolerable side effects caused by the administration of spironolactone or trilostane (gynecomastia, loss of libido, impotence, etc.).

The surgical removal of an APA leads in almost all cases to a permanent normalization of electrolytes and the production of aldosterone. A long term normalization of blood pressure after the removal of adrenocortical adenomas, however, can not be achieved in all patients: after a longer or shorter period of latency, about a third of the patients develop renewed hypertension, which however can be controlled well through the use of the usual antihypertensive agents.

Long-term drug treatment is prominent in cases of inoperability or in patients unwilling to consent to an operation, which does not differ in principle from the therapy for IHA (Table 34.2).

34.5.4 Therapy for adrenocortical carcinoma

The therapy for an aldosterone-producing adrenocortical carcinoma also consists primarily of the complete removal of the affected adrenal gland.

In the presence of metastatic spread, a surgical reduction of tumor mass should be considered necessary, but in these patients − as well as in cases of inoperability − chemotherapy treatment with o,p'-DDD (mitotane) is emphasized (Table 34.2). o,p'-DDD, an isomer of the insecticide DDT, leads to a selective necrosis of the adrenal gland. Although five-year survival spans have been reported with the use of this therapy, the prognosis for carcinoma of the adrenal gland is extremely bad.

34.5.5 Therapy for primary aldosterone-producing hyperplasia of the adrenocortical organ

Primary aldosterone-producing adrenocortical hyperplasia (PAH) is a very rare subgroup of primary aldosteronism, which exhibits the morphological criteria of hyperplastic changes in the adrenal gland, but with regard to biochemical characteristics resembles APA. Operative removal has, so far, led to a permanent normalization of blood pressure and concentrations of aldosterone and potassium in the few described patients (Table 34.2).

Summary (Section 34.5)

- Aldosterone-producing carcinoma and adenomas of the adrenal gland should primarily be removed by surgical procedures.

- Bilateral idiopathic adrenocortical hyperplasia should categorically be treated with medication (spironolactone; or if unsuccessful, prospectively dihydropyridine calcium antagonists or inhibitors of steroidogenesis).

34.6 Therapy for Cushing's syndrome

The treatment of Cushing's syndrome displays specific differences in accordance to its genesis − pituitary ACTH-dependent Cushing's syndrome (Cushing's disease), ectopic Cushing's syndrome (ectopic ACTH or CRH syndrome) or primary adrenal Cushing's syndrome (primary adrenal hypercortisolism).

34.6.1   Specific therapy for Cushing's syndrome

34.6.1.1   Treatment of pituitary ACTH-dependent Cushing's syndrome (Cushing's disease)

The therapy of choice for Cushing's disease is transsphenoidal microadenomectomy. If the adenoma can not be localized, it is recommended that 80−90% of the anterior pituitary be removed. If the patient wants children, a primary radiation therapy (cobalt-60) should be carried out; if this is not successful, it is recommended that the adrenal glands be removed bilaterally. The disadvantages of a bilateral adrenalectomy are manifested firstly in the life-long, obligatory substitution of glucocorticoid and mineralocorticoids, and secondly in the postoperative reformation of pituitary adenomas (accompanied with an excessive build-up of ACTH and hyperpigmentation) (so-called Nelson's syndrome) in about 15% of the cases after a few years.

The cure rate, defined as undetectable morning plasma cortisol concentrations, amounts to 70−80% following the first operation in specialized centers; the results following a second operation are significantly worse. − Patients treated successfully must receive postoperative treatment with glucocorticoid substitutes until the hypothalamic-hypophyseal-adrenal axis has functionally recovered (about 6−12 months).

In 40−50% of the patients who can not be cured by operation, hypercortisolism can be corrected through radiation therapy of the pituitary gland. The success rate among children is 85%, so that some specialized centers prefer radiation therapy over an operation for this population. − Since the success of radiation treatment only sets in between 3−12 months after treatment, hypercortisolism can be treated with the administration of medication to inhibit the synthesis of steroids (Section 34.6.3).

34.6.1.2 Treatment of primary adrenal forms of Cushing's syndrome

Therapy for primary adrenal forms of Cushing's syndrome (corticoadrenal adenomas and carcinoma) aims at the removal of the tumorous adrenal gland, whereas micronodular or macronodular hyperplasia of the adrenal glands requires a bilateral adrenalectomy.

The benign forms of primary adrenal Cushing's syndrome are almost always curable, whereas carcinoma of the adrenocortical organ exhibits an extremely bad prognosis. A relapse after the operative removal is common and largely resistant to radiation or chemotherapy, so that, as a final measure, the administration of steroid synthesis inhibitors and o,p'-DDD (mitotan; see Section 34.5) can be offered to the affected patient as a palliative therapy (Section 34.6.3).

34.6.1.3 Treatment of ectopic Cushing syndrome / ectopic ACTH and corticotropin-releasing-hormone (CRH) syndrome

Whereas a permanent cure has been achieved in rare cases following the complete removal of ectopic CRH or ACTH producing tumors, this form of Cushing's syndrome usually evades curative treatment due to the advanced stage of the disease and an often unknown localization of the primary tumor. The bilateral removal of the adrenal glands will relieve patients with non-resectable tumors from the symptoms of hypercortisolism; as an alternative or in cases of inoperability, a drug treatment with the adrenal steroid synthesis inhibitors can be attempted (Section 34.6.3).

34.6.2   General therapeutic measures for Cushing's syndrome

34.6.2.1 Preoperative treatment of Cushing's syndrome

The goal of preoperative preparations for the surgical treatment of Cushing's syndrome is the correction of a diabetic metabolic condition through the administration of insulin as well as the (parenteral) correction of any potential hypokalemia. A reduction in hypertensive arterial blood pressure values should ensue with spironolactone (25−100 mg), whereby a decrease in blood pressure to systolic values under 150 mmHg should be avoided due to the risk of intra- and post-operative hypotension.

34.6.2.2 Postoperative treatment of Cushing's syndrome

Patients who have undergone a bilateral adrenalectomy require mineralocorticoid and glucocorticoid substitution for the rest of their lives. The therapy is initiated on the day of operation with the continuous, intravenous administration of 400 mg hydrocortisone/24 hours − at best in a glucose-saline (0.9%) solution (2:1) − and, after reducing the dose to 200 mg hydrocortisone per day, continued during the first days following the operation. On the third or fourth day, a conversion to oral substitution (for example cortisone-acetate 150−200 mg distributed over four single doses daily) should ensue. A gradual reduction in the dose after six weeks to the maintenance dose of 25−50 mg per day is desirable. The additional administration of 0.1 mg fludrocortisonacetate per day is necessary for the substitution of mineralocorticoid.

A provisional postoperative substitution of steroids in gradually reduced doses (lasting in some cases up to a year) is necessary following the unilateral adrenalectomy of glucocorticoid-producing adrenal gland adenomas or carcinomas due to the suppression of the healthy adrenal gland normally observed.

Postoperative care following the transsphenoidal, selective removal of an adenoma in hypophyseal-hypothalamic Cushing's syndrome (Cushing's disease) also requires steroid substitution due to the suppression of physiological ACTH production, which is, as a rule, however, temporary in nature.

34.6.2.3 Drug treatment of Cushing's syndrome

A drug treatment of hypercortisolism is indicated in cases of inoperability (metastatic or non-resectable adrenocortical carcinoma, non-localized or far advanced ectopic Cushing's syndrome, poor general condition of the patient), and should primarily aim at inhibiting cortisol synthesis.

The adrenostatic effect of aminoglutethemide (orimetene) is explained by the inhibition of 20α-hydroxylase. This prevents the conversion of cholesterol into 20α-hydroxycholesterol, eliminating the preliminary stages necessary for the formation of cortisol (and aldosterone). The treatment with aminoglutehemide should ensue in low doses and − when ensuing as monotherapy − should not exceed a maximum dose of 2 g per day (distributed over 4 individual doses). Side effects (giddiness, adynamia, ataxia, gastrointestinal complaints, hypothyroidism) often require that this substance be discontinued or the dose reduced.

Metyrapone also blocks the synthesis of cortisol and aldosterone (inhibition of the 11-α-hydroxylase). Subjective side effects (gastrointestinal complaints, hypotensive circulatory complaints) have also been observed with methyrapone primarily with high doses (maximum dose 3 g per day).

Our experience has been that a combination therapy with methyrapone and aminoglutethemide with a corresponding reduction in the doses of individual substances should be given preference over monotherapy with high doses, since this can achieve a sufficient inhibition of cortisol synthesis and significantly reduce the rate of side effects. O,p'-DDD (mitotane), an isomer of the insecticide DDT, leads to a largely selective necrosis of the zona reticularis and the zona fasciculata of the adrenocortical organ. Furthermore, mitotane is known to have a direct inhibitory effect on the glucocorticoid synthesis. A therapy with the maximum recommended dose of 10 g per day is only accomplished in the fewest of cases due to the often intolerable side effects (gastrointestinal, neurological and psychological disruptions). Due to the possibility of a failure of the adrenal gland, every adrenostatic treatment requires repeated checks of the plasma cortisol concentrations as well as a substitution therapy with glucocorticoid (0.5−1.0 mg dexamethasone or the equivalent amount of a different glucocorticoid).

Suramine, a substance that initially was used for the treatment of parasitic diseases and later tested in the treatment of AIDS, also appears to inhibit the adrenal steroid synthesis and exercise a specific destructive effect on the adrenal tissue as well. This substance could possibly be seen as a further alternative in the drug treatment of metastatic, cortisol-producing carcinomas of the adrenal gland; at this point in time, however, it can not be recommended, since there is only a very limited extent of corresponding therapeutic experience.

Summary (Section 34.6)

• Primary therapy for Cushing's syndrome aims at the surgical removal of the cause, i. e.:

  − Adrenalectomy for adenomas, hyperplasia or carcinoma of the adrenal gland,

  − transsphenoidal, selective adenoma removal for hypophyseal-hypothalamic Cushing's syndrome (Cushing's disease), and

- tumor extirpation for ectopic Cushing's syndrome (ectopic ACTH or CRH syndrome).
- Preparations for an operation for Cushing's syndrome include compensating for a diabetic metabolic condition, hypokalemia and the reduction of hypertensive blood pressure values.
- Postoperative measures of steroid substitution are required temporarily, or life-long for patients having had a bilateral adrenalectomy.
- A curative surgical treatment is often not possible for ectopic Cushing's syndrome and carcinoma of the adrenal gland, so that drug treatment of hypercortisolism in these patients is desirable.
- A radiation therapy for Cushing's disease should only ensue in adults after the conclusive failure of operative measures; for children, however, radiation therapy is recommended as a primary measure because of the high curative success rate.

34.7   Therapy for primary hyperparathyroidism

34.7.1 Therapy for hypertension in primary hyperparathyroidism

Therapy for the often moderately increased arterial blood pressure values in primary hyperparathyroidism without secondary, renal damage is usually unproblematic and does not differ significantly from the normal drug treatment for primary hypertension (see Chapters 19–30). However, the administration of thiazide diuretics to stimulate the renal-tubular reabsorption of calcium can lead to an increase in hypercalcemia, and should be avoided.

For asymptomatic patients with hypertensive blood pressure values without evidence of any restriction in renal function (and without any essential osteal manifestations), an operative removal of the pathologically altered parathyroid gland(s) should be taken into consideration, since, firstly, this can cure the hypertension and, secondly, can prevent any (hypertension-related?) renal damage. It should be noted, however, that most specialists feel that hypertension (which can be controlled well with drugs) in asymptomatic, primarily normocalcemic patients with primary hyperparathyroidism and no evidence of end-organ damage is only indicated for surgical procedures where regular follow-up inspections can not be assured (see below). The decision therefore must be made dependent on the individual case.

34.7.2 Principle therapeutic procedure for primary hyperparathyroidism

Reference must be made to textbooks on endocrinology for detailed therapeutic procedures concerning primary hyperparathyroidism.

The previous section has already made reference to the relative indication for operations in asymptomatic, primarily normocalcemic patients, whereby the assurance of regular monitoring is a "conditio sine qua non" for the non-surgical treatment in order to register any potential progression of the disease (renal or osteal changes) in a timely manner.

For symptomatic patients, there is an absolute indication for operative procedure. The goal for adenomas is the removal of the affected parathyroid gland, whereby the intraoperative, histological examination of at least one further gland is recommended to rule out multiple affection. Hyperplasia of the parathyroid gland generally extends to all accessible parathyroids, so that, in such cases, an almost complete resection with retention of one half of a gland is desirable.

Summary (Section 34.7)

- Drug therapy for hypertension with hyperparathyroidism does not principally differ from the treatment of primary hypertension, but the administration of thiazide diuretics (increase in hypercalcemia) should be avoided.

- Hypertension with primary hyperparathyroidism is usually curable through the operative removal of the diseased parathyroid gland(s).

- Asymptomatic patients (with or without hypertension) − with assured follow-up inspections − represent a relative indication for operation.

- Symptomatic patients with primary hyperparathyroidism must receive surgical treatment.

34.8 Therapy for other forms of secondary hypertension

Therapy for the other secondary forms of hypertension does not differ from normal antihypertensive treatment, so that there is no need to provide a specific description here.

The treatment of pregnancy-specific hypertension pregnancy was already covered in Section 33.3.3.2.

Literature (Chapter 34)

Auda SP, Brenan MF, Gill JR. Evolution of the surgical management of primary aldosteronism. Ann Surg 1980; 191: 1−7.

Averbusch S, Streakley C, Young R, Gelmann E, Goldstein D, Stull R, Keiser H. Malignant pheochromocytoma: effective treatment with a combination of cyclophosphamide, vincristine and dacarbazine. Ann Intern Med 1988; 109: 267−273.

Benoit G, Moukarzel M, Hiesse C, Verdelli G, Charpentier B, Fries D. Transplant renal artery stenosis: experience and comparative results between surgery and angioplasty. Transplant Int 1990; 3: 137−140.

Bravo EL, Gifford RW. Pheochromocytoma: diagnosis, localization, and management. N Engl J Med 1984; 311: 1298−1303.

Deutsche Liga zur Bekämpfung des hohen Blutdruckes e.V. Deutsche Hypertonie Gesellschaft. Renovaskuläre Hypertonie, Heidelberg 1992.

Ganguly A. Glucocorticoid-suppressible hyperaldosteronism: an update. Am J Med 1990; 88: 321−324.

Gifford RW, Manger WM, Bravo EL. Pheochromocytoma. Endocrinol Metab Clin N Am 1994; 23: 387−404.

Groth H, Vetter H, Neyses L, Stimpel M, Vetter W. Trilostane − a new and effective drug for primary aldosteronism. In: The adrenal gland and hypertension (eds.: Mantero F, Biglieri EG, Funder JW, Scoggins BA), 443−448, Raven Press, New York 1985.

Groth H, Vetter W, Stimpel M, Greminger P, Tenschert W, Klaiber E, Vetter H: Adrenalectomy in primary aldosteronism: a long-term follow-up study. Cardiology 1985; 72 (suppl 1): 107−116.

Guo J, Gong L, Chen S, Luo B, Xu M. Malignant pheochromocytoma: diagnosis and treatment in fifteen cases. J Hypertens 1989; 7: 261−266.

Krempf M, Lumbroso J, Mornex R, Brendel AJ, Wemeau JL, Delisle MJ, Aubert B, Carpentier P, Fleury-Goyon MC, Gibold C, Guyot M, Lahneche B, Marchandise X, Schlumberger M, Charbonnel B, Chatal JF. Use of m-131-iodobenzylguanidine in the treatment of malignant pheochromocytoma. J Clin Endocrinol Metab 1991; 72: 455−461.

Lafferty FW, Hubay CA. Primary hyperparathyroidism. A review of the long-term surgical and nonsurgical morbidities as a basis for a rational approach to treatment. Arch Intern Med 1989; 149: 789−796.

Manger WM, Gifford RW. Pheochromocytoma: current diagnosis and management. Clev Clin J Med 1993; 60: 365−378.

Orth DN. Cushing's syndrome. N Engl J Med 1995; 791−803.

Pelegri A, Romero R, Reguant M, Aisa L. Nonresectable phaeochromocytoma: long-term follow-up. J Hum Hypertens 1989; 3: 145−147.

Pommier RF, Brennan MF. An 11-year experience with adrenocortical carcinoma. Surgery 1992; 112: 963−971.

Ramsay LE, Waller PC. Blood pressure response to percutaneous transluminal angioplasty for renovascular hypertension: an overview of published series. Br Med J 1990; 300: 569−572.

Rosenthal T. Drug therapy of renovascular hypertension. Drugs 1993; 45: 895−909.

Russo D, Andreucci VE, Iaccarino V, Niola R, Dal Canton A, Conte G. Percutaneous renal embolisation in renovascular hypertension. Br Med J 1988; 296: 1160−1161.

Sandler LM, Richards NT, Carr DH, Mashiter K, Joplin GF. Long-term follow-up of patients with Cushing's disease treated by interstitial irradiation. J Endocrinol Metab 1987; 65: 441−447.

Semple PF, Dominiczak AF. Detection and treatment of renovascular disease: 40 years on. J Hypertens 1994; 12: 729−734.

Stimpel M, Vetter W, Groth H, Greminger P, Vetter H. Captopril before and after spironolactone therapy in primary aldosteronism. Klin Wochenschr 1985; 63: 361−363.

Stimpel M, Wambach G. Therapie des Phäochromozytoms. Dtsch med Wschr 1987; 112: 1426−1427.

Stimpel M, Ivens K, Wambach G, Kaufmann W. Are calcium antagonists helpful in the management of primary aldosteronism ? J Cardiovasc Pharmacol 1988; 12 (suppl 6): S131−S134.

Stimpel M. Treatment of primary aldosteronism. [In German]. Dtsch med Wschr 1992; 117: 947−949.

Tyagi S, Singh B, Kaul UA, Sethi KK, Arora R, Khalilullah. Balloon angioplasty for renovascular hypertension in Takayasu's arteritis. Am Heart J 1993; 125: 1386−1393.

Vetter W, Robertson JIS, Grim CE, Lüscher TF, Malborough J (eds). Renovascular hypertension. In memoriam Andreas Grüntzig. Cardiology 1986; 44 (suppl 1): 1−114.

Weibull H, Bergqvist D, Jendteg S, Lindgren B, Persson U, Jonsson K et al. Clinical outcome and health care costs in renal revascularisation − percutaneous transluminal renal angioplasty versus reconstructive surgery. Br J Surg 1991; 78: 620−624.

Working Group on Renovascular Hypertension. Detection, evaluation, and treatment of renovascular hypertension. Final report. Arch Intern Med 1987; 147: 820−829.

Yamakita N, Chiou S, Gomez-Sanchez CE. Inhibition of aldosterone biosynthesis by 18-ethynyl-deoxycorticosterone. Endocrinology 1991; 129: 2361−2366.

Young WF Jr, Hogan MJ, Klee GG, Grant CS, van Heerden JA. Primary aldosteronism: diagnosis and treatment. Mayo Clin Proc 1990; 65: 96−110.

Index